Ə11

Theory of
Fertility Decline

Theory of Fertility Decline

JOHN C. CALDWELL

Department of Demography
The Australian National University, Australia

1982

ACADEMIC PRESS
A Subsidiary of Harcourt Brace Jovanovich, Publishers
London   New York
Paris   San Diego   San Francisco
Sydney   Tokyo   Toronto   São Paulo

ACADEMIC PRESS INC. (LONDON) LTD.
24/28 Oval Road
London NW 1

United States Edition published by
ACADEMIC PRESS INC.
111 Fifth Avenue,
New York, New York 10003

British Library Cataloguing in Publication Data

Caldwell, J. C.
Theory of fertility decline.—(Population and social structure)
1. Family size—Social aspects—Underdeveloped areas
2. Family size—Economic aspects—Underdeveloped areas
I. Title   II. Series
304.6′3   HQ776.5.U/

ISBN 0–12–155080–X
LCCCN   81–68983

Text set in Linotron Times by Deltatype, Ellesmere Port,
and printed and bound by T. J. Press (Padstow) Ltd.

Editor's Preface

Jack Caldwell is a maverick. His wealth flows theory of fertility decline may be, indeed like any scientific theory almost surely is, wrong in some respects. Where he is almost surely right is in his trenchant critique of traditional statistical, economic explanation in demography. Western social science is replete with examples of overgeneralization from defective data on the European bourgeoisie to explain the rest of the world. The elegant econometrics of fertility change are no exception.

Good economic demographers would probably agree with the critique of their history (although not necessarily with the proposed theoretical replacement). What seems most important in this debate is Caldwell's insistence on tough empirical research to understand the true foci and conflicts of familial maximization. The people having the children seem not always to be interested in the goals that economists posit for them; they are striving for something else. Finding out what that is requires an understanding of the lives they live—of their personal struggles to fill prescribed roles and achieve dignity, to win a place in the hereafter that is social memory, to defend those who have gone before and those who will come after against social and political, not only economic competition. It requires the researcher to observe this life struggle in context—with time, with determination, with compassion, and with a cast-iron stomach. Caldwell's work is squarely in the natural-history tradition of anthropology and his book an illustrious addition to a series devoted to that tradition.

Dec 1981   E. A. Hammel

Acknowledgements

All the research described in this book has been carried out with my wife, Pat Caldwell, and also with a range of collaborators from the countries studied. Throughout the entire period, two institutions have played an indispensable role in all the work. One is The Australian National University which has employed me during much of the time, and provided funding and conditions for research and extended leave. The other is The Population Council which has provided by far the largest share of funds and also employment for important periods. Both institutions have provided intellectual inputs.

In addition, I have worked in a considerable number of institutions in the Third World where I have always found congenial and stimulating collaborators who were an important source of information about their cultures. These institutions include The University of Ghana, in Nigeria, the Universities of Ibadan, Ife and Nigeria (Nsukka), the University of Nairobi, the Cairo Demographic Centre, the United Nations Desertification Conference programme, and the Population Centre in Bangalore, India.

Two journals have played particularly important roles in allowing this debate to take place. The *Population and Development Review* has generously allowed me to republish the papers that appear as Chapters 4, 5, 6 and 10. *Population Studies* has been equally generous in permitting the republication of the papers that form Chapters 3, 7 and 8. Permission has been obtained for the republication of Chapter 2 by the *Journal of Comparative Family Studies* and from Julian Simon and JAI Press for the republication of Chapter 9. Chapter 11 was presented to an International Union for the Scientific Study of Population workshop in 1980 and Chapter 12 to the International Conference of Rural Sociologists in the same year. Permission has also been obtained from my co-author, Lado Ruzicka, to republish Chapter 6.

A very substantial contribution to the editing has been made by Pat Quiggin and assistance with the papers forming the book has also come from Jennie Widdowson, Nancy Kuskie and Wendy Cosford. A great deal of typing has been done by Barbara Addison, Pat Mooney, June Steele and Carol Casey.

Dec 1981   John C. Caldwell

vii

Contents

C. The Construction of a Theory 113

D. Testing the theory in historical context 181

A

Introduction

1

The development of the theory

The Development of "Wealth Flows" Theory

The papers in this book record the development of the "wealth flows" theory of fertility decline. As they were written, they were increasingly made to conform to a design so that a coherent publication could be put together.

Thus, they begin with the problems that beset field demographers attempting to employ pre-existing theory. Next a possible alternative theory is elaborated and tested against what is now known of Third World populations. Subsequently, efforts are made to test it against Western historical data. Then, certain difficulties are identified and explored. Finally, there is a summary of the situation at the beginning of the 1980s and an attempt to distinguish the way forward to a more general theory.

Necessarily, this volume omits much of what it rests upon. First, there is the research experience and the research papers arising directly from research with only limited short-range generalizations. Secondly, there are papers which had a considerable theoretical content but which either presented research findings in too much detail (e.g. Caldwell and Caldwell, 1978) or dealt with different but related topics such as child mortality (e.g. Caldwell, 1979). Nevertheless, a brief description of this experience is probably necessary for a full understanding of the argument.

My wife and I began Third World demographic work in Thailand in 1959. In the 22 ensuing years we have lived and researched in developing countries for approximately half the period, and have spent most of the balance analysing such data in the industrialized world or working on the demographic history of the latter area. In 1960 we were in Malaysia (then Malaya), 1960–2 in Ghana, 1968–1970 and 1973, together with shorter periods in 1971–2 and 1974–5, in Nigeria, and in 1970 in Kenya. Some time in 1972–3 was also spent in the region of the Sahelian drought. Over the whole time we have worked for shorter periods in Egypt and during the 1970s, for increasingly longer spans in India.

The dates are significant. We began work in Thailand just as the most detailed and influential application of Notestein's demographic transition theory to individual countries became available (Coale and Hoover, 1958). The theoretical papers are a product of the latter 1970s and early 1980s, following the disagreements of the 1974 World Population Conference in Bucharest, where the author presented a paper in the opening session of the Tribune protesting that the discussion of the advantages of fertility decline was being carried out in a too simple and unreal way (Caldwell, 1975c), and the presentation to a 1975 conference of an influential paper claiming to show that high fertility was invariably a disadvantage amongst peasant agriculturalists (Mueller, 1975 and 1976).

The work upon which the theory is based belongs to an extreme wing of the demographic research tradition. Most demographers work on large data sets, often with little contact with the people whom the statistics describe. Fortunately, in early 1962 it became clear that the 1960 Ghana Census was not going to yield material quickly enough to absorb my time. We thereupon used our limited funds for cheap and relatively small scale investigations which meant borrowing methodology from the anthropologists (and reading them) and becoming intimately acquainted with each village and its families in turn. For a demographer with traditional training, the experience was illuminating—so illuminating that we have attempted to use similar methods ever since.

Certain research experiences were of particular significance. In the 1962–4 period in Ghana, three were especially noteworthy in that they revealed aspects of the society which demographers were not led to expect. One was a fairly large survey of rural–urban migration with the emphasis on rural families (Caldwell, 1969). Although it was not the focus of the work, the data seemed to show fairly clearly that members of large families were not economically worse off than members of small ones and that their future prospects were not relatively less. One puzzle that immediately arose was why such findings were not regularly reported—or alternatively were denied—by those who carried out Third World surveys. Subsequently, we were to study the elite in Ghana's four largest urban centres (Caldwell, 1968a). Here again, parents seemed little disadvantaged by their fertility. We were fortunate in becoming acquainted with these families just at a time when some of their children had not been educated while others were in school. It became clear that the fact of a child's schooling had immense implications for family relationships and for the family economy. This theme persists throughout all our later work. Intrigued by these findings we undertook a survey of the fortunes of aged persons in rural areas (Caldwell,

1966) and this confirmed that low fertility had not brought relative gains, while at the same time demonstrating that the education of children often ultimately did so.

During the next dozen years, the complexity of the impact of fertility was to be brought home by two other experiences. The first was work during 1969 (Caldwell and Igun, 1970, 1972) in Nigeria which showed that rural populations were most unlikely to use contraceptives even when they knew about them and had access to them. The second was the experience of the Sahelian drought in 1972–3 (Caldwell, 1975d, 1981) which demonstrated just how important were family links when coping with periodic disasters.

From 1973 a systematic attempt was made to investigate some of these problems in the Changing African Family Project (Okediji et al., 1976) which spanned twelve African countries, while in 1974–75 the Nigerian Fertility Study[1] examined wealth flows within families in Nigeria.

Finally, the period 1977–78 was spent in Southwest and South Asia examining the nature of peasant families in the region.

Section B, *Problems and Reality*, of this book sets out the problems as well as providing sufficient knowledge of one society, the Yoruba of Southwest Nigeria, to allow the reader to perceive that the patterns of Western society cannot be assumed to exist everywhere. There were problems in showing the nature of Yoruba society, and a variety of approaches, including the use of proverbs and everyday sayings, was adopted. The research discovered that the Yoruba, far from believing that high fertility undermined the strength of a family, equated family size with success.

An examination of every family in Ibadan (Caldwell and Caldwell, 1978) revealed that even in a city of almost a million inhabitants only a small minority of the middle class restricted family size, and that they did so precisely because the nature of their family relations had changed so as to render children an economic disadvantage and not because they were the first to perceive the economic burden of children.

Chapter 3 sets out the intellectual dilemma of the author and other demographers at the time. Demographers in developing countries often did feel a species apart—understood by audiences in industrialized countries but hesitant about explaining their views and beliefs to anthropologists or other social scientists in the Third World, let alone to the local residents. It began to dawn upon us that we might be the kings without clothing. Part of the gulf was a product of the use of statisticians and statistically oriented economists in a field where the only possible approach was a social scientific one which would yield an understanding of individuals and families. Part was the use of large-scale surveys and computers, and part was a sheer refusal of many to read what other disciplines had discovered, seeming at

---

[1] For a description of the Study, see Appendix to Chapter 2.

times to justify their lack of knowledge of the Third World on the grounds that they were there to help the transformation to a developed world as soon as possible. Demographers often acted as delegates from another world.

Because they were written for different audiences at about the same time, some paragraphs and footnotes in Chapters 2 and 3 are similar, but have been allowed to stand here, in preference to altering papers already published.

Section C, *The Construction of a Theory*, presents the attempts from 1976 onward to offer an explanation that would fit in with Third World experience. The wealth flows theory was deliberately constructed with a view to its testing in the field, although devising a complete range of tests has proved difficult. The term "wealth flows" was adopted because it became clear that most economists, let alone others, did not usually understand "income" to include everything covered here by wealth. It is possible that "benefit flows" would have been preferable, because of the definition of wealth as a stock. The theory emphasizes the fundamental nature of social and economic relations within the family and how subtle changes in the former can have a profound effect upon the latter. It also emphasizes the importance of micro-studies to demographic theory.

The argument is taken further in Chapter 5, written two years later. This paper, produced after further work in the Middle East (P. Caldwell, 1977) and South Asia carries the argument from lands of shifting cultivation to the great peasant societies. It also emphasizes the need for applying scientific method to the study of fertility transition—namely, that it is essential that the conditions of stable high fertility should be understood before offering an explanation for the onset of fertility decline. In this paper the first examination is made of the familial mode of production and of its survival in industrial society in the form of household production (derived from the ongoing work on the nature of the Australian transition). It is argued that the cultural superstructure lags behind changes in the means of production and hence the parents of large families experience no economic disadvantage long after familial production has been substantially transformed. This is a very different argument from Notestein's "props" where it was argued that cultural forces obscured the realization that high fertility was uneconomic or made it irrelevant. In this paper there is also a greater concentration on the advent of mass education as a specifically destabilizing force.

Section D, *Testing the Theory in Historical Context*, presents three attempts to look at the dynamics of change. Chapters 6 and 8, examine the Australian fertility transition, which we had been researching, but the implication is that the findings are probably representative of a range of similar countries. The work on late nineteenth century Australia showed just how important was the cost side of the equation: children were cheap because of a culture that ensured that this should be so. The paper also explores the sequence of change: the persistence of domestic production, and the final collapse of suburban society. It demonstrates just how fast different groups followed each other to successively lower fertility levels, thus throwing very substantial doubt on economists' analyses based on apparently substantial fertility differentials at a specific time. Evidence is produced to show that changes in the marrying age had very little relation to any conscious decision to limit the ultimate size of the family, but were rather based on the degree of difficulty in setting up a household.

Chapter 7 takes a more general look both at the Western fertility decline and at three Third World societies, Taiwan, Turkey and Mexico, where fertility has fallen to different extents. In terms of family change, some emphasis is placed on alterations in the relative position of the sexes as well as on that of the generations. This approach is continued in Chapter 8 which follows the Australian fertility transition through until the present day with implications for the future. It argues that even post-transitional fertility decline must be seen as a succession of stages in changing intergenerational and sex relationships.

Section E, *Specific Difficulties*, takes up two themes which were too broad for the specialized theory Chapters. The first, Chapter 9, is another version of the isolation of the demographer. Why is it necessary to provide a separate theory for demographic transition? Why should it not be possible, and even preferable, to employ more general theories of social and economic change? The investigation ends up by casting doubt on these more general theories and wondering whether their inability to explain demographic change is not a symptom of a deeper weakness. It also finds that they have had an adverse effect on demographic theory in their reluctance to identify Westernization for what are primarily non-scientific reasons.

Chapter 10 takes up a theme noted in passing in several chapters, the role of mass education in both the historical West and the Third World. It should be emphasized here that the argument is not that mass education alone can produce fertility decline but that it can affect its timing by decades if the wealth flow is close to the equilibrium point. A distinction is made between education in the West, where the ingredients came mostly from the society itself, and in the Third World where it arrived from elsewhere. Stress is placed on the change in economic and other relationships within the family that arise from education.

This argument is applied also to the field of infant and child mortality in a paper which could not be included here because its focus is not directly on fertility (Caldwell, 1979). Yet that paper is of fundamental importance to the argument. If high fertility were not disadvantageous to parents in traditional society, then why did fertility decline so frequently in societies where child mortality had fallen? Evidence is adduced in this paper to show that it may well have been the same changes in intrafamilial relations that drove down both child mortality and fertility.

In the final Section, F, *Recapitulation and Broader Implications*, Chapter 11 summarizes the theory as it stood by 1980. However, Chapter 12 places it in a broader theoretical framework which is as yet only a sketch. This chapter draws heavily on yet another paper which could not be included here because its specific focus was not fertility theory. That paper (Caldwell, *et al.*, 1981a) is an examination of relative family labour inputs in a range of social situations in Bangladesh. It has important implications, nevertheless, for understanding why family relations change, with all that implies for potential fertility decline, as productive relations are transformed.

This book rests, then, on the assertion that parents have not been economically disadvantaged by high fertility for most of the world's history. Therefore, some explanation for fertility transition must be found other than either the withdrawal of cultural approbation for high fertility together with taboos against low fertility or the decline in mortality. The matter is of crtitical importance, because the industrialized world would have been a very different place if fertility had not begun to decline a century ago, and the nature of the global society of the future depends greatly on the timing and pace of future fertility declines.

B

Problems and Reality

2

Fertility and the household economy in Nigeria

It has widely been argued that rapid population increase, arising from high fertility, is disadvantageous to economic growth in developing countries even as measured by the expansion of the whole economy but particularly as measured by the rise in per capita incomes.[1] Such a demographic-economic relationship is likely to be important in inducing fertility decline only so far as governments are sufficiently convinced of the correctness of the analysis to exert themselves in providing antinatal services and in persuading people to use the services. It is probable that even these activities will have a significant impact on fertility only to the extent that the demographic-economic relationship within the household has moved towards rendering high fertility disadvantageous. The household economy is not necessarily merely a miniscule national economy which when aggregated with multitudes of others of its type will produce the national economy reflecting the same characteristics on a much larger scale.

Studies of the economic value of children in the household context in non-industrial societies are rare. The best attempt at applying rigorous analysis to the information that exists is probably Eva Mueller's "The Economic Value of Children in Peasant Agriculture" (1975). It is because this paper is quite outstanding and not because it is an obviously defective member of its species, that it is singled out here as an example of the type of analysis which can be misleading and which often tends to place stress upon weak data while ignoring the implications of more obviously solid data.

Mueller set herself the task of investigating "to what extent in peasant agriculture male and female children contribute to household expenses, earnings and savings" both while children and in later life. She concluded that "children have negative economic value in peasant agriculture. Up to the time when they become parents themselves, children consume more

[1] See for instance Coale and Hoover (1958), van de Walle (1975), Enke (1966) and Ohlin (1971).

than they produce" (ibid. p. 66). "The work contribution of children is not large enough to prevent them being an economic burden on peasant societies" (ibid. p. 50), and in fact "it would appear that in most LDCs children under 15 do relatively little market work" (ibid. p. 19) and "children of either sex consume substantially more than they produce until they reach the 15–19 age bracket" (ibid. p. 42). Alternatively children may do productive work, but in this case it tends to be substitute and not additional work: "Adult men may gain leisure by having large families, or the women may be freed from the market place. In the limiting case, work by children may be merely a substitute for work by others in the household" (ibid. p. 32). Finally, "raising a large number of children would seem to be an expensive method of providing for the relatively minor aggregate burden of old age support" (ibid. p. 46).

The approach and the conclusion are worrying. Work over the last fifteen years in West Africa, and acquaintance with other parts of the developing world, lead me to the conclusion that the situation described here is not reality as most of the peasants, and even their relatives in the towns, know it. In fact one can accept the analysis only by assuming that simple peasants do not understand the economic realities of their own lives, or that they are inhibited from responding rationally by a load of inherited taboos and quasi-religious attitudes which they carry through life[2], or that insufficient access to antinatal measures makes it impossible to respond rationally. It is impossible to live and carry out research in a peasant society for any sustained period and retain this outlook. Peasants, once the language barrier has been overcome, turn out to be extraordinarily hard-headed about things that affect their own interests. Nor is ignorance the essential explanation: in Nigeria, farmers have been shown to be only one-fifth as likely to turn contraceptive knowledge into practice as are townsmen (Caldwell, 1975b, p. 84).

It is possible to argue that Mueller's approach and data are fundamentally defective, as they almost certainly are. It is difficult to establish the probable level of a peasant's income, because he has no employer and no wage scale, although the market prices for staples and his area of cultivation may be a guide to receipts for staples. However, his supplementary income may be substantial, difficult to detect and almost impossible to assess. In Nigerian research, employing survey techniques which yielded plausible answers to most responses and data that survived tests by matching against data collected by independent systems, we have not been able to show satisfactory relationships between stated income and other characteristics of respondents of provable accuracy such as occupation or education. McDevitt, after a long period of intensive survey work in rural Nigeria,

[2] See for instance Butz (1972).

concluded that most of the money data were of little value (1975, pp. 8–10) and pointed out that the rural businessman does not make a distinction between his household and his business economy (ibid. p. 5). Taylor, working in rural Kenya, employed an unusual research strategy to show that there is a declining likelihood of income being revealed as its source becomes less respectable or less derived from personal exertion and more from investment: the statement of income derived from coffee-growing was more complete than that from a share in a truck let alone a share in a bar or takings from prostitution.[3] The failure to disclose all earnings, investment and expenditure to interviewers is conventionally explained as fear of taxation authorities; yet our experience in Africa suggests that a much more potent fear is that the responses will be overheard by relatives and others who have never been certain of the amount of money dispensed by the respondent and who have claims on his care and may have received different assistance from that given to others. Mueller attempts to circumvent the inadequacy of money data by employing an approach based on labour-inputs into the growing of staples. This has two major weaknesses. First, it underestimates the complexity of peasant economies, which is particularly unfortunate in the context in her type of analysis because a particularly high proportion of children's inputs is into work other than the production of staples and because the question of the value of children's work is likely to become a real issue in modernizing economies were diversification is taking place. Secondly, it is based upon measurements of labour inputs and consumption, which are suspect, at least in the case of the latter where none are clearly derived from adequate measurement in the developing world.[4]

However, the fundamental weakness of this type of approach is that it employs survey data of questionable value while ignoring much more certain information which should be the logical starting point for any economic and social enquiry. The truth is that the peasant societies of Africa and Southern Asia all have high fertility levels, except for certain areas such as a region of Middle Africa where infertility arising apparently from disease is widespread, and that few people believe that they would benefit by having a family of the size now found in industrialized countries. Mueller is aware of this but appears to regard it as a misapprehension by the rural population of their own position: "the idea that raising children has some net economic

---

[3] Frazer Taylor (Carleton University, Ottawa, Canada), personal communication. Taylor, when interviewing, employed only English and Swahili, and did not disclose his knowledge of Kikuyu, thus enabling him to listen to the discussion in Kikuyu as to how much should be revealed to him. Our experience in Nigeria has been that even the income recorded in this way would substantially understate all income because of an unwillingness by the respondents to reveal their total incomes to each other.

[4] Mueller, (1975 p. 10–11). Those which appear to be based on measurements from the developing world, such as Lorimer's and Epstein's, turn out when checked to be derived measurements.

benefit to parents seems to be widely held among the peasants themselves" (ibid. p. 1).

The first task of the social scientist should be to investigate these societies to discover how their economies are structured so that the less fertile are not rewarded by their restraint. This will be attempted in this chapter by focusing on a single society, Yoruba society in the Western and Lagos States of Nigeria, employing primarily data from a research programme which has continued since early 1973, but using supplementary evidence on Yoruba and other West African societies from research over the previous decade in Nigeria and Ghana.[5] While the economy of these people is much more complex than those analysed by Sahlins, some insight into earlier conditions which helped to frame it can be derived from his assertion that "primitive economic behaviour is largely an aspect of kinship behaviour, and is therefore organized by means completely different from capitalist production and market transactions" (1960, p. 391). Some insight into the condition of many of our economists and other social scientists can also be gained from his charge that our understanding has often been obscured by projecting our ethnocentric view of an economy and of life aims.

The emphasis in this chapter will be on the rationality of Yoruba fertility behaviour and beliefs given the existing society and economy, although stress will also be placed on continuing change and its implications for fertility. This approach should not be confused with the argument that high-fertility families (Simon, 1974, p. 98) or societies (Boserup, 1965; Clark, 1967) do not suffer from population growth because their extra numbers and needs are themselves the stimulus for the greater production necessary—a challenge and response view. Nor is it the approach that argues that only the higher rural incomes resulting from successful technological innovation in farming can improve living conditions and create a more modern life style to a point where social expectations reach a threshold where faster advance is seen to lie through lower fertility (Kocher, 1973, pp. 56–92). The argument in this chapter is that social change can alter social and economic organization and ends and that as these ends change so will fertility control and fertility; the response is a rational response to the ends and does not dam itself irrationally against a wall of tradition until a threshold pressure is reached sufficient to make the wall crumble.

The purpose of this chapter will consequently be to examine Yoruba society, to demonstrate its levels of fertility and fertility ideals, to ascertain the economic ends and other desires of the population, and to adduce the value of children in this context.

---

[5] See Appendix (and note nomenclature which will henceforth be used to identify the source of data obtained from this programme).

The Yoruba

The demonstration that the fertility values of a peasant society still play the dominant role in Yoruba society is of considerable interest as the Yoruba have come a long way from the nearly homogeneous society of peasant cultivators living in small villages.

Cocoa farming began around 1900 and has been the dominant form of cash farming in all but the drier areas since the 1920s. Ultimately it covered so much land that many Yoruba areas imported yams and other food (Bascom, 1969, p. 23–24). In the last generation land has become less plentiful, as is evidenced by a marked decline in farming land available for permanent lease; and, over the same period, farming has become more capital intensive largely because of the need for spraying equipment to suppress diseases attacking the cocoa trees (Vanden Driesen, 1971).

Yorubaland has long exhibited extraordinary levels of urbanization, having one city, Ibadan, in the mid-nineteenth century with perhaps 150 thousand people, and probably accounting until the end of the century for one-sixth of the urban population of tropical Africa (Caldwell, 1980). By 1963 over one-third of the population of the Western State and almost two-fifths of that of the Western and Lagos States combined lived in urban areas; by 1975 the latter proportion may well have been closer to half with over one-quarter living in two centres, Lagos with about two million residents and Ibadan with around one million.[6] The towns, especially the smaller ones, house great numbers of farmers and others with substantial interests in farms. Nevertheless, their existence is evidence that the Yoruba have long had other economic interests as well, predominantly in commerce. In the 1850s Bowen commented on the number of women specializing in the public sale of prepared food[7] while over half of all women now describe themselves as traders (1963 Census volumes; CAFN 2) they belong to one of the few ethnic groups in tropical Africa where the women do not do most of the farming (Boserup, 1970, p. 15–36).[8] By 1963 less than half the male labour force described themselves as farmers and by 1975 the proportion may have been little over one-third (1963 Census volumes; CAFN 2).

In the last generation, schooling has spread rapidly so that almost half the population over seventeen years of age has had some education with the proportion reaching seven-tenths for persons in their twenties (CAFN 2).

[6] The 1963 urban proportions are from Nigeria Federal Census Office, *Population Census, 1963: Western Nigeria*, 11, and *Population Census, 1963: Lagos*, 11, Lagos, undated. Although the census was undoubtedly an overcount, the proportions given here may not have been far astray. The 1975 estimates are made by prorating 1973 estimates from CAFN 1 and CAFN 2.

[7] Quoted in Bascom (1969) p. 25.

[8] See map on p. 18 from Baumann (1928).

Statistically the society is divided by religion, the 1963 census recording Christians as 50% Moslems as 44% and others, mostly older people adhering to the traditional religion, as 8% (1963 Census volumes). Such divisions mean less than they do in almost any other society and there are no marked geographic or socioeconomic distinctions between Christians and Moslems, although the historic tendency of Christianity to provide schooling does mean that Christians are on average better educated and more likely to secure high-status, urban employment.

The Yoruba family, and presumably the family in many other non-European societies, is less similar to the Western family than many social scientists realize. Even when such social scientists concede the importance of relationships and obligations beyond the nuclear family, their subsequent analysis frequently overlooks the concession (this problem seems to beset the KAP surveys and their interpretation). Yet an understanding of the family is the basis for an understanding of the household economy and of traditional fertility.

In 1973 about half of all Yoruba women were in polygynous marriages (CAFN 2), which means that a considerably higher proportion would spend some of their married lives in such marriages. There is evidence from one rural Division of a considerable decline in Yoruba polygyny over the last generation (Vanden Driesen, 1972, p. 49–53). This may be related to the increasing levels of female education, for more highly educated women are much less likely to be found in polygynous marriage (CAFN 1, CAFN 2, NF 1).[9] There is evidence from the surveys that polygynous marriages can cause trouble in rural areas now that there is money to be distributed and extra demands such as education on resources: one respondent explained about a friend, "because he is rich his problem is not financial but because the children are from different mothers there is hatred in the family (CAFN 2, Vol. 2.1, respondent 2159). Salient characteristics of the Yoruba conjugal and familial relationships will be left to a more detailed discussion below which will justify the above assertion. There is no intention of implying here that polygyny determines most of the characteristics of marital relationships, but the institution is one that lends itself readily to statistical measurement.

Fertility and Desired Fertility

Yoruba fertility is high and there is as yet no certain evidence of decline in any part of the society. The evidence from the 1973–75 survey programme

[9] In CAFN 2, 7% of polygynously married women had any secondary education while 35% of monogamously married women did.

was that the adjusted total fertility ratio for all surveyed women was 7·4 (CAFN 2 corrected by the Brass technique) and that there was no statistically significant fertility differential between women of completed fertility by size of centre of residence or by other socio-economic characteristics. However, the average number of children borne by women 17–29 years of age was only two-thirds as much in the two cities as in villages with fewer than 20 000 inhabitants, although the difference fell to only 5% for women 30–39. The explanation lies partly in a higher proportion of very young women in the city, partly in later marriages there and probably partly in a greater predilection for unmarried or childless young women to leave the village for the city; but these explanations do not seem to cover the whole gap and it is possible that the beginning of fertility decline, at least in the city, is now being observed. Evidence from a larger sample drawn entirely from the city of Ibadan (CAFN 1) reveals that the average number of children borne by women over 45 years of age declines by one child from women with only primary school education, through those who did not proceed beyond secondary schooling to the relatively small number with tertiary education.[10] No other socioeconomic characteristic yields an indisputable differential or one that is unlikely to be explained by the educational differential.

Little attempt is made to control fertility, and the major constraints upon it are very substantial periods of sexual abstinence by women after birth and a high frequency of female terminal abstinence which probably begins in many cases before the onset of infecundity. These controls are rarely explained in terms of the economic difficulties resulting from high fertility but the former is almost always justified in terms of preserving the infant's health (NF 2) and the latter for personal reasons such as being too old now for the worry of raising more children (NF 3) (Caldwell and Caldwell, 1977). But those women who have at any stage attempted any antinatal practice except continence numbered by 1973–5 only 16% in the city of Ibadan (CAFN 1), 4% in the villages of Ibadan's rural hinterland and 2% in the villages of the less urbanized Ekiti Division (Orubuloye, 1975, 1981), figures which were nevertheless higher than those recorded 4–6 years earlier.[11]

[10] However, women with no education recorded lower fertility in Ibadan than women with primary education (CAFN 1). David Lucas has reported the same finding from his survey research in Lagos (1976, Table 9.6, p. 218). It is possible that illiterate women may be more affected by sterilizing disease (some of them are probably prostitutes but the ramifications of ill-health are undoubtedly much wider than this); they may also be more likely to adhere strictly to long periods of post-natal sexual abstinence. However, it is also probable that they reveal a lower proportion of diseased children while undoubtedly experiencing a higher level of mortality among the children.

[11] Caldwell and Igun (1970) recording a survey carried out in March–April 1969 when levels in Ibadan were around 8% and in the rural areas 1%. Levels of rural contraception as low, or usually lower, are the rule in tropical Africa (see Caldwell, 1975b, p. 87).

Nevertheless, there is very little evidence that family planning is securing a rural toehold: further investigation of the few women practising contraception in villages around Ibadan or in Ekiti showed that they were mostly the wives of school teachers or of men with white collar jobs in the distant towns (Orubuloye, 1975 and 1981).

In 1973 (the following analysis is entirely from CAFN 2) the proportion of all women in the Western and Lagos States who had ever used any antinatal method other than sexual abstinence was 11%, which was subdivided into 5% currently using modern contraceptives (apparently largely pills, condoms and IUDs in that order), 5% who had used such contraceptives in the past and 1% employing rhythm or withdrawal (CAFN 2).[12] The use of contraception rose steeply with education and occupation and was markedly higher in the larger urban centres and amongst younger adults. Women with education exceeding three years secondary schooling and with husbands in white collar occupations[13] made up only 11% of the sample but 55% of the current users of modern contraception; such women living in Lagos or Ibadan formed only 3% of the sample but 35% of current users.

The high level of fertility was not primarily the inevitable and unwanted result of so few women being able to use contraception. It was in fact in line with the views and desires of most of the community as can be seen from the responses to survey questions set out in Table 1. Analysis of responses by a large number of socioeconomic characteristics suggests that the most important are education, occupation (or occupation of husband), age and size of centre of residence in that order. Each of these characteristics shows a statistically significant association with the distribution of almost every response in the table. Because these characteristics are interrelated, all the analysis in this chapter has also been carried out with the whole four taken in combination. Where relevant, parity (the number of live births to the respondent) has also been included in the analysis. The tables are presented by sex, largely because the reader will expect it and nothing less will demonstrate the astonishing lack of differentials by sex.

It is clear that the community as a whole still wants the seven live births it has been achieving. In fact, given the high mortality conditions of Nigeria, the average Yoruba respondent may prefer eight or more live births, for the interviewees have undoubtedly been discussing desired numbers of surviving children. There is an abhorrence of childlessness and a surprisingly

[12] The separate question of past use of various methods, and other evidence from the survey programme, suggest that current use of rhythm and withdrawal is probably understated and these are probably at least 2% and 1% respectively.

[13] White collar occupations are defined here as all professional, administrative, clerical and other indoor occupations which are non-manual and necessitate literacy. It includes military and police officers and even government messengers (partly because these people will otherwise misstate the nature of their job to interviewers). Most of these people do not work in collars.

TABLE 1
Fertility attitudes in Yorubaland 1973;
Selected responses to specific questions by sex (percentages of total respondents)

Question	Response	Percentage giving that response			Significant deviations
		Females	Males	Both sexes	
(1) What do you think is the best number of children to have?	1–3	1	2	1	(1) A majority responded under 5 only amongst female respondents under 30 married to WC workers and living in centres with over 2000 inhabitants.
	4	16	16	16	
	5	18	17	17	
	6	24	22	23	
	7+	11	16	14	
	Up to God	29	26	28	
	No response	1	1	1	
					(2) A majority responded under 6 amongst females under 50 married to WC workers.
					(3) Up to God responses are mostly from traditional farming population where amongst illiterates, who are the majority, it reaches 43%.
(2) Do you think a woman should have as many children as possible?	Yes	23	23	23	(1) There is no longer a majority in any subgroup; the highest Yes is amongst male farmers over 50 where it reaches 44%.
	No	71	72	71	
	Don't know	6	5	6	
					(2) The most marked age break is amongst the farming population where Yes amongst females under 30 is 26% and amongst males under 30 it is 29%.
(3) Agreement/ disagreement "Bearing children is the most important thing a woman can do".	Agree	92	91	92	
	Disagree	7	8	8	

TABLE 1 (Continued)

Fertility attitudes in Yorubaland 1973;
Selected responses to specific questions by sex (percentages of total respondents)

Question	Response	Percentage giving that response			Significant deviations
		Females	Males	Both sexes	
(4) Agreement/ disagreement "I love children—nearly all children".	Agree Disagree	90 8	88 10	89 9	
(5) A husband and wife have five daughters and no sons and wonder whether this is enough children. What would you do in this situation?	Have more children	57	60	58	There are majorities for having more children amongst all groups in centres with fewer than 20 000 residents and in farming families irrespective of the size of the centre.
(6) (Only those married respondents where the wife (or wives) is fertile and has had no child for 2 years). Would you like to have another baby within a year?	Yes	72	76	74	(1) Only amongst females married to WC workers in Lagos does Yes fall to 50% for those with less than secondary schooling and under 50% for those with more education.
					(2) Many of those answering No in traditional society had babies 2–3 years before and believe the time since is too short for sexual relations to resume.
					(3) Analysis by parity reported in text.
(7) What are the good things about having no children at all?	No good things at all	95	92	93	

TABLE 1 (Continued)

Question	Response	Females	Males	Both sexes	Significant deviations
(8) Agreement/ disagreement "A parent with many children is surely happy?"	Agree Disagree	56 41	52 42	54 41	(1) Majorities no longer are found in the cities or amongst those with extended education. (2) In the farming sector agreement is about 70%.
(9) Agreement/ disagreement "A man with twelve children is blessed"	Agree Disagree	51 45	49 47	50 46	Comments as for (8).

Source: CAFN 2
Note: (1) Certain responses are not shown in this and subsequent tables and No response is never shown.
(2) WC = white collar occupation; the occupation, unless otherwise noted, when discussing families is that of the husband.
Throughout the tables, extended education means at least three years secondary schooling.

large proportion of those women in a position to have another child who wish to do so straight away. This desire amongst women who had not borne a child for two years to become pregnant again is even more revealing when the analysis is carried out by parity: for those with less than three live births the proportion wanting another within a year was almost 90%, for those with three live births it fell to 75% with four or five live births to 66%, and thereafter stablized at about 60% so that the majority of even high parity women wanted a baby.

In rural areas almost half the unschooled farming population, who still form the majority of the populace, may reply to some questions that the determination of the matter is "up to God". This is neither an evasive nor a superstitious reply and such respondents are perfectly happy to discuss what they mean, which is really that these are matters over which they have little control and that to attempt more control would probably achieve little while bordering on the impious.

Nevertheless, some scepticism of high fertility and more of high-fertility values is creeping in. The change is fostered by western schooling and by life in the large cities and the smaller family (i.e. four or five children) is often thought of, both by the highly educated and by peasant farmers, as a pattern

TABLE 2
Advantages and disadvantages of high fertility, 1973:
Selected responses to specific questions by sex (percentages of total respondents)

Question	Response	Percentage giving that response			Significant deviations
		Females	Males	Both sexes	
(1a) If you did have another child this year, would you be richer or poorer in the future?	Richer	25	25	25	There are no associations with any of the characteristics of the respondents
	Poorer	19	20	19	
	Same	34	35	34	
(1b) (Question put to male household heads in NF 1 who by definition already had considerable families and were middle aged or older) Would you have been richer with another child?	Yes, richer	37			
	Qualified Yes (i.e. richer in specified circumstances)	1			
	No (all other answers except don't know, i.e. proper and same)	44			
(2) Agreement/ disagreement "A man with ten children is a fool"	Agree	37	39	38	(1) The strongest association is with age; a majority of all respondents under 30 now agree.
	Disagree	58	57	57	
					(2) Strong associations also with education, occupation and living in a city.
					(3) Agreement ranges from over half in Lagos and Ibadan to just over one-quarter in traditional farming areas.
(3) The best thing about having many children is . . . ?	Nothing good	36	37	37	
	Guaranteed descendants	13	13	13	
	Support in old age	11	11	11	
	Economic advantages	10	11	11	
	Social advantages	9	12	10	
	A good and happy thing	9	9	9	

TABLE 2 (Continued)

Question	Response	Females	Males	Both sexes	Significant deviations
(4) Do you think a woman should have a lot of children? Is it possible to have too many? What would you say would be too many?	Under 6	4	6	5	
	6	10	12	11	
	7	9	7	8	
	8	13	13	13	
	9	3	2	2	
	10	14	13	13	
	11+	8	9	9	
	No, she should have as many as possible	10	10	10	
	Up to God	21	20	21	
	No response	8	8	8	
(5a) Do you agree with the (Yoruba) proverb: "Lots of children, lots of misery".	Yes	74	73	74	(1) Strong associations with education, occupation and age. (2) Weaker association with size of centre.
(5b) How many children do parents have before they begin to feel this misery?	Under 6	4	5	5	The only group where the modal number chosen falls persistently below 11+ is women with husbands with white collar occupations. This appears to be a stronger influence than age or size of centre (and includes nearly all women with extended education). The numbers most frequently quoted by wives of white collar workers are 7 and 8.
	6	8	9	8	
	7	10	7	9	
	8	13	10	11	
	9	3	3	3	
	10	11	13	12	
	11+	11	12	12	
	Either "a great number" or "no number" would make them miserable.	18	18	18	
	Depends on their income or circumstances	22	22	22	
	No response	0	1	0	
(6) (For those who did not want another child: 19% of female respondents and 15% of male respondents) Can you tell me any reasons why you might not want another child?	(Percentage of respondents who wanted no more)				
	Widowed, separated, too old	36	21	29	
	Economic reasons, mainly schooling	21	28	24	

TABLE 2 (Continued)

Question	Response	Females	Males	Both sexes	Significant deviations
	Economic reasons—other	11	18	14	
	Had enough children	21	19	20	
	Health, dislike of childbirth	6	5	6	
	Social reasons —freedom, mobility	1	2	2	
(7) Agreement/ disagreement "Money is the elder brother and children the younger brother"	Agree	80	78	79	

Source: CAFN 2 except for question (1b) which is from NF 1.

of life not of universal applicability to the country but suited to, and perhaps increasingly necessary for, the educated middle classes of the cities and large towns.

That there are believed to be some economic limitations to unrestricted fertility is clear from the responses shown in Table 2.

It is quite clear that the Yoruba population do not believe that families can be indefinitely large and a majority of the population agree that more than ten children per family is excessive. But it is far from clear that the ceiling is largely imposed by economic circumstances. The most significant aspect of this research, and a finding that can probably be replicated widely in tropical Africa, is that only 20% of the respondents believe that the marginal child makes the family poorer. Indeed more believe that the addition makes it richer. Perhaps more surprising to those who bring their ideas and methods of analysis from very different cultures and economies the belief (almost certainly borne out by experience) that larger families do not impoverish is held by most residents of the city even amongst the educated white collar families. It will be the main purpose of this chapter to show why.

When asked to name the best thing about a large family only one-ninth of the respondents answered in terms of current economic gain and another ninth in terms of future support. Non-economic motivations predominate as they do also when considering the childless or very small family or when debating the desirability of more children. When respondents were asked what would be bad about having another baby during the year, only one-ninth gave a reason that was in any way economic, and, even if the respondents were restricted to females who agreed that there were drawbacks and were not worried about the period that had elapsed since the last child, the fraction does not rise above one-third (CAFN 2). The case for a woman having no further children (Table 2:6 and more extensively in NF 3) is more often personal or social rather than economic: there are too many children or too many young children now that she or her husband are beginning to feel old; she has become a grandmother and should not have competing emotional loyalties between children and grandchildren of similar age; childbirth has become increasingly feared or sexual relations increasingly burdensome.

The contrast between western society and rural (and, but probably to a lesser extent, non-rural) Nigerian society is not that, as the number of children grows, the family in the former society becomes increasingly more impoverished because the only value of the child is as a consumption good while in the latter it increasingly prospers because the child is mainly a productive agent. The evidence seems to be that the economic wellbeing of the Nigerian family does not change very much with family size and hence the social advantages of eight children outweigh those of four and completely eclipse the horrors of the no-, one-, or two-child families. Beyond about ten children (and beyond a smaller number for certain more educated or urbanized subdivisions of the society) most of the community feel that there are few more social gains to be made by increasing the sheer number while psychological wear and tear, and, for some families, financial strain mount rapidly. Certainly four-fifths of the respondents agreed with the sentiments of a popular song being danced to and sung in Yoruba in the nightclubs of Lagos and Ibadan at that time that repeatedly stated that "Money is the elder brother and children the younger brother", which meant that money was the more important and implied that if a choice had to be made it would be chosen—but, in contrast to foreign social scientists and probably to the song-writer and most of the bright young things who danced to it, it would appear that few of the respondents could understand why such a choice would ever present itself.

For reasons that will become clearer as the chapter proceeds, there is an apprehension of having a small family and a profound fear of having none. Such a fate can arise from infecundity, although a man will amost invariably blame one or even a succession of wives for being childless and will employ both polygyny and divorce followed by remarriage to attempt to overcome it. But, as the whole community knows in a high-mortality society, it can also arise from unwisely having too few children only to have all or most die. The intensity of feeling on this issue is plumbed in Table 3.

Table 3 provides an excellent illustration not only of the intensity of the fear of being left without descendants but of the degree to which important

TABLE 3
Feelings about dying without living descendants, 1973:
Selected responses to specific questions by sex (percentages of total respondents)

Question	Response	Percentage giving that response			Significant deviations
		Females	Males	Both sexes	
Agreement/ disagreement (for all questions)					
(1) "A man lives on through his sons."	Agree	98	97	98	
(2) "Children are still needed to do services for the ancestors."	Agree	86	84	85	Agreement is least among Lagos men with extended education in white collar employment, but even in this group it is 81% and is no lower amongst those under 30 years old in this category
(3) "The real dead are those who die without descendants."	Agree	92	92	92	
(4) "A woman without children might as well never have been born."	Agree	62	62	62	

Source: CAFN 2.

aspects of the traditional culture have survived the almost complete conversion of the society to Islam and Christianity and also the impact of western education. In the traditional religion of most of tropical Africa the dead survive as spirits only in so far as their descendants remember them, carry out services for them and indeed try to contact them. Without such descendants the spirits fade away and death is complete. Given this kind of belief, and it is clearly present in Table 3, one cannot take one risk in a hundred, perhaps not one in a thousand, of being left without descendants—and, at the present level of mortality in Yorubaland, reducing one's risks to these levels would mean having 4 children and 6 or 7 children

TABLE 4
Desires and ambitions, 1973:
Selected responses to specific questions by sex (percentages of total respondents)

Question	Response	Percentage giving that response			Significant deviations
		Females	Males	Both sexes	
(1) Think of all the things that might happen to you if you were very lucky. What would be the best thing that could possibly happen to you?	a) Acquiring a great deal of money and/or many possessions	36	42	39	Money and possessions was the most frequent response in all subsections of the population.
	b) Being able to educate the children further	19	14	17	
	c) Getting a better education or job	8	12	10	
	d) Having more children	10	4	7	
	e) Having both more children and more money or possessions	6	4	5	
(2) If someone gave you 100 naira (50), what would you do with it?	a) Put it into business or farm (including stock for petty trading)	55	39	47	(1) Among white collar respondents with extended education business/ farm falls to 14% compared with 58% for those in farming and manual occupations.
	b) Spend it on education of children or self	18	22	20	(2) Among white collar respondents with extended education saving is conspicuously important, and education and clothing more important than in other groups.
	c) Buy clothes	10	8	9	
	d) Spend it (unspecified)	5	11	8	
	e) Save it	6	9	7	
	f) Spend it on house	4	7	5	

TABLE 4 (Continued)

Question	Response	Females	Males	Both sexes	Significant deviations
(3) If you won the lottery or the pools and won an enormous amount of money (say 20 000 naira or 10 000), what would you do with it? (First choice responses only)	a) Spend it on house	39	37	38	(1) There are very few differences between the sub-sections of the population largely because the sum of money is so great that even the urban white collar respondents with extended education feel that they would also have to invest in a business while all groups feel that they could both afford a house and educate their children.
	b) Put it into business or farm (including buying a taxi)	26	25	26	
	c) Spend it on education of children	23	21	22	
	d) Save it	4	5	5	
	e) Spend it on own education	2	4	3	(2) Those under 30 would spend relatively more on their own education.
	f) Spend it (unspecified)	1	2	2	
	(First preference only)				
(4a) What would you like to have in the following list if you could afford only one? If you could afford a second, what would it be? What about a third? 1. a new car 2. a second-hand lorry 3. a new house 4. another child 5. a lot of new furniture 6. a university education for one of your children 7. a trip to England 8. more education for yourself 9. a lot of new clothes	a) a university education for one of your children	43	40	41	(1) Amongst those under 30 with any education (and among manual workers under 30 with no education) education for oneself dominates.
	b) a new house	22	26	24	
	c) another child	14	7	10	(2) Amongst most other groups a university education for their child is most important.
	d) more education for yourself	8	15	12	
	e) a new car	7	8	8	
	f) a trip to England	2	2	2	(3) A new house comes second to education for all traditional farming groups.
	g) a second-hand lorry	1	2	2	
	h) a lot of new clothes	1	1	1	(4) A new car is not an important first choice in any group, not even Lagos white collar workers with extended education.
	i) a lot of new furniture	0	0	0	
	(Total of percentages for 1st, 2nd or 3rd preference)				
	a) a new house	81	82	81	
	b) a university education for one of your children	77	78	77	

TABLE 4 (Continued)

Question	Response	Female	Male	Both sexes	Significant deviations
	c) a new car	49	52	51	
	d) more education for self	18	27	23	
	e) another child	26	16	21	
	f) a trip to England	16	16	16	
	g) a lot of new clothes	17	9	13	
	h) a second-hand lorry	9	10	9	
	i) a lot of new furniture	7	9	8	
(4b) Respondents who pointed out in Question (4a) that one does not have to afford a child and who hence did not include it in their list of preferences		29	29	29	
(5) What job or position would you most like to have or (for the oldest group) have had?	a) Business man/woman	64	62	58	(1) Farmers and urban non-WC all aspire to be business men or women.
	b) Professional or white collar	21	29	25	(2) White collar respondents with extended education largely aspire to be professional or other white collar.
	c) High position in traditional society	5	6	6	
	d) Skilled job	2	5	4	
	e) Higher position in present employment	1	2	2	(3) White collar workers with lesser education are split between those wishing to be business men/women and those wanting to have professional or other white collar jobs.
(6) What job or position would you most like one of your sons to have?	a) Professional (other than doctor) or white collar	47	49	48	
	b) Doctor	37	38	37	
	c) Business man	4	5	4	
	d) High position in traditional society	1	1	1	

TABLE 4 (Continued)

Question	Response	Female	Male	Both sexes	Significant deviations
	e) Skilled position, craftsman	1	1	1	
(7) What job or position would you most like one of your daughters to have?	a) Nurse b) Professional (other than nurse or doctor) or white collar c) Doctor d) Business woman e) Skilled position f) High position in traditional society	39 30 12 8 2 1	36 31 14 8 2 1	38 31 13 8 2 1	(1) Professional or other white collar jobs dominate among white collar workers and other urban population. (2) Nursing is equally important among farmers.
(8) If someone offered you a good job for three years but you could only take it if you put off having a baby for that time, would you be prepared to try to stop having a baby for three years?	Yes Perhaps No	64 7 27	67 7 24	65 7 25	Proportion saying yes highest among white collar workers with extended education. For white collar females with extended education it becomes 85%.
(9) What is the minimum level of education for your children that would satisfy you?	No Schooling Primary schooling Secondary schooling University or other Tertiary education			2 6 46 38	(1) Only 1% give a level (by the categories employed here) below their own. (2) Only 10% give the same level and they are mostly parents with at least secondary education. (3) 89% say higher level.
(10) Would you be happy if your child became a farmer?	Yes Qualified Yes (usually specifying a farmer with capital, trained manager of a government farm etc) No			17 20 56	No was 66% among illiterate farmers.

Source: CAFN 2, question 1–8; NF 1, questions 9 and 10 (note that NF 1 was asked only of male household heads).

respectively, although white collar workers with extended education living in Lagos or Ibadan might do it with 3 and 4 or 5 children respectively.[14]

What do People Want out of Life?

It is impossible to understand the working of the traditional village society and economy, a society and economy which still largely determines that of the large towns and cities and probably will do so for many years to come, without an appreciation of what people want to do with their lives and how they want to spend their money. The failure to investigate this matter has been a major weakness of fertility studies; KAP surveys have asked all kinds of questions about fertility ideals without bothering to investigate other ideals, some of which might well be competitive with desired fertility. In Table 4 some data on desired expenditures and ambitions for the respondents themselves and their children are tabulated partly to see if there is conflict here.

Yoruba society is strongly commercial, and realistic dreams are of money and what money can do.[15] Particularly noteworthy is the extent to which suggested extra income, beyond the normal income which covers most day-to-day living costs, is thought of in terms of investment: business and stock for business, education and housing. The table by concentrating mainly on larger outlays may overlook individual desires for transistor radios and bicycles, but the truth is that village society, at least, is not conspicuously consumer-orientated except perhaps with regard to clothes.

One major expenditure, virtually amounting to a consumption good, is not revealed by this type of survey question. However, when we recorded biographies of the success and expenditure of those who had emerged from the traditional society to attain economic success (NF 4 and NF 5) we found that the expenditure which brought the greatest pleasure was that on relatives and even non-relatives. Extended family obligations can be worrying if money is short. Most western observers have brought to the field the reactions and emotions of their own society and have usually referred to the burden of the extended family. But, in the biographies, the emphasis was again and again on the growth of love and respect with this expenditure and the joy that this reaction brought to the spender. Even from the western

[14] The Coale-Demeny "North" set of model life tables are employed (Coale and Demeny, 1966) and the assumption is made that sons should survive to 30 years of age and daughters to 25 to ensure that they have living descendants. An expectation of life at birth of 45–50 is employed for the whole population (based on P. O. Olusanya, 1975) and one of 57½–60 years for the children of city white collar workers with extended education, the socioeconomic and rural–urban differential being estimated from child-survival data in CAFN 2.

[15] Here and elsewhere I have been helped by discussions with Peter Morton Williams, now Head of the Sociology Department, University of Cape Coast, Ghana.

point of view, this may well be a rational outlook given the necessity for purchasing security which is discussed in the next section.

The willingness to spend on education is a remarkable feature of the table, as is the clear appreciation that this is the way out of the traditional economy. The desire for more children is also a conspicuous feature of the responses, especially when it is realized that many of the respondents could not imagine a child being a competitive expenditure—29% said as much but many more just omitted children from their lists while failing to make the protest which was noted only if it were spontaneous and recorded by the interviewers (it was not on the questionnaires and interviewers had not been instructed to record it).

Consumption expenditure is not high in the list of first preferences and rises when successive preferences are totalled only because some expenditures are ruled out for many respondents: there is a ceiling on university education because some families' children already have educational records which clearly will not get them there; further education for oneself is restricted to the young and especially those with some education; more children is an unlikely or impossible choice for older women.

What is clear is the two-generational nature of the planned attainment of the benefits of the modern society. Most adults know that they lack the education, or the opportunity for it, needed to reach the urban professional and white-collar classes—the undoubted goal of all, the positions of prestige and power where men and women work indoors, direct others, use the telephone with assurance, seldom suffer feelings of deprivation and are able to help their relatives. But, with some luck and savings, even the middle aged can take up trading or other business and a few do really well. The biographies are full of reference to the guidance of God or of wise parents, other relatives or friends who suggested the right course at the right time or of fellow lodge members or others who helped to provide access to scarce goods for sale. Success is not easy, but this is the route. Children, however, can be educated directly for complete success, especially if they can be kept at school or sent to the right schools. This can be done by farmers, but a successful business makes it much easier. The urban white-collar classes and the farmers almost all want their children to be educated for as long as possible to reach the professional classes and they are willing to make very considerable sacrifices to ensure this. Amongst both the skilled and unskilled workers of the large urban centres there is more doubt about this credo (NF 1); these parents are already in the town themselves and are trying to improve their own positions there without all their earnings being eroded by asssistance to children. Perhaps their respect for the extended family system of obligations is beginning to crumble; perhaps too there are the beginnings of class war and some scepticism about helping their children to join the bourgeoisie. The move towards sharing the benefits of the modern world means a flight from farming or at least from peasant farming. One-fifth of all respondents would be willing for their children to be large-scale mechanized farmers or managers or agricultural advisers in state farms but they draw the line at traditional farming. Only one-sixth were prepared to see their children peasant farmers, and the fraction was no higher amongst parents from farming families. Indeed the fraction was as high as it was because urban white collar workers either feel some guilt about denying the traditional life or cherish what may well be romantic illusions.

Most would be willing to make considerable sacrifices to ensure occupational and economic success. Between two-thirds and three-quarters would be willing to defer births in order to achieve or hold on to good jobs. The reason that such attitudes do not result in fertility decline is not in most cases that such resolves could not be carried through but that there is in fact little conflict between high fertility and economic advancement. The great majority of women are in no position to be offered such a job choice. Even women in professional positions usually do not feel particularly pressured by a large family, partly because employers are still attuned to the high fertility culture, but largely because families or the home village can still supply young girls, often with little education, as inexpensive nurse girls (NF 5). The latter situation may be passing, largely because schooling is reaching an increasing proportion of the population.[16]

Traditional Needs and Wants

Observers from far more atomized societies often fail to realize the strengths and constraints of village life. There is an intimacy and interdependence in the small traditional community which the observer from the modern society finds difficult to credit. In a world of simple poverty where the possibility of riches and comfort hardly arose but where disasters were frequent and risks to life or to minimal comfort commonplace, it was important that people, especially relatives, should guarantee each other help particularly in times of real need. The emphasis in tropical African and other Third World societies tends to be far more on security and on being guaranteed survival through time of duress than it is on maximizing the profit in good times.[17]

[16] See the work being done in Ghana by Christine Oppong, especially Oppong (1975a and 1975b).

[17] See Caldwell (1975d), pp. 46–47, on West African rural life, and Garlick (1971), pp. 110–118, on urban life.

TABLE 5
The value of the family 1973:
Selected responses to specific questions by sex (percentages of total respondents)

Question	Response	Percentage giving that response			Significant deviations
		Females	Males	Both sexes	
(1a) (For respondents over 40 years of age) Have your children allowed your family to be connected with a lot of other families by marriage?	Yes	62	56	58	
(1b) (For respondents who replied Yes to 1a) Is this a good thing?	Yes	97	94	96	
(1c) (For respondents who replied Yes to 1a) Can you ask these relatives by marriage to help you in a way that you could not ask non-relatives?	Yes	65	64	65	
(2) Agreement/ disagreement "I can ask even relatives by marriage, for things or services that I cannot ask non-relatives."	Agree	84	83	83	
(3) Agreement/ disagreement "A man with many grown up children has a lot of power in society."	Agree	62	63	62	(1) Strong associations with working in the traditional sector and having no schooling. (2) Weaker association with being in a small centre. (3) In traditional farming communities with less than 100 000 inhabitants agreement reaches 72% while among white collar workers with extended education in Lagos and Ibadan it falls to 40%.

Source: CAFN 2.

Such security was gained by establishing a network of personal relationships—perhaps at times even buying obligations. The most important network was that with relatives, which in size was largely dependent on the extent to which one's fertility (and that of one's relatives) overcame the ravages of mortality and on the extension of the network of relatives made possible by marriage. It is little wonder that high fertility and early marriage were highly esteemed. Contemporary reaction to these matters is explored in Table 5.

Even many respondents over 40 years of age, especially males, were still too young for their children to have made *many* marriages. Some were subfertile and others were reluctant to concede that three or four marriages were either *many* or sufficient. However, there is no real disagreement, even in the most modernized sectors of the society, that the building up of one's network of relatives by reproduction and marriage is a good thing. One respondent echoes many: "It is good to have relatives on both sides—connection through the marriage of the girls is very good" (CAFN 2, Vol. 2.1. Respondent 2159). There is a feeling, doubtless based on experience and evidenced by the discrepancy between the responses to Questions (1c) and (2), that one cannot seek as much assistance from relatives by marriage as from blood relatives.

The traditional Yoruba community is a lot more than a mutual aid association. It is a highly structured society where one's power and prestige are partly determined by the number of adult supporters (especially, in the case of males, adult male supporters) one has. To this end, much depends on the number of one's relatives, but much more particularly on the number of adult sons.

In such a society there is a real problem about how one becomes more affluent, especially in terms of markedly increasing personal or household consumption, and how one enjoys the benefits brought by an industrializing world. The old way has been to seek high positions in the traditional hierarchy, but, as can be seen in Table 4, few any longer make even chieftaincy their goal (except as an honour bestowed or bought for success in other spheres) and fewer still have such aspirations for their children. Chiefs, in fact, receive wealth and disburse wealth, and are surrounded by the appurtenances of chieftaincy but are often poor in terms of the tempting possessions of the modern world.

The villager often has trouble markedly increasing his income. He can call on relatives for help in times of trouble or even to keep a child at school, but he can hardly exert the same pressure to buy a transistor radio. Even if he has the money there are real problems about spending it in conspicuous consumption. Such expenditure would certainly suggest wealth and would inevitably mean greater demands for assistance that would be harder to resist than if one's circumstances were demonstrably humble. In any case the village has a traditional way of life which places contraints upon the behaviour of the humble if they do not hold high traditional office or have not demonstrably separated themselves from the society by education, occupation and perhaps residence. The villager does have access to the modern world and its consumer society but it is more often indirect than through personal purchases and consumption in the village. This chapter will attempt to show how that access is achieved.

Nor does the villager find it easy to invest profitably any money which does come his way.[18] Raising money for small businesses is usually thought to be more a matter of personal saving by the person going into business, for trading success depends very much on individual ability and exertion. Apart from the now necessary cocoa spraying equipment it is by no means yet clear how small-holder farming can be made more capital intensive and what the return on such invested capital would be.

As long as the system of extended family obligations can be maintained, and as long as large differentials exist between farming and white collar incomes, then investment in the education of relatives may show the best returns. Certainly it is a return that might survive the passing of the years with all the inflation and other economic and political vicissitudes which that may bring. Perhaps the investment is not particularly profitable as seen by a western economist; perhaps, through his eyes, it is not profitable at all. A balance sheet of this type will be attempted later in the chapter. But it may purchase security and it may be more profitable than expenditure on an old or sick relative. Furthermore the returns may be in a form that the village cannot or is reluctant to acquire directly. An earlier study in Ghana showed that most villagers believed that investment in education was the best investment open to them (GA).

Villagers usually resent the analysis of educational expenditure as investment and talk instead of family ties. As will be seen below, they may be right in the sense that the expenditure is more a general investment than a specific one. The returns are not in proportion to the amount spent and not necessarily closely related to whether expenditure could or could not be made in an individual case—the system depends more on attitudes to familial relationships than it does to the proper return to an investor.

---

[18] See Galletti, Baldwin and Dina (1956), pp. 571–2, who concluded that little of the windfall gains made from the cocoa boom of the early 1950s was invested or spent by the farmers. They concluded that a little might have been paid into deposit accounts or *ESUSUS* (a kind of revolving fund where each depositor is given all the deposits of one round—see Bascom (1952) and NF 6—but could not account for the remainder. It would seem a reasonable supposition that some was accounted for by understatement in expenditure and that the rest was being hoarded as money.

The analysis of the value of children in the village household economy often completely fails to understand the subsistence nature of village services even when it does comprehend the subsistence nature of the consumption of goods. This is the more surprising because foreign technical aiders in Africa, especially those living in smaller communities, discover that in non-industrialized societies, wants are more frequently satisfied by services than goods. In their own societies much of their expenditure is in fact on goods which are not of particular aesthetic value in themselves but which merely occupy space while providing services. Vacuum cleaners pick up the dust; mowers keep down the grass; washing-up machines clean the dishes and washing machines the clothes; hot water systems provide hot water; electricity, gas and water reticulation systems carry fuel and water to the house; telephones and telegraph services get messages to the people; cars can be used for bringing home goods or for getting rid of rubbish; refrigerators and freezers make it possible to bring perishable goods into the household less frequently. In a society where nearly all these consumer durables are vastly expensive and difficult or impossible to maintain, the services are largely provided by either cheap labour or more frequently by family subsistence labour. The technical aider notes that his own household is run by great inputs of labour, but often assumes that this is solely because he is demanding a way of life which does not fit in with the existing economy; he often fails to see that all households run this way even on a lesser scale. Messages, fuel and food are carried, food often daily to prevent it perishing, while people with fairly rudimentary equipment pick up refuse, cut grass and heat water. In terms of the availability of cheap or ostensibly free labour, the farmer would be irrational who forced himself and his family to produce ever more crops for sale (assuming that a market existed) to buy expensive gadgets to supply the services he could get directly. Some day his world will become more complex: the gadgets will be cheaper and maintenance will be available, labour will be dearer, and children will feel that childhood is for games and not work. Until then, family work is producing more staples for the market and usually a more efficient way of maintaining or raising living standards. Furthermore, there is a division of labour. Children do many tasks not as an inferior supplement to adult labour (as Mueller implies, although admittedly restricting the analysis to the production of staples) but as a form of specialization in work that adults would find painful to do. Often the youngest do the specialized tasks, such as carrying messages or looking after even younger siblings. Such tasks are done outside the home as well as in it. It is easy to fall into the trap of thinking of most outdoor rural exertion as being digging, planting and harvesting. In fact a great deal takes the form of carrying goods, fuel, water and messages, or walking long distances to the nearest road with a passenger lorry or bus. Rural work of this kind will eventually be reduced not by farm machinery but by more roads, wells, dams and tree plantings and evenly piped water. In the meantime there is indispensable work to be done by children, as is affirmed by Table 6.

TABLE 6
The importance of children's work, 1973:
Selected responses to specific questions by sex (percentages of total respondents)

Question	Response	Percentage giving that response		
		Females	Males	Both sexes
Agreement/disagreement (1) "Small children save adults from menial (lowly, painstaking, little) tasks."	Agree	89	87	88
(2) "Children are important because of the help they give in the home."	Agree	94	92	93

Source: CAFN 2

Table 6 and the role of children's work can be fully understood only if it is realized that one of the services provided by children is the ability of their parents to enjoy more leisure. Galletti *et al.* (1956, p. 286) emphasized the Yoruba enjoyment of leisure and grace, and Jones (1968) emphasized that leisure in terms of social obligations is a very real thing in Africa and competes with cash-earning activities.

The Nature of the Family

The kind of economic ends and the support for high fertility depend fundamentally on the nature of the family. That nature is often misinterpreted in KAP surveys and other analyses, even when questions are included on polygyny and extended family obligations, to suggest an economic unit similar to the western nuclear family. In point of fact, Yoruba separation of the sexes, in the sense of independently going on with one's own way of life and economic concerns, is so great that one anthropologist concluded that one could not speak of a single society but of separate male and female

TABLE 7
The nature of the family, 1973:
Selected responses to specific questions by sex (percentages of total respondents)

Question	Response	Percentage giving that response			Significant deviations
		Females	Males	Both sexes	
(1) (Married respondents with children only) Who do you feel closest to (i.e. who do you have the strongest emotional bond with) your husband/wife, your children or your brothers and sisters?	Spouse Children Siblings	30 63 7	30 61 9	30 62 8	(1) Siblings are of more importance in rural areas but in no rural subsection of the population does this response rise much over 10%. (2) Amongst males the Spouse exceeds Children in the case of those with extended education living in the two big cities; amongst females Children is the most common response in all subdivisions of respondents. (3) In the traditional rural sector in centres with less than 20 000 inhabitants preference for children over spouses is for males 2·7:1 and for females 4·4:1. (4) Education is a much more important factor than degree of urbanization or occupation in changing the balance of these relationships.
(2) (Currently married only) Do you usually live with your husband/wife? Do you sleep in the same room or house or compound?	Same room Elsewhere in same house Same compound, but different building Elsewhere	35 51 4 10	35 53 5 7	35 52 5 8	
(3) (Currently married only) Do you and your husband/wife eat together?	Yes Occasionally No	31 21 48	30 22 48	31 21 48	

TABLE 7 (Continued)

Question	Response	Percentage giving that response			Significant deviations
		Females	Males	Both sexes	
(4) Agreement/ Disagreement "The costs of children should be mainly borne by the mother"	Agree	17	15	16	
(5) Do you want to have any more children?[19]	Yes			51	The response ranges by education from 59% for males with no education to 37% for those with secondary education.
(6) Do you want to have any more wives[19]	Yes			19	The response ranges by education from 31% for males with no education to 7% for those with secondary education.

Source: CAFN 2, Questions 1–4; NF 1, Questions 5–6.

societies (and economies) which existed in the same place and time but rarely intersected each other (Marshall, 1970, p. 181). Some facets of this society are brought out in Table 7.

Almost certainly the social and emotional distance between spouses has some relationship to polygny: the institution is easier to organize when there is some separation between spouses and the the possibility of the husband taking extra wives means that the emotional bond between a woman and her children is the most secure. However, the pattern of feeling and behaviour is not merely a reaction to the fact of polygny: the pattern of responses varied little between monogamous first marriages and all other types of marriage. There is evidence that in traditional agrarian cultures confined to monogamous marriages the parent-child bond may have been strong relative to that between spouses.[20]

[19] *Note:* This survey was of men with a number of children who were adults or near adulthood. Hence the men are fairly old as in many cases is the wife or wives.

[20] In a survey of married women in Melbourne, Australia, reported in Australian Family Formation Project (1972), it was found that agreement to the proposition that the bond between spouses was closer than that between mothers and children was agreed to by seven-tenths of the native-born and of the immigrants from Northern Europe but only by four-tenths of those from Southern Europe.

In polygynous families in societies where there is no proscription of women working there is likely to be a high degree of economic segregation in the household, with each wife and her children working as a semi-autonomous productive and financial unit. This helps to explain why polygamous husbands do not regard each extra child as adding solely to their own economic load—to a very considerable extent monogamous husbands also react in this way. It also helps to explain why emotional and financial matters are not tightly confined to the family of husband plus wife or wives and the children of the unions. Once this type of family is not a relatively closed economic unit, then much of the reasoning about the extra burden of high fertility shouldered by the father falls down. Admittedly only a small proportion of the society any longer feels that the mother should bear all the costs of the children. This change has occurred partly because of new costs unknown to the traditional society, particularly those related to education and examined at length later in this chapter. Even with regard to education, it should be emphasized that the assertion that financial responsibility is not wholly the mother's affair, does not imply that the full cost must be borne by the father—although he does seem to be increasingly the organizer of the support for education.

The Role of Education

This organization of support for education tends to be complex and supported by strong moral suasion. In one large survey of Yorubaland (CAFN 2) 98% of respondents agreed to the proposition, "An older brother should help his younger brothers' and sisters' children if the younger brothers and sisters are poorer". The survey showed that 35% of families had other children living with them of whom five-sixths were relatives, mostly the husband's or wife's siblings, nephews and nieces or grandchildren. The main reason for children staying was given as: education, 61%; being cared for (often grandchildren whose parents were working elsewhere), 30%; household helps, 9%—although it should be realized that these categories overlap and many children could really be placed in all three. In urban white collar households in the city, two-thirds have other children in them while among farming households in the small centres the proportion falls to one-quarter. In the same survey it was shown that 40% of farmers' families in small centres had children living elsewhere, three-quarters for education, compared with only 21% of city white collar workers' families from which just over half the children were away for education. It might be noted that education as used here included both schooling and apprenticeship although the former makes up 86% of the total, the proportion of apprentices being highest among the children of urban manual workers and lowest among the white collar workers. One reason that economic gains from fertility are limited is that the smallest families are seen to be those that can most easily take in and help other children; thus a study in neighbouring Cameroon showed that help for outside children declined as the number of the families' own children increased (CAFC).

There is then a massive informal educational support system supplementing the state provision of schools. Usually it involves children going from smaller to larger centres and from poorer and less well educated families to related richer and better educated ones. Some children go even from the latter families but it is more frequently for personal reasons such as joining grandparents for a period.

This system does not ensure that all children can get support or that all stay at school. Another survey of the same region (NF 1) showed that of sons with some schooling (now the great majority), three-quarters had some financial help from their fathers, one-quarter from their mothers and smaller fractions from siblings and other relatives. In the case of daughters the fractions of fathers and mothers helping fell to under one-quarter and one-fifth respectively. The support does not necessarily last. The same survey showed that only 19% of the children reached what they and their parents regarded as a satisfactory level, 21% pressed to leave at an earlier stage and were allowed to do so, 5% were refused permission to continue by the school, and 55% had to discontinue their education because of lack of money either in the sense that the money for their support could not be found or that the family could not afford to have them not earning. Most Nigerian children wish to stay at school because of the great gains ultimately to be made by doing so, but many fear to do so because of the Murdstonian nature of many of the schools (NF 4 and NF 5); nevertheless many of those who left school by choice may have done so because of pregnancy, widespreadly feared in West Africa as a distruptor of female education—justifiably according to recent evidence from the Cameroon (CAFC).[21]

On the face of it this looks a simple case of large families costing parents more to educate them and hence making high fertility uneconomical. So it may eventually turn out to be. Certainly all tropical African surveys show that parents are acutely aware of educational costs.[22] But, for the time-being, the position is not nearly as simple as this. Relatives are unlikely to help unless the parents are already helping, so one investment encourages others. There is rarely such a thing as a common household budget; the

[21] One quarter of all females in the sample who had terminated their education during primary school and one-third of those who had terminated it during secondary school reported that they had done so either because they were pregnant or because they married.

[22] Caldwell (1968c), Table 3, p. 603, where 13 surveys or regional divisions of West African surveys showing the educational financial burden separately are presented.

mother may help more, often raising the extra money by trading for long hours, not by arrangement with her husband but because her son has told her that the husband is not meeting the costs.

However, the institution that most weakens the direct relationship between high fertility and education costs is the sibling educational–occupational chain. If a child has been educated far enough to secure the kind of urban high-income position that such education leads to, then it is almost inevitable that he will meet the expectation of helping with the education of his siblings. A son who breaks through into the professions may well give such assistance for twenty years thereafter, sometimes obviously feeling pressed but usually not appearing to be resentful and clearly enjoying the gratitude of his brothers and sisters. Of 140 sons of this type surveyed (NF 1), 80 were giving financial support for their siblings' education, while some others were providing accommodation and keep; many of the balance had no siblings who needed educational help. The owner of a timber mill explained that it was the first children who were expensive and that his maximum outlays occurred when he was educating four children, none of whom had begun work; now, with eight children, they were educating each other and from now on additions to his family would bring him nothing but prosperity.

Even this explanation does not touch upon the greatest gains to be made by educating children and, to a lesser extent, other relatives. The educated provide a window to the modern world and a means of sampling its pleasures. The peasant farmer cannot hope to become an accepted resident of the wealthier suburbs of Lagos or Ibadan; but he can help his son to get there and can go and stay with him, being introduced at parties to the "big men" of the town. He can boast at home about the son's success, restrained only by a realization of how much jealousy is being aroused. While the father or mother do find some limitations on how much money they can splash in the village on frivolous consumption goods, the same limitations do not apply to what the successful son can bring home to them, and in any case there is more joy and excitement about receiving presents. Another informant pointed out that it is obvious in the village when a man's son secures white collar employment in the city; after the first return visit of son the parents will be seen in better clothes, after the second the father may be seen listening to a transistor radio, and so on. The son will inevitably bring more general honour upon the family by contributing, perhaps handsomely, to village ceremonial occasions and to the celebration of weddings and funerals; he will also be an important person on these occasions. He will bring new intellectual skills and outside contacts to the village, and his father will promise that his advice can be sought during the next visit. Indeed, in spite of their busy lives, it is the successful children who visit the village most often (Adepoju, 1974, pp. 385–387), partly because they can afford it and partly because they are pressed to do so. Much of what successful children can bring to a village is a blend of outside money, knowledge and attitudes; in a study of two centres it was found that wells and latrines had been provided for individual houses almost solely by educated children working in distant places (Orubuloye and Caldwell, 1975). The same children often improve the houses, perhaps first the room they stay in on their return visits, followed later by adding rooms or strengthening walls. They may have a concrete area built which is better for drying the cocoa than the usual hard earth. Eventually they may add to the village itself by building a splendid house, often left vacant or housing poorer relatives in one or two rooms as caretakers. If the son is successful enough he may well have sufficient influence to persuade authorities to pave the road to the village or to establish a school or a dispensary or to provide a permanent source of water.

The outsider finds it difficult to convince the villager that the education of children is all financial sacrifice and that the sacrifice could be limited by restricting fertility. Nevertheless, the outsider is almost bound to conclude that the returns on education described above accrue solely to the villager and result from the large urban–rural differential in income, and that his argument will describe the position of the urban middle class. As it will be seen later, this does not at present seem to be the case. The familes of the urban middle class understand the ladders to success in the modern sector of the ecomomy and are in a financial position to educate their children to the point where (together sometimes with the help of a little influence) they can secure large incomes, establish really successful sibling educational–occupational chains and see that the wealth diffuses through the whole family.

One other factor little mentioned in research reports but frequently mentioned in the villages, is the view that not all children are sufficiently gifted to give an adequate return on educational investment or to achieve sufficient success to provide their parents with a channel to the modern world. It is very much of a lucky dip. Hence, high fertility is needed to shorten the odds on success in the lucky dip (see Table 10 where the emphasis is on survival to participate).

The Cost of Children

Children undeniably incur costs even in the village, and this is increasingly so as the village economy becomes more monetized. That such costs, financial and physical, are realized is shown in Table 8.

The interpretation of responses to Question 1 in Table 8 is beset by two problems. One is that there was some confusion between whether the

TABLE 8
The cost of children, 1973:
Selected responses to specific questions by sex (percentages of total respondents)

Question	Response	Percentage giving that response		
		Females	Males	Both sexes
(1) At what age do children who have not been to school earn enough or produce enough to make up for what has to be spent on them?	Under 10	1	1	1
	10–14	18	18	18
	15–19	26	25	26
	20	25	26	25
	Other responses (especially "when training finished")	30	30	30
	Median of age (numerical responses only)	16	16	16
(2) Agreement/disagreement "The rel financial worry about children is schooling."	Agree	92	92	92
(3) Agreement/disagreement "A woman with many children has to work harder than one with few."	Agree	91	91	91
(4) Agreement/disagreement "It is difficult for market women who have many young children."	Agree	78	82	80

Source: CAFN 2.

balance of expenditure referred to the current balance or the lifetime one. The other is precisely the problem that causes economists to misunderstand the value of children from survey data on such societies. The question suggests a monetary balance, indeed it expresses itself in terms of "earning", and disregards the service of children which would otherwise have to be bought or substituted for by adult effort. Nevertheless, children do give rise to monetary difficulties which are dominated by costs of schooling.

There is equally no doubt that children, particularly when young, cause additional work, at least to their mothers. The weight of opinion seems to be that this burden is on the increase as the society becomes more commercial, children more infected by ideas from school and village society more segmented and less of an entity. Women engaged in full-time activity away from the home, especially in the larger centres, increasingly find it difficult to have their smaller children adequately cared for. Help is still available on a scale unknown in the west (NF 5) and can be organized by relatives and fellow villagers, but schooling is reducing the once vast pool of available illiterate girls, and educated mothers are becoming unprecedently worried at having their children minded by illiterate village girls.[23]

It is dangerous to translate other costs too readily from western to African economies. In much of the society, especially that of the villages, the growing of food to supplement the staples is done in kinds of gardens by the mothers usually assisted by children. The staples, such as yams, maize, cassava (manioc) and cocoyam (taro), are largely grown by the fathers (in striking contrast to the position in most of tropical Africa (Boserup, 1970, pp. 15–36)), but boys, even young ones, assist with many of the tasks. Cloth for clothing is often provided not for individuals at specific times of need but by the father, or perhaps a son working elsewhere for a high income, in the form of a whole bolt to be shared out amongst the family as a way of celebrating an occasion marked by a communal festivity or as a sign of respect for attendance at a funeral or wedding.[24] A larger family does not necessarily mean a larger house; nor are the occupants of a house necessarily confined to husband, wives and children. Nor is housing by any means wholly within the monetary sector of the economy. Traditionally families of the whole community in cooperation built their own houses with the walls and roofs made respectively out of the lateritic earth and the palm fronds or grass which surrounded them. An increasing proportion of the roofs are iron but most people, even in the city of Ibadan, still live in houses with walls and floors made of the free earth and rental is probably the dominant form of tenure only in Lagos.[25] Significantly, however, even in the villages there has been a movement away from communal and family labour to specialist construction.

Yet the above discussion had omitted what may well be the most significant aspect of the cost of children, an aspect which nowhere seems to enter analyses of the value of children. Traditional society has been

[23] For a study of these problems at perhaps a more advanced stage see Oppong (1975a).

[24] This point has been stressed by I. H. Vanden Driesen in a personal communication.

[25] c.f. Douala, the largest city of neighbouring Cameroons where 64% of households pay no rent (CAFC).

segmented in terms of roles and expenditure. What is spent on male heads of households is determined by what is spent on other male heads of households; children's peers are their models for how a child should be treated. Children, except perhaps those with a substantial amount of schooling, do not look at their fathers' food, clothing, possessions, entertainment, travel and other aspects of life to see what they might rightly aspire, and do not clamour for such things citing their fathers' possession of them as an example. Nor do fathers, or even mothers, feel guilty about assuming consumption patterns that are not shared with their children. This is made easier, of course, by the somewhat financially and emotionally divided nature of the family. Much of the expense on children in the modern, western, nuclear family arises from a movement towards equality in expenditure patterns within the family; this is largely the product of recent decades, and almost certainly children in most families (even in the nuclear family it might be noted) were relatively much less expensive than adults when there was a greater emotional distance between father and child and when it was held to be "good for a child" to live austerely.

The Returns from Children—During Childhood

As argued above, it is necessary to drop the largely artificial distinction between children's money-earning activities and their services. Even when children do earn money on their own (in contrast to helping with the production of the farm or business), they often become just another budgetary segment of the household raising their own living standards, sometimes by quite frivolous expenditure. If an investigation is to be of value then, it must be into all tasks done by children and their importance. A painstaking effort has been made (CAFN 2) to investigate all children's activities in Yoruba society, and some of the findings, grouped into general categories, are reported in Table 9.

Table 10 is not as comprehensive as it should be. We were deterred from formally examining the work of children under 7 years of age by the number of writers who feel children's work to be unimportant under 10 or even 15 years of age. In retrospect it is clear that they must be referring to the production of staples, and probably to such major operations as clearing, digging, planting and harvesting. Experience in the field showed that the minimum age should have been dropped to no more than five years, and that the position was similar to that described for the Dagomba in Ghana by Oppong:

TABLE 9
Children's activities grouped, 1973, by sex, centre size, age and schooling status (percentages of all activities)

Sex	Age	Schooling	Centre	Farming	Household	Minds Children	Carrying and Communication	Marketing	Apprenticeship	Other	Nothing	Total
Males	7–10	Never	Under 2th	16	36	0	40	4	0	3	1	100
			2-20th	18	43	0	29	5	1	2	2	100
			20-100th	17	35	0	39	3	1	3	2	100
			100-500th	16	39	1	32	5	1	4	2	100
			Ibadan	9	37	0	46	2	0	6	0	100
			Lagos	4	39	2	46	7	0	1	1	100
		Past	Under 2th	12	39	0	42	3	0	3	1	100
			2-20th	11	48	1	32	3	1	2	2	100
			20-100th	14	39	0	40	2	0	3	2	100
			100-500th	12	39	1	35	5	2	4	2	100
			Ibadan	8	41	0	43	2	0	6	0	100
			Lagos	2	41	2	45	6	0	1	3	100
		Current	Under 2th	5	44	0	44	2	0	2	3	100
			2-20th	9	47	0	34	2	0	5	3	100
			20-100th	6	43	0	43	1	0	3	4	100
			100-500th	3	43	1	41	4	0	5	3	100
			Ibadan	4	43	0	44	0	0	7	2	100
			Lagos	0	40	1	48	2	0	3	6	100
Males	11–14	Never	Under 2th	42	23	0	15	6	8	6	0	100
			2-20th	38	23	1	16	7	10	4	1	100
			20-100th	44	19	0	14	5	10	8	0	100
			100-500th	35	23	1	16	6	12	6	1	100
			Ibadan	23	31	0	13	9	17	7	0	100
			Lagos	16	29	0	20	11	19	5	0	100
		Past	Under 2th	36	27	0	18	6	6	7	0	100
			2-20th	28	33	1	18	5	10	5	0	100
			20-100th	36	23	0	17	5	9	10	0	100
			100-500th	27	28	1	18	9	10	7	0	100
			Ibadan	22	37	0	14	8	12	7	0	100
			Lagos	11	35	1	24	12	12	5	0	100
		Current	Under 2th	23	30	0	27	3	0	16	1	100
			2-20th	14	48	0	26	4	0	7	1	100
			20-100th	26	31	1	27	5	0	9	1	100
			100-500th	15	42	2	24	6	0	10	1	100
			Ibadan	14	46	0	30	4	0	6	0	100
			Lagos	5	45	1	34	8	1	3	3	100
Males	15–18	Never	Under 2th	51	13	0	6	7	14	9	0	100
			2-20th	40	16	1	5	9	15	11	2	100
			20-100th	40	10	0	7	6	19	17	1	100

TABLE 9 (Continued)

Sex	Age	Schooling	Centre	Farming	Household	Minds Children	Carrying and Communication	Marketing	Apprenticeship	Other	Nothing	Total
Males	15–18	Never	100-500th	32	18	0	7	10	20	12	1	100
			Ibadan	27	29	0	4	9	19	12	0	100
			Lagos	17	23	0	8	12	18	20	2	100
		Past	Under 2th	47	16	0	7	7	14	9	0	100
			2-20th	34	23	2	7	6	16	11	1	100
			20-100th	34	14	0	9	5	21	17	0	100
			100-500th	28	20	0	8	10	20	13	1	100
			Ibadan	27	26	0	7	9	15	16	0	100
			Lagos	12	28	2	9	11	22	15	1	100
		Current	Under 2th	38	29	1	8	5	1	15	3	100
			2-20th	24	42	2	10	3	1	13	5	100
			20-100th	33	24	1	16	3	1	22	3	100
			100-500th	23	31	1	13	10	2	16	4	100
			Ibadan	19	42	0	17	10	1	9	2	100
			Lagos	9	38	1	24	9	0	15	4	100
Females	7–10	Never	Under 2th	5	51	0	30	6	1	7	0	100
			2-20th	3	57	0	24	11	1	2	2	100
			20-100th	2	49	0	35	8	1	4	1	100
			100-500th	4	49	0	26	11	3	6	1	100
			Ibadan	1	44	2	43	5	1	4	0	100
			Lagos	1	51	0	32	11	1	4	0	100
		Past	Under 2th	3	52	2	32	8	0	3	0	100
			2-20th	2	56	0	26	9	2	3	2	100
			20-100th	1	50	1	37	7	1	1	2	100
			100-500th	2	53	3	29	8	2	2	1	100
			Ibadan	0	48	0	43	5	0	3	1	100
			Lagos	1	50	3	32	12	1	0	1	100
		Current	Under 2th	1	54	1	34	5	0	3	2	100
			2-20th	1	55	1	29	5	0	6	3	100
			20-100th	1	51	1	36	4	0	4	3	100
			100-500th	1	51	2	31	5	1	6	3	100
			Ibadan	0	50	0	42	1	0	4	3	100
			Lagos	0	51	2	37	3	0	2	5	100
Females	11–14	Never	Under 2th	10	43	3	11	22	7	4	0	100
			2-20th	5	50	2	9	18	11	4	1	100
			20-100th	5	50	1	12	19	7	6	0	100
			100-500th	7	46	3	10	16	12	6	0	100
			Ibadan	1	51	3	7	20	12	6	0	100
			Lagos	2	58	2	5	20	10	3	0	100

TABLE 9 (Continued)

Sex	Age	Schooling	Centre	Farming	Household	Minds Children	Carrying and Communication	Marketing	Apprenticeship	Other	Nothing	Total
		Past	Under 2th	7	48	3	12	22	6	2	0	100
			2-20th	3	52	2	11	20	11	0	1	100
			20-100th	5	54	1	11	16	8	5	0	100
			100-500th	4	47	4	12	17	13	3	0	100
			Ibadan	0	54	1	8	19	10	8	0	100
			Lagos	1	54	4	7	23	8	3	0	100
		Current	Under 2th	4	60	2	19	11	0	4	0	100
			2-20th	1	61	2	21	9	0	5	1	100
			20-100th	2	59	2	19	8	1	8	1	100
			100-500th	2	60	2	16	11	1	8	0	100
			Ibadan	0	72	2	15	6	0	5	0	100
			Lagos	0	70	3	14	9	0	3	1	100
Females	15–18	Never	Under 2th	9	37	4	4	24	9	13	0	100
			2-20th	4	38	6	2	22	10	17	1	100
			20-100th	4	41	2	7	21	11	14	0	100
			100-500th	4	33	4	6	19	16	18	0	100
			Ibadan	2	55	3	2	17	11	10	0	100
			Lagos	2	42	3	2	21	10	18	2	100
		Past	Under 2th	7	40	5	6	21	12	9	0	100
			2-20th	2	45	7	3	18	16	8	1	100
			20-100th	3	42	2	5	20	13	15	0	100
			100-500th	3	38	4	5	21	16	13	0	100
			Ibadan	2	59	3	2	13	10	11	0	100
			Lagos	1	45	7	3	21	15	7	1	100
		Current	Under 2th	5	59	5	8	14	2	6	1	100
			2-20th	2	65	6	5	9	1	9	3	100
			20-100th	4	61	3	9	11	2	9	1	100
			100-500th	2	57	5	7	15	2	10	2	100
			Ibadan	0	78	5	3	10	0	3	1	100
			Lagos	0	70	4	9	9	1	5	2	100

Source: CAFN 2. Detailed tables have been reproduced in *The Changing African Family, Nigerian Segment, Project 2, The Value of Children: Work Performed by Children in the Western and Lagos States of Nigeria*, Demography Department, Australian National University, Canberra, 1974.

Note: These figures differ somewhat from those given in *The Changing African Family, Nigerian Segment, Project 2, The Value of Children: Marginals for Three Categories of Interviewees*, Demography Department, Australian National University, Canberra, 1974, partly because they are re-aggregated here from very detailed data, but largely because the activities listed here are *all activities* and not the *major activity* specified by each respondent for each category.

"Children begin to learn to help in house and farm at a comparatively early age, from five years onwards, tasks usually being commensurate with their ability and size. Their services are in many cases indispensable, for, by carrying out the more monotonous, time-consuming tasks such as bird-scaring, cattle-herding, baby-minding, water-carrying, they give their parents and guardians leisure to pursue their specialist activities; to attend market or just to do more arduous chores. . . ." (Oppong, 1973, p. 51).

Amongst the Yoruba, as amongst the Dagomba, young children copy the activities of their parents in play and it is hard to distinguish a borderline between such play and subsequent useful work. A Yoruba respondent describing the activities of somewhat older children said:

"Sons encourage daddy by going on errands willingly; [they] buy clothes, [palm] wine, medicine and bring clothes when needed, and send firewood. [They] help mother bring vegetables from the farm, fetch firewood and bring water when she needs it. Daughters can help father carry yams from the farm and they are usually helpful during the cocoa season in removing beans from the cocoa pods and in drawing water for spraying Gamalin 20 [They] help mother in the kitchen and help her sell things in the market" (CAFN 2, vol. 2.1., respondent 2160).

In Table 10 the category, *farming*, includes both work generally described as that and also more specific descriptions such as *weeding, making mounds, harvesting, planting* and *loading. Housework* includes both work generally described in this way, but also *sweeping, washing dishes, washing clothes, ironing, cooking, cleaning* and *splitting wood*. With increasing age, the balance of work within this category changes: young children can sweep and wash dishes, their older siblings, especially their big sisters, are much more likely to be washing clothes, ironing, and, above all, cooking. *Minding children*, is mostly subsumed under the heading *housework*, but some children, especially older girls, were specifically described as spending much of their time doing this—either *looking after children* or *teaching children*, the latter being confined to those with a substantial amount of schooling. *Carrying and communication* covers *running errands, carrrying messages, carrying wood* for fuel and *carrying water*. The educated are more likely to carry messages or to go on certain types of errand where literacy or an ability to cope with the modern world of officials is an advantage. *Marketing* includes *traditional marketing* as well as working in shops, which is more important in the bigger centres and among those who have had some schooling, *wholesaling parents' produce* and *selling own produce. Other* includes general references to *physical work* or *earning money* (sometimes in such Yoruba occupations as plaiting hair), *hunting, fishing, reading to* [illiterate] *parents* and *washing cars. Nothing* includes not only that specific description itself but *reading* and *studying* and hence is highest for those currently at school.

The *never at school* category is the closest approximation we have to the division of children's labour before the arrival of mass schooling. It is clear that housework and carrying were the work of the young and that, with increasing age, carrying declined amongst both sexes and housework among boys, while sons did ever more farming and daughters more marketing as adulthood approached.

The impact of schooling has been the same on children's work as on adults' work: there is less likelihood of doing as much farming or marketing, and those children who have been to school are more likely to be working in the house or going on errands, and more likely to be doing these things if they are still at school. The other impact of modernization separated out here, the size of the centre of residence, is not nearly as great, although children of city families are less likely to be farming.

The *household* work category includes helping in production for the market. Children, especially daughters, are called upon from a young age to help those mothers who specialize in preparing palm or kernel oil, gari (from cassava), cooked maize products, beans (cow peas) or in weaving, spinning and dyeing. All these activities are profitable and hired labour may have to be used if children are not available. Children may also participate in such profitable activities as washing clothes for others or plaiting hair. Sons, as well as adults seeking products for sale or home consumption, can gather fuel or wild plantains from the forest—in fact the possibility of any able-bodied person being able to collect and sell such products determines, according to Vanden Driesen, a floor wage level for unskilled workers in farming.[26]

As long as such floor wages exist and as long as society encourages children to pick up work when it is available, children can contribute substantially to their own support. There are labour-demand peaks in farming in June–August and to a lesser extent in March–April when extra help has to be hired, usually both in the form of immigrant workers and local labour. The latter are often local children, especially the older ones, and, although the wages paid for local labour are not always the same as those for immigrant labour, the rates tend to move together (Galletti *et al.*, 1956, p. 305). There is of course a continuing problem in that the demands for household and wage labour coincide.

A listing of the individual tasks performed by children does not bring out fully the economic reasons for the satisfaction frequently expressed by the fathers of large families. From the point of view of the father, one of the advantages is undoubtedly the ability to do one's own farming and other work without having to worry about help from more distant relatives,

[26] Personal communication from I. H. Vanden Driesen referring to his field research in the Ife Division of the Western State during 1968–69.

neighbours and hired labour during periods of peak demand or crisis or when some task requiring a lot of muscle power at one time is to be undertaken. There are, however, advantages in having a large family that go beyond this and which have been explored by Reyna (1975b) in that part of Chad which is adjacent to Nigeria. The large family can not only cope with its own tasks but it often has excess labour which can be used to make windfall gains when sudden demands for other labour are required or even to meet more constant demands; in Yorubaland excess labour from the larger families appears to be disproportionately important in meeting the peak farming labour needs, providing servants for those women engaged in such household industries as dyeing or extracting palm oil, and bringing fuel from the forest. Findings in Ghana (Caldwell, 1968b, pp. 371–373) suggest that they might also be disproportionately important in providing labour for urban areas, especially the nearest large towns. It might be noted that these tasks beyond the family confines, carried out in a society where a great deal of rural production and consumption is subsistence, often provide a significant fraction of all cash flowing into the household—and remove a significant proportion from those smaller families who are forced to hire labour.

Undoubtedly the analysis of children's labour and earnings is not a simple matter of computing total returns and averaging them out over the whole family. Even if a large family were to exhibit lower per capita consumption than a small one, its patriarchal head might well enjoy a higher level of consumption than the neighbouring head of a small family, might work less, and might enjoy the power of heading a much larger operation. The mother has gains to make (or serious needs) at times or under certain circumstances: 93% of all respondents agreed with the proposition, "Sons are really important when fathers are working far away"—a situation which is increasingly common.

On the other hand, schooling, although offering the possibility of considerable returns when children are employees elsewhere, has disrupted the rural labour pattern. This does not seem to arise wholly, or even perhaps largely, from the fact that children are absent in schools. The truth seems to be that school children have experienced another way of life, have absorbed ideas from other cultures, have often been spoilt at home by illiterate parents who are a little apprehensive of them (Caldwell, 1968a, pp. 107–110), and are loth to undertake hard agricultural labour. There is some evidence that the first generation of school children regarded such labour as necessary for keeping them at school (S. A. Aluko, personal communication), but 20 years ago Galletti reported that parents were so apprehensive about ordering school children to work on the farms during vacations that they begged the schools to instruct them at the end of the term to do so (1956, pp. 78–79). At the same time, there has been a decline in the pride that parents of large families feel about the numbers of their offspring, at least during childhood but perhaps not after they have grown up. Less than half of all Yoruba respondents in a 1973 survey (CAFN 2) agreed with the proposition, "Having more children somehow makes you feel more powerful and more respected than having only a few".[27] However, agreement was greater in rural than urban areas, greater among the uneducated than the educated, and somewhat greater among males than females, so that among men with no education or education limited to primary or lower secondary school working in traditional occupations outside the two large cities, agreement was one-and-a-half times as common as disagreement.

The Return from Children—When They Grow up

Nor can the returns be worked out for the present alone. It is a fallacy to think of the value of grown-up children being merely equivalent to an insurance policy against old age and sickness. Even in terms of financial help, most parents receive continuing assistance from adult, married children irrespective of their state of health or feebleness. In fact, as Galletti points out, many old men still own farms and benefit from them even though they are entirely worked by grown-up sons or by hired labour financed by the marketing activities or wives or grown-up daughters (1976, p. 350).[28] But Nigerians increasingly feel that the Europeans disapprove of parents receiving returns from children except when in need, especially resulting from ill-health or old age, and accordingly are ever more likely to respond to surveys in these terms.

A preliminary investigation into reactions toward adult children and the returns from them is made in Table 10, although this will be supplemented later by an attempt to quantify such returns.

Half the community still believe it necessary to have a *very* large family, while many of the remainder believe it necessary to have a large family. A typical respondent replied: "One has to have as many children as possible because some may die, some may turn out to be failures in life" (CAFN 2, Vol. 2: 1. respondent 2062). Certainly there are more exponents of the very large family in rural areas where mortality is still very high and where the traditional way of life has changed least; yet the most striking fact about the differential between the rural areas and the cities is not that

[27] Agreement = 46%; disagreement = 50%; don't know etc. = 4%.
[28] Most of the "owned" land is land where the title is held by the community but *de facto* ownership does exist (see Vanden Driesen, 1972).

TABLE 10
Ensurance of sufficient adult children and the roles they perform, 1973: Selected responses to specific questions by sex (Percentage of total respondents)

Question	Response	Percentage giving that response			Significant deviations
		Females	Males	Both sexes	
(1) (Respondents over 40 years of age only) Do you think it is necessary to have a very large number of children					
(i) to ensure that any grow up?	Yes	48	53	51	Strongest agreement in the high mortality traditional sector specially among respondents 30–49 years old, who were old enough to feel such worries but not old enough in most cases to discover whether their children were surviving to adulthood.
(ii) to ensure that there will be one or two who will be willing to help?	Yes	51	55	53	Strongest agreement in the high mortality traditional sector among respondents over 50 who are beginning to worry about help in old age.
(iii) to ensure that there will be one or two bright enough to be able to earn a lot?	Yes	49	53	51	Strong agreement in the traditional sector where two-thirds of respondents agree but minority agreement elsewhere falling to one-third amongst white collar workers in the city.
(2) Agreement/ disagreement "Grown up children no longer relieve their parents of hard physical work."	Agree	61	60	61	There are no significant differentials: family experiences seem to differ in all parts of society.

TABLE 10 (Continued)

Question	Response	Females	Males	Both sexes	Significant deviations
(3) Agreement/ disagreement "Children are important because of the help they give to parents when they are old."	Agree	95	96	95	
(4) When people are old, do they need their own grown-up children to do hard physical work for them, or will other people help just as well?	They need their own children	41	41	41	The view that people need their own children is somewhat stronger amongst the old and in the traditional sector, but is held by half the respondents only amongst those over 50 years of age working in the traditional sector in villages with less than 2000 inhabitants.
	Other people help just as much	56	57	57	
(5) Agreement/ disagreement "A widow, even if she has no adult sons, always has someone to defend her and her property."	Agree	86	87	87	
(6) (Respondents over 40 years of age only) How many of your children give you real assistance when they grew up?	All of them	31	18	24	Those most likely to receive no assistance are the city white collar workers with extended education. No significant differentials by age of those parents who have grown-up children.
	Nearly all of them	21	25	23	
	Only one or two	22	21	22	
	None	17	27	23	
(7) Agreement/ disagreement "A man with many grown-up children has a lot of power in society."	Agree	62	63	62	Strongest agreement from those with no schooling, but strong agreement from all in traditional occupations. Less strong agreement according to smallness of the centre. Among illiterate farmers in centres with fewer than 100 000 inhabitants over two-thirds of all respondents agree compared with two-fifths of city white collar workers with extended education.

Source: CAFN 2.

it exists but that it is so slight. Large numbers of city dwellers believe that big families are necessary as guarantees against a series of risks for the same reasons as villagers do. The exact reason for favouring high fertility may well not be very important: there is an almost complete correlation between giving one reason for believing it necessary to have a very large family and giving another reason. This does not mean the reasons are not believed or are irrational; it means rather that children can yield various benefits and that there are real disadvantages if mortality substantially erodes their numbers. Family and communal assistance are still plenteously available nearly everywhere as is evidenced by the responses to the question on widowhood, but they do not replace the physical or financial assistance that children can provide. The greater emphasis on this in rural areas does not mean that there is less community assistance there but merely that all forms of assistance are needed more in villages.

The really important response is that on assistance given by children: nearly 70% report assistance and most of the rest either have no adult children or are demonstrably so well off as not to accept assistance. More significant still is the fact that assistance is not associated with the age or apparently the health condition of the parent; money and goods are given to healthy, fully employed parents in the prime of life and are given by children of all ages and marital conditions. It may well be that the economic return on the large family will outlast the social return. The kind of prestige and power (very much interlinked in the traditional community) that the illiterate farmer derives from having a considerable number of grown-up children in the village has no counterpart among the white-collar workers of the town; they derive their prestige from their education and job, the size of their house, and from throwing parties and other conspicuous expenditure.

An attempt was made (CAFN 2) to adopt a life cycle approach to children's help to parents, following through four streams—sons helping fathers, sons helping mothers, daughters helping fathers and daughters helping mothers—from assistance given when they lived as dependent children until they were in their prime and their parents were at least partially dependent aged. The results are given in Table 11.

The work done by children is the same as our analysis has previously shown. It does bring out the fact that daughters are often important to their fathers because they wash their clothes (the task only just failed to get on to the table in the case of the aged), apparently more than their wives do. In fact, when a man needs specifically female assistance he may well turn to his closest female relative: his daughter rather than his wife. The assistance to the aged is overwhelming in the form of support: financial assistance, now the dominant need even where the economy is still closest to the traditional subsistence one, taking them into the children's households, or, where their

TABLE 11
Major assistance given by children to parents at extreme ends of the life cycle, 1973 (Responses in order of frequency and all responses given by more than 5% of respondents recorded)

	Sons' help for fathers	Sons' help for mothers	Daughters' help for fathers	Daughters' help for mothers
A. When children are at least partially dependent minors	(1) Farming (2) Household work (3) Physical work (4) Help in business	(1) Household work (2) Physical work	(1) Household work (2) Washing clothes (3) Farming (4) Physical work	(1) Household work (2) Help in marketing (or business) (3) Physical work
B. When parents are at least partially dependent aged	(1) Financial assistance (2) Taking him in (3) Farming (4) Physical work	(1) Financial assistance (2) Taking her in (3) Household work	(1) Financial asistance (2) Taking him in (3) Household work	(1) Financial assistance (2) Household work (3) Taking her in

Source: CAFN 2.
Note: Physical work is made up of carrying and communications plus splitting wood and other heavy tasks.

own households still exist, helping them there. The latter, for sons aiding aged fathers, may still include keeping their farms going.

The Balance of Cost and Return

The 1973 Nigerian research carried further a research approach first employed ten years earlier in Ghana (GRH). In field research there is always wisdom in hindsight. In Ghana it became clear that the whole idea of looking at separate categories of children could have been conveyed better if this section of the questionnaire had been preceded by a battery of simpler questions virtually teaching the respondents how to think in such terms. This was done in Nigeria (the questions in part (b) of Table 12 are some of those that came before the questions in part (a) in the actual questionnaire). We knew by the end of the Nigerian research that the questions still carried too much implication that we were interested in cash balances during childhood and were excluding subsistence services and possibly subsistence production. The initial question that elicited the information in Table 12 category by category was: "The last question was probably hard to answer because we included together all kinds of children—old ones and young ones, girls and boys, children who go to school and children who do not. In the next questions we try to separate them into different groups. In each case we want to know if children of this kind have to have more money spent on them than the value of their work and earnings (i.e. their parents are worse off) or if their work and earnings are worth more than the money spent on them (i.e. their parents are better off)." Responses to this question took four forms—money spent is greater, earnings and work are greater, cost and return are much the same, and don't know or no response (a very small

TABLE 12
The current balance of cost and return on children, 1973:
Respondents claiming expenditure greater by sex, age and educational
status of children (percentages of total respondents)

(a) *By detailed subdivisions of children*

Age	Daughters			Sons		
	Never at school	At school in past	Currently at school	Never at school	At school in past	Currently at school
7–10	76	80	93	78	81	93
11–14	43	54	95	45	57	95
15–18	11	18	86	12	16	88

(b) *Cost and return by various dichotomies of children*

Category 1	Category 2	Expenditure		Returns	
		Category 1 greater	Category 2 greater	Category 1 greater	Category 2 greater
(i) older children	younger children	41	49	84	11
(ii) school children	children not at school	91	5	25	69
(iii) girls	boys	27	42	23	52

Source: CAFN 2.

group of responses). The real dichotomy in a society where there are not strong social pressures to reduce family size and where fertility would presumably begin to change only under fairly clear economic pressure is between the first category and the remaining three categories and hence the analysis in Table 12 has been treated this way. As, somewhat surprisingly, there were few significant differentials between the responses of fathers and mothers, the responses are not subdivided by the sex of respondents (while the area where an important difference occurs is discussed in the text).

At least in terms of a balance which may be largely, and perhaps somewhat unrealistically, a cash balance, the responses show a clear pattern. Children are always a drain on the pocket as long as they stay at school and children under ten are also a net drain even if they do not go to school. The position is a little ambiguous in the case of 11–14 year-olds not currently at school, but the very ambiguity shows that they are unlikely to prove a decisive net loss.

Several points should be noted both in the Table and in other analyses of the same data and data elsewhere.

The patterns found in the table are not capricious depending on small changes in the wording; if the data collected in Ghana a decade earlier are re-analysed in the categories employed here and for a similar region of Ghana (i.e. Divisions 2 and 3 of that analysis—the coast and forest, but excluding the savannah woodland to the north) then the percentages found in the various cells are almost identical—changing education levels over the years being irrelevant because of the analysis by separate educational categories (GRH).

The net loss on school children 15–18 is not entirely, or perhaps even mainly, because of their withdrawal from productive work. Not everyone agrees that they cannot do such work, and this is particularly the case in the rural areas where farming is available for the boys and marketing for the girls. The most serious problem is that schools demand expenditure on clothing and possessions, that school children exert a demand for possessions not traditionally the right of children, and that parents, especially illiterate ones, are more apprehensive, or at least more undecided, about refusing these demands than they would be for illiterate children who are supposed to conform to the established patterns. This conforms with the findings of a more detailed study of these matters in Ghana (Caldwell, 1968a, pp. 107–110).

Once again it should be emphasized that when respondents are weighing these questions they do not have in mind a common household budget, but instead fathers and mothers are thinking separately of the kind of work and the kind of expenditure that they themselves do. Thus mothers consistently rated daughters' productive work higher than fathers did. When asked the general question, "who earns more or does more productive work—boys or girls of same age?" one quarter as many males said girls as boys, but the fraction rose to two-thirds among females.

Respondents can be asked directly to assess the return on investment in children. The results of such attempts are shown in Table 13. The higher

TABLE 13
The return on investment in children, 1973:
Selected responses to specific questions by sex (percentages of total respondents)

Question	Response	Females	Males	Both sexes	Significant deviations
(1) (Respondents over 40 years of age with at least one child who has reached adulthood). Have your children produced more wealth and given you more assistance than the money you spent on them as children?					
(a) (Respondents with at least one child who did not go to school) Those who did not go to school?	Yes	46	30	37	Yes exceeded No amongst respondents of each sex over 50 years of age.
	No	38	43	41	
	About the same	16	27	22	
(b) (Respondents with at least one child who did go to school) Those who did go to school?	Yes	46	35	40	Yes exceeded No amongst respondents of each sex over 50 years of age; the margin was greatest amongst traditional population—rural, farming and where parents were illiterate.
	No	39	49	45	
	About the same	14	16	15	
(2) Agreement/ disagreement "The best investment is in the education of one's children (or relatives)."	Agree	97	98	97	

Source: CAFN 2.

TABLE 14
Economic implications of family size, 1973:
Selected responses of specific questions by sex (percentages of total respondents)

Question	Response	Females	Males	Both sexes	Significant deviations
(1) If the Government (or anyone else) said that they would pay you money not to have any more children once you had four living children, how much money would it take before you would agree?	Under N2000 ($3000)	13	9	11	
	N2000–N20 000 ($3000–$30 000)	16	16	16	
	Over N20 000 ($30 000)	42	45	44	
	Would not accept money	26	29	28	
	Could not prevent pregnancy	3	1	2	
(2) (Currently married only)					
(a) What would be the good things about having a (another) baby this year?	Pleasure at having a baby	29	28	28	
	Pleasure at having larger family	19	22	20	
	Other positive responses	9	9	2	
	Nothing good	33	30	32	
(b) What would be the bad things about having a (another) baby this year?	Too old	6	4	5	
	Nursing last baby	17	11	14	
	Economic problems	7	14	10	
	Prevent wife from working	2	1	2	
	Wife's ill health	2	1	2	
	Other	4	4	4	
	Nothing bad	52	54	53	
(3) If you had another baby this year, would it inconvenience you? Would it stop you doing things which you would otherwise have done? What things?	No inconvenience	42	50	46	All inconveniences greater among those in white collar occupations, with extended educations, and living in large cities
	Work	16	7	12	
	Social life	8	8	8	
	Studies	5	5	5	
	Travelling	1	1	1	
	Financial problems	1	2	1	

TABLE 14 (Continued)

Question	Response	Females	Males	Both sexes	Significant deviations
4(a) Why is it important to have some boys?	Major support of family in father's old age or after his death	37	35	36	No signficant differentials.
	Maintaining family name	26	31	28	
	Remain part of family while daughters marry out	17	15	16	
	Inherit property	9	8	9	
	Do hard physical work	5	5	5	
(b) Why is it important to have some girls?	Help in keeping the household going	34	32	33	Looking after parents slightly more important in traditional areas and linking families slightly more important in non-traditional areas.
	Looking after parents in old age	27	16	22	
	Marriage linking family with other families	16	21	19	
	For reproduction	8	15	11	
	They are kinder, gentler, more sympathetic	8	6	7	
(5) Which of the following statements do you most agree with?					The greatest differentials were in choosing (iv) which was chosen by more than 25% among white collar workers in the two cities and centres with more than 200 000 inhabitants but by only 6% of respondents in rural farming families.
(i) Children are better than wealth.	(i) Children are better than wealth	25	24	25	
(ii) Children are wealth.	(ii) Children are wealth	56	51	54	
(iii) Children are almost as good as wealth.	(iii) Children are almost as good as wealth	9	12	10	
(iv) Children use up wealth.	(iv) Children use up wealth	9	12	11	

TABLE 14 (Continued)

Question	Response	Females	Males	Both sexes	Significant deviations
(6) Agreement/ disagreement "Children in big families are:					
(a) less well fed than children in small families.	Agree	63	60	62	There was a very strong association between agreeing with one statement and agreeing with another (even though the three were well separated in the questionnaire). Agreement was highest among city white collar workers and lowest in traditional rural families even though both are apparently discussing the latter.
(b) not as well dressed as children in small families.	Agree	64	59	62	
(c) more likely to get into trouble than children in small families."	Agree	69	67	68	

Source: CAFN 2.

affirmative response levels in Table 13 amongst females than males is almost certainly solely explicable in terms of the fact that the respondents are of approximately the same age whilst fathers are on average much older than their children than mothers are; hence a smaller proportion of the males had children who had been adults for very long. By the age of 50, the returns are beginning to be greater for each sex, and, not surprisingly, greatest for farmers who have educated their children. Certainly there is no real feeling in the society that other investments would be better than educating children—and here "better" is almost certainly understood by most respondents in terms both of monetary and other returns. Similar questions in Ghana have evoked agreement from most that the best investment is in education (Caldwell, 1966, p. 19).[29]

In Table 14 an analysis is made of more general questions on the same topic—questions which attempt to gauge reactions without assessing money flows.

[29]   In a survey of persons over 60 years of age, only 18% and 35% respectively of urban and rural residents reported that they had received back less from children than they had spent on them.

Table 14 reinforces earlier doubts about using an ethnocentric Western approach in Nigeria for relating fertility and economic ends insofar as we assume those ends to be the maximization of family consumption. There is an identification of children with wealth that is deeply believed—it is not an artifact of poor communication or translation, as repeated interviews in depth proved. Evidence of this type deeply disturbs conscientious economists who begin to wonder about the universal application of their science. The problem is probably less one of the universality of western economics than of understanding the logic behind the economic and social ends of villagers when seen through the eyes of an observer reared in a western city.

Apart from the identification of children and wealth, the advantages and disadvantages of children are thought of largely in social terms or as guarantees of security. Only a small minority think of an increase in family size imposing greater economic hardship, and this presumably is a reasonable assessment of the position. It is significant that the belief that the children of large families are less well off is held most strongly by the better off families of the city; it is tempting to suspect that they, and the outside observer, really feel that the rural poor are squalid. It is a salutary lesson to the outsider to find that Africa's peasantry rarely regard themselves or their children as being wretchedly poor.[30] Certainly few regard themselves as being so poor that they would sell their right to higher fertility. The amounts of money required from the Government before ceasing reproduction may be a vague hope or an expression of defiance—there is evidence from elsewhere of respondents quoting vast sums rather than allow governments to dictate fertility levels.

An Investigation into the Inputs into Children and the Returns from Adult Children and from Education

In 1974–5 an attempt was made to measure the inputs into children and the returns in Nigeria's Western State (NF 1). As with all investigations of this type, there was a good deal of apprehension about the questions and

[30] When respondents in CAFN 2 were asked "If you were very poor, how many children would you have?" after having been asked earlier other questions about their child preferences, none replied that this extra question did not make sense because they were in fact very poor, and the majority cited a number smaller than they had previously quoted as the number they wished to have themselves as their ideal family size. For a further illustration of this point in the case of a population that most of the world regards as indisputably wretchedly poor, namely the nomads and farmers of the Sahel during the drought of the early 1970s, see Caldwell (1975d), *passim.* *c.f.* the responses in a survey of married women in Melbourne, Australia, reported in Australian Family Formation Project (1972), only 15% of respondents reported that the payment of even very large child endowments and 21% the payment of a permanent salary would encourage them to have an extra child.

TABLE 15
Financial return to parents from working children 1974–75

(a) *Investment in education by parents and financial assistance from working children*

(Financial assistance to parents)

(in percentages of all working children)

Monetary help from parents with education	All working children N.	%	Money sent both regularly and in emergencies	Money sent regularly only	Money sent in emergencies only	No money sent
Help given	392	100	34	4	35	27
No help	149	100	17	0	61	22
All cases	541	100	29	3	42	26

(b) *Parent giving assistance and financial assistance received from working children*

Parent receiving assistance from children

(in percentages of all working children)

Parent giving Assistance	All working children N.	%	Both parents	Father	Mother	Neither
Both parents	115	100	65	4	7	24
Father only	249	100	58	9	2	31
Mother only	3	100	33	0	0	67
Neither	151	100	63	13	2	22
All cases	518	100	61	9	3	27

(c) *Annual monetary returns compared with parents' annual income from all sources* (expressed as percentages)

Returns as percentage of parents' income

Income earner	Total	None	Under 10%	10–20%	20–30%	30–40%	40–50%	50–60%	60–70%	70–80%	80–90%	90–100%	Over 100%	Median percentage return
Father	100	22	32	23	6	3	3	0	0	2	2	2	5	approx. 10
Mother	100	24	19	16	8	5	3	2	1	1	3	0	18	approx. 15
Whole household	100	22	31	21	11	2	1	2	0	1	0	1	8	approx. 10

TABLE 15 (Continued)

(d) *Financial assistance from children according to their sex and occupation* (Percentage distributions)

(i) *Sons*

			Financial help for parents			
Occupation of sons	All working sons N.	%	Money sent regularly	Money sent in emergencies only	No money sent	Direct financial help to siblings for education
Farmers	22	100	0	73	27	45
Manual workers	159	100	23	50	37	49
White Collar Workers	146	100	51	36	13	60
All working sons	327	100	34	45	21	54

(ii) *Daughters*

			Financial help for parents			
Occupation of daughters	All working daughters N.	%	Money sent regularly	Money sent in emergencies only	No money sent	Direct financial help to siblings for education
Farmers	4	100	0	75	25	75
Manual workers	118	100	17	53	30	39
White collar Workers	49	100	65	25	10	53
All working daughters	171	100	30	46	24	44

Source: CAFN 1.

inevitably understatement of income and other money received. This did not prevent us from obtaining a clearer picture of the whole process than was previously available.

Of all children over 15 years of age at the time of the survey, 75% of sons and 78% of daughters were no longer living with either parent (the higher proportion for daughters being explained by earlier marriage). About one-fifth of those living with parents had been away for work elsewhere at some stage but had returned. Just over half the sons were working, most of the balance still being educated; while only two-fifths of the daughters were in some kind of remunerative occupation, the balance being housewives, waiting for marriage or at school. A comparison of the education and occupations of parents and children served as some measure of the vast socioeconomic change underway. Two-thirds of fathers had never been to school, but only one-quarter of their sons lacked any education; over five-sixths of mothers compared with less than half of daughters had no schooling at all. Less than half the proportion of sons were farmers as were their fathers; while three times the proportion of daughters were urban white collar workers as were their mothers. Private and public investment in education had helped to bring about a social and economic revaluation in the community as a whole. Table 15 attempts to assess the financial return at the level of the individual parent.

Table 15 shows quite clearly that the system depends for its working on the concept of extended family and communal help: those who can help usually do so. Most parents who did not give any assistance were unable to do so and were not blamed for their failure. At least they were not blamed sufficiently for it to result in any restriction of subsequent assistance from their children—if anything, their greater need provoked a little more assistance. Similarly those children who do not help are mostly those who can least afford to do so—the predicted revolt of the educated in favour of a western type of system of obligations has not yet occurred on any significant scale.

Investment in children is probably an investment in the real sense of the term. But this does not come about because there is any correlation between giving assistance to a specific child and receiving help back from that child. It comes about because greater financial help to capable children—and this qualification is clearly understood by the parents—may allow them to reach the urban white collar occupations, and perhaps even the professions, with high and regular incomes. If they reach such heights they will in most cases return more money and remit it more regularly.

Children on average are reported to remit money to parents equal to 10%, or a little more, of both fathers' incomes and household incomes; among those who remit at all the reported proportion is around 15%. For perhaps half the population the number of remitters may eventually be three or more (see Table 10) thus increasing parental income by half. Such an analysis is illuminating but misleading. It hides most of the returns on the investment. First, the monetary return is probably understated. Second, the non-monetary returns may well outweigh the monetary ones (speaking only in terms of goods and not of other gratifications). Third, the successful investment buys security; the main aim is that the child should obtain employment with guaranteed tenure and regular salary that will permit help to be given to parents no matter what disaster should strike them—blighted cocoa crops, drought, flood, cholera, urban unemployment, a succession of funerals or many other domestic or village crises.

Perhaps the most surprising finding to emerge from the research—a finding of which we became increasingly aware during the field work—was that the returns on the investment in children are proportionately greater for urban residents than rural residents and that the white collar workers, even the professional classes, reap a great deal from the system. The reason is that incomes rise disproportionately rapidly with education and the urban white collar families have both the money and the necessary understanding of the system to keep their children moving up the educational ladder—they even manage to organize the most complete sibling assistance chains so that it is rare for any but their youngest children not to help their brothers and sisters. Thus the whole family—often a family much larger than a nuclear one—prospers and becomes known.

Alternative Investments—Both Economic and Social

For most farmers—indeed for most Nigerians—there are only two other forms of investment that may raise living standards, increase security and raise prestige. Housing is excluded as not being a productive investment. Forest farming is at present also largely ruled out because, apart from necessary herbicides, it is not clear to farmers or observers how to make a profit on investment—except by acquiring more land (increasingly difficult now in parts of the Western State) and using more labour. If more labour is needed then the same problems arise as are mentioned below for the small trading business.

One form of investment is the small business: trading, a retail shop, selling goods from one market to another, wholesaling from factories, small craft workshops and so on. However, it is usually assumed that such businesses will only flourish and certainly that they will only return a profit to the investor if a relative, and a capable one at that, is involved. In fact there would be strong family disapproval of the employment of a non-relative if such spare money was available.

The other is polygyny, which may help solve the labour problem both for extra farming and for a business. The surveys (especially NF 1) showed that family income increased with the number of wives, partly because of their additional productivity, but partly too because richer husbands can acquire extra wives more easily.[31]

[31] Vanden Driesen explains this partly because of the greater ease in the polygynous family of working land holdings which are far apart (1972) p. 53. Certainly the same explanation can be offered with regard to urban businesses.

These are the economic realities of Yoruba life as a random selection of responses to questions demonstrate.

(NF 5) "Nigerian men are quite unlike their counterparts in other parts of the world [this means Europe and America, especially England]. Even when they have enough money to cater for the family, they would not give it out; instead they marry another wife or wives. Any Nigerian woman who has a means of livelihood should work or else she might be disappointed the day her husband would turn his back on her" (biography 10). (CAFN 2 on the spending of N 20 000) "I will build a house, invest some in a transport business and open a beer parlour for my latest wife" (Vol. 2.1., respondent 2055).

(CAFN 2 on the spending of N 100) "I may use it to start a new building or I may marry a new wife" (Vol. 2.1., respondent 2081).

(NF 5) "I happen to come from a polygamous family myself and because of this I realized the importance of getting something going because the husband will not be able to give much attention to each child. The mother has to substitute sometimes" (biography 7).

(NF 5) "My children are very small and there is nothing they can do at present, but I think they will render some help when they are able" (biography 2).

A Society Without a Real Appreciation of Money

It is easy to conclude that Yoruba society is not yet fully oriented towards maximizing income or consumption or that children are regarded as such

TABLE 16
Choices between money and children, 1973:
Selected response to specific questions by sex (percentages of total respondents)

Question	Response	Females	Males	Both sexes
Agreement/disagreement (1) "A rich man with a few children is more important than a poor man with many children."	Agree	81	82	82
(2) "Having lots of money is more important than having lots of children."	Agree	65	68	66
(3) "A brother who has four children and is able to study and travel is wiser than his brother who has eight childen and has to work all the time."	Agree	85	85	85

Source: CAFN 2.

valuable consumption goods that they are not felt as alternatives to other consumption goods. That this is not so is clear from Table 16 and from the reaction already recorded in Table 2 to the assertion that "Money is the elder brother and children the younger brother".

The Yoruba reaction is not an irrational one to either money or fertility, but merely that in few households do these two desires conflict; probably in the great majority of households the pursuit of money is still assisted by the pursuit of high fertility, at least if the measurement is made from the stance of the parents.

What Does it all Mean in Terms of the Present and in Terms of Change?

Perhaps the first lesson is that social science is often extraordinarily ethnocentric especially in the area of the family as an emotional, social and economic unit. It is not merely *western*; it is usually specifically northwestern European, or even English-language or sometimes American middle class to the extent of being WASPish. In the area of fertility research it treats the extended family as if it really were an extension of nuclear family obligations and not that a man might have prior obligations to his sister over his wife, or a woman to her married daughter over her husband or even young son. This often leads to its being blind. Against overwhelming evidence that few people in West Africa believe that high fertility leads to their economic undoing, the usual reaction of foreign demographers has been neither to ignore it and thereby the possibility of analysing the economy so as to show why the reaction might be a rational one or to treat the belief as a sign of the conservatism of a traditional society and therefore as an indication of the need for identifying the progressive groups in the society.

If the demographer does plunge into the economics of fertility, the chances are that he will err in his analysis and conclusion for two reasons.

The first is obvious and therefore not very serious. The economic data collected in the field are probably far more deficient than the social and demographic data obtained. Money is a sensitive matter and people are used to giving wrong information about it; many expenditures and some sources of income they find difficult to recall or even embarrassing to mention. Painstaking field research will probably slowly improve the position partly by determining something close to national accounts for each community: by objectively measuring the supply of goods and services, consumption and production.

The second is much subtler and can, for an outsider, be positively esoteric. The demographer is likely at first to measure the family economy in terms of his own society. He will assume that consumption expenditure is rationally that spent on goods and that the most satisfactory end is the accumulation of large objects owned by a family. He will tend, perhaps like the populace itself, to regard general feeding almost as a cost of production rather than as an economic end in itself—but then he may err in regarding ceremonial consumption in the same way. He will most often regard expenditure on those outside the nuclear family as a type of enforced expenditure—which it sometimes is—and will ignore the purchase of respect and affection which compete with other forms of consumption. He will have great difficulty with these expenditures disentangling the purchase of esteem in the community, the value of which he will almost certainly underrate, from the safeguarding of security which he will equate with paying insurance premiums in his own society. He will think of purchases being made for the family, almost invariably the nuclear family, and will have difficulty distinguishing both the extent to which the purchases are the property of a single person or group of persons—the husband or the wife or the wife and her children—and the extent to which they are meant for the admiration and use of a much wider circle of people.

There is no point in carrying out an economic analysis if the researcher substitutes his own society's economic ends. Fundamentally economic ends are social ends, although these social ends may over a long period have been at least partially determined by material circumstances—the means of production, the type of residence and settlement, the degree of security, the political institutions and so on. In Yorubaland one cannot in the analysis downgrade such traditional objectives as gaining prestige in the community or being owed obligations or achieving a high place in the community hierarchy or being responsible for a splendid reburial ceremony; nor should one lay insufficient stress on such modern or transitional ends as having a child with an advanced education or occupying a position of prestige and power in the new national economy or political structure. Nor should the researcher ignore the extent to which the possession of a large family can contribute to achieving these ends.

The analysis is rendered more difficult because the society and economy are experiencing rapid change—change which will alter economic ends only as fast as it alters social ends. Given that qualification, I should remark that nothing I have experienced in West Africa suggests that there is any cultural lag—any delay in recognizing how to achieve new objectives arising from traditional ways of looking at things and an inability to do things in a new way—in adjusting to new economic ends that are determined by changed social ends. The rate of social change determines economic change and this in turn determines the value of children and hence fertility change.

The social demographer working in the Third World is probably handicapped more by coming from western society with its perhaps unique familial and social structure than he would be if he came from any other major society. The characteristics of the modern West which are so marked in this context are: the strong nuclear family with little financial or other assistance given to more distant relatives, even to the spouses' siblings or to married children and grandchildren; the strong bond between spouses, which is frequently not incompatible with more occupational differentiation and greater subordination of wives than is found in some traditional societies; a common household budget and pool of possessions; a feeling that the scale of expenditure on one member of the household helps to determine what is spent on another member, and an increasing relative expenditure on children accompanied by a decline in moralizing about what is good for them; security guaranteed increasingly by the State and with little hope of securing it from relatives beyond the nuclear family; respect (even from relatives) arising almost wholly from achievements in the society as a whole rather than the community—examination success, jobs gained, salaries paid etc.; property, even farming land, purchased on an open market largely regulated by the State with little effective community pressure; a good measure of respect for conspicuous consumption even when one's siblings or neighbours are conspicuously poorer; a growing belief by both adults and children that childhood is for games and education; a declining belief that social success or even hobbies should rival concentration on occupational achievement by husbands, and so on.

Some of this list are recent occurrences in the West and perhaps the inevitable consequence of modernization: the reluctance to ask children to work, the expenditure of relatively more on each child compared with what is spent on the father, and a concentration of one's interests in one's occupation, at least in the middle classes. Some have a much longer and peculiar history and owe something to the fact that Western Europe has not proceeded rapidly or even directly from food gathering to peasant cultivation on communal land to the urban, industrial economy of our own times; there are roots in the Protestant Reformation, in the Catholic Church, in feudalism and perhaps in the Roman Empire. Western European literature, long before the social security systems of modern governments, shows that adequate help from relatives outside the nuclear family or from the village as a whole was not assured; monogamy, a common budget, a relatively strong husband–wife bond (and certainly eating and sleeping together) and little hesitation about spending existing money on household possessions have a very old history; while freehold land dates back to the decay of feudalism.

This aside has been necessary to make two points. Even before the nineteenth century European culture had many ingredients that predisposed children to being an economic burden with the growth of urban, industrial society with mass schooling. This has not been the case in Nigeria and probably in many other parts of the Third World. Nevertheless, with economic development, Nigerian fertility will probably fall. It will do so not because this is inevitable in the early stages of modernization but because that modernization has been imported from Europe and its social aspects (often dependent for their implementation on the changes in the economy) are as powerful as its economic ones. By far the most powerful influence has been mass secular schooling, which has been even more westernizing and universal than mission-borne Christianity; there is nothing in the above list of aspects of western culture which the schools and the Christian Church do not lean towards.

Traditional Yoruba society, like peasant society nearly everywhere, was a relatively permanently settled community of people most of whom were either related to each other or were descendants of people who had long lived together. There was an understanding, especially amongst the elders, as to how traditional government, law and the apportioning of land worked. One had a place in the world, a guarantee against disaster, and a guarantee that one would not be relatively too much impoverished or destitute unless the whole community met with disaster. Such guarantees meant reciprocal guarantees, which meant that everyone lived much the same way of life; extravagance and conspicuous consumption were largely a matter of the festivals and the ceremonies or associated with chieftaincy. In the circumstances there was no sudden cut-off point in degrees of relationship or responsibility; the blurring of the family edges was made more certain by the widespreadness of polygyny and by the extent to which mothers were responsible for seeing to the material well-being of the children. Fertility was not an economic question, except insofar as a better-off man might acquire more wives and hence more children. The limits of female fertility were almost entirely psychological, physiological and social as they largely still are. Childlessness, even if brought on by infant and child mortality, exposed a woman to practical difficulties and to all kinds of suspicions including those of being a witch or being possessed by one. Indeed the birth of a still-born child or of a sickly child doomed soon to die could be evidence that this bewitched foetus had lain an unnatural time in her womb—perhaps years.[32] By the time a woman had given birth seven or eight times it was likely that she would give up sexual relations because she was a grandmother and hence it was inappropriate or menopause had indicated that she was too old or indeed that she or her husband felt that she was (Caldwell and Caldwell, 1977, p. 201). It was a society with an *open family* system and great interdependence; people worked but they valued leisure more and ceremony most.

[32] Personal communication from O. Adeyeye. C.f., on Sierra Leone, Harrell-Bond (1975, pp. 482–3).

The world that produced this society is passing. The towns are growing; most men now work outside farming; and the economy is becoming increasingly monetized. The colonial and independent national administrations, together with the great range of new occupational opportunities, significant in their incomes, power and location outside the home centre, have largely destroyed the prestige of traditional office. Sex roles in the family and outside are changing; although women traditionally did the bulk of the non-farming jobs, the new public service, professional and business managerial posts are most commonly offered to men; educated children often make illiterate parents unsure of themselves and thus change the nature of the parent–child bond; educated wives have much the same effect on the marriage tie. Rural–urban migration often tends to produce nuclear families in a residential sense and frequently moves in that direction in an emotional sense; wives and husbands are no longer integrated units in the female and male sides respectively of traditional village life and may be much more dependent on each other.

These changes have been used by some demographers to argue for at least temporary higher fertility in Nigeria's urban areas (Morgan with Ohadike, 1975, pp. 194–197) and by others to show that the burden of children must be greater in the towns and that fertility must fall. There appears to be little evidence that either is happening to any marked degree or very quickly. Fertility has not risen because a good deal of postnatal abstinence is practised in the towns; polygyny still exists on a large scale and husbands can find other women more easily than in the village (Caldwell and Caldwell, 1977)—and what this does not explain, increased use of contraception probably does. But the failure of fertility to fall in this essentially transitional society is a more complex story.

The whole Yoruba society is at present transitional in the sense that the direction and rate of change can be sustained for only a comparatively short time, perhaps to the end of the century. By that time the population which depends directly and predominantly on farming for its livelihood will have been reduced to a point where the impact of rural–urban migration will only be a minor aspect of the town labour market and where the rural–urban income differential will be a significant lure for only the small residual rural population. By that time the farming population might make up only 10–15% of the population of the Western and Lagos States. Indeed its very smallness might reduce the rural–urban income gap by substantially raising the selling price of food, although this might prove to be impossible because of competition from more distant and rural parts of Nigeria. Perhaps more significant will be the reduction of the educational gap between the generations and almost certainly the income gap. The present parental generation is the last in which a majority of the fathers will be illiterate; by

1990 a majority of children of secondary school age will have fathers with some schooling; by the end of the century most children at primary school will probably have fathers with either some secondary schooling or at least completed primary and mothers with a substantial amount of primary schooling. Two changes related to education and urban life are likely to prove decisive in terms of the value of children. One is that the educated children will successfully press for an ever larger proportion of family expenditure thus reducing the intergenerational gap in consumption. The other is that they will become more reluctant to give substantial assistance to reasonably comfortable educated parents in urban white collar occupations—a reluctance that will almost certainly be encouraged by wives claiming a right to a greater interest in their husbands' expenditure than is now the case. As the pool of illiterate or uneducated and underemployed potential nurse girls dries up, the minding of children while the mother works will become more difficult and more expensive. With these changes it seems inevitable that contraceptive use will increase and fertility will decline.[33]

In the meantime—perhaps for another generation—educational investment is still profitable for the urban middle class and large families are no particular hardship. By the contemporary standards of the West, children are brought up very strictly indeed. They know their place; they do not dominate the household; they do not press particularly hard for expenditures beyond a conventional, but rising, minimum; they are looked after to a considerable extent by siblings or poorer relatives; they study hard. The situation is made easier by the extroversion of Yoruba society and by the pleasure felt in having a lot of people in the house—expensive ceremonial occasions are a feature of town as well as rural life. Educated children help each other financially with their education and they help their parents. If they did not, they would still feel a family and community resentment, and even a shutting of doors, that would scar them. But this is not the fundamental reason for conformity. As long as the system lasts, as long as no one breaks the chain letter, the rising educated generation will in turn benefit. They will probably receive assistance and gifts from even better educated and richer children. However, the position in the urban middle class is increasingly more complex than this. The educated children have much to gain as long as domestic budgets remain open and are not identified with the nuclear family—as long as brothers can help each other without their wives querying considerable outlays of this type. An open family system with financial help, assistance in getting high positions and the

[33] C.f. Caldwell (1975b, p. 95), where it is argued that projected trends in anti-natal practices in such cities as Lagos and Ibadan are likely to result in measurable falls in fertility by 1980. A similar argument based on the projected increases in anti-natal practices in rural areas leads to the conclusion that fertility change by 1980 in rural areas is likely to be of little significance.

TABLE 17
Priority research topics of the value of children

Area	Research	
	Emphasis on understanding the usual position in the society	Emphasis on understanding direction and rate of change
(1) Work done by children.	Hour by hour measurement of the activities of village children not at school.	Hour by hour measurement of the activities of urban children who attend school.
(2) Division of labour and income.	(a) Range of activities performed by large families (joint families with high fertility) in rural areas. (b) Specific returns and advantages to fathers of large families as distinct from family per capita returns.	Economic ramifications of urban elite families and assistance given to each other in terms of education and jobs.
(3) Money flows.	More exact work on all money flowing to persons in family and all outflows from them.	Money flows in (i) rural–urban migrant households and (ii) elite households.
(4) Feelings of financial responsibility.	Towards helping parents on their farm or in their business to earn income.	(a) Towards education of siblings. (b) By adult children of healthy parents (i) when children are unmarried, (ii) when children are married.
(5) Budgeting.	Extent to which husbands and wives (and children?) keep separate budgets and have separate financial responsibilities. Extent to which there is accurate knowledge of each other's budgets.	Impact of urban life. Extent of consolidation of a single household budget and knowledge of each other's budgets amongst (i) rural–urban migrant households, (ii) elite households.
(6) The concepts of security and mutual obligations.	(a) The normal working of the system and the relative importance of relations and of the increase in the network of relations by means of fathers' marriages and children's marriages. (b) The working of the system during a community disaster.	(a) The importance of mutual obligations in the urban areas as a defence against disaster. (b) The importance of the giving of assistance to relatives and others as a competitive consumption expenditure. The buying of respect.

TABLE 17 (Continued)

Area	Research	
	Emphasis on understanding the usual position in the society	Emphasis on understanding direction and rate of change
(7) Community festivals and similar activities.	(a) The expenditure on festivities; the extent to which this is competitive consumption expenditure. (b) The role of festivities. (c) The concept of leisure and of non-occupational enjoyment; the limits on time and energy that can be put into production.	(a) Contributions towards such festivities in home villages and in the town in (i) rural–urban migrant households and (ii) elite households.
(8) Changing treatment of children.	(a) The meaning of childhood; attitudes towards children's work and leisure.	(a) The meaning of children in (i) rural–urban migrant households, (ii) elite households. (b) Changing consumption demands of children. (c) Changing ratio of expenditures on parental generation to expenditures on child generation. (d) The changing treatment of children; changes in moral expressions about how children should be treated and how they should behave.
(9) Consumerism.	Consumer expenditure—its nature and its limits.	Consumer expenditure in the town—its nature and its limits.
(10) Extended family obligations and corruption.		Extended family obligations in the modern environment: assistance with jobs and the extent to which this can be regarded as corruption.

TABLE 17 (Continued)

Area	Research	
	Emphasis on understanding the usual position in the society	Emphasis on understanding direction and rate of change
(11) The small family and marked restriction of fertility.	(a) The situation of early adopters of modern contraception. (b) The clientele of family planning clinics.	(a) The situation of early adopters of modern contraception. (b) The clientele of family planning clinics. (c) The achieved small family in urban areas; its nature and the reason for its existence. (d) The adoption of contraception in urban areas over time.
(12) Studies in depth of financial flows in individual families (virtually with participant observation).	Rural household.	(i) Rural–urban migrant household. (ii) Elite household.
(13) The impact of education and its effect in changing traditional family relationships and attitudes to fertility and fertility control.		Studies in depth of young educated women with special regard to attitudinal and behavioural change with regard to marriage, fertility and family relationships.

probability that one's brother will put in a good word for one with people of authority has economic and social advantages and is not lightly cast aside. Eventually much of this will begin to look like corruption and government and private administration will be increasingly subject to waves of self-cleansing. This will be a sign of the passing of the open family system and of the declining value of children. It is this delayed, two-generational, effect on fertility of urban life which has blurred some research findings and which led to the conclusion in an important comparative study that "studies failed to provide an understanding of the manner in which urban life discourages large families" (Loewenthal and David, 1972, p. xii).

An understanding of the value of children in contemporary Nigeria and similar societies and of the likely direction and rate of change together with the implications for fertility requires a great deal more sophisticated research in the area of social demography and its economic borderlands than has yet been attempted anywhere. In Table 17 an attempt has been made to sketch some research priorities.

It is not suggested that all the 40 projects outlined in Table 17 should be separate undertakings. Frequently several could be fitted into a single investigation. But nothing less than this programme will give an understanding of why fertility remains high in Yorubaland, why it will not fall quickly, and what socioeconomic changes are likely to presage fertility decline.

A good deal of anthropological work already throws some light on these questions, but demographers have rarely incorporated these findings with their own.[34] Other projects are underway, especially on the achieved small family (CAFN 3), the adoption of contraception in urban areas over time (CAFN 1) and the study in depth of the familial and other condition of early contraceptors.[35] Something has also been done about the users of family planning clinics.[36]

Appendix

Research cited by initials

GRH and GA *Ghana Rural Household Survey* (description in Caldwell, 1967) and *Ghana Aged Persons Survey,* Caldwell (1966) based on the Demography Programme of the University of Ghana; field work 1962–64; research financed by the University of Ghana from a Population Council grant; research workers included J. C. Caldwell, Pat Caldwell and P. J. Caldwell; GRH sample was of 709 households throughout rural Ghana, and the GA sample was of 400 males and 400 females throughout Ghana.

CAF *Changing African Family Project* (Okediji; *et al.*, 1976); based on the Sociology Department, University of Ibadan, Nigeria, with the co-operation of the Demography Department, Australian National University; field work, 1972 onward; research financed by the Population Council; Directors, F. O. Okediji and J. C. Caldwell, Field Director, Helen Ware.

CAFN *Changing African Family Project—Nigerian segment* (Caldwell, 1974); based on field work 1973; surveys and volumes held by the Demography Department, Australian National University, are: CAFN 1, "The Beginning of Family Limitation", and volumes of papers and responses 1·1 and 1·2; sample of 6606 Yoruba females aged 15–59 in Ibadan; CAFN 2, "The Value of Children", "Work Performed by Children", and volumes 2·1, 2·2, 2·3, 2·4 and 2·5; sample

---

[34] Partly because the findings were often not adequately quantified. Research on changes in fertility control as a result of rural-urban migration is being undertaken in Togo (CAFT).

[35] In the rural Western State of Nigeria by I. O. Orubuloye.

[36] In Lagos and Ibadan by J. G. Ottong.

of 1497 Yoruba males and 1499 Yoruba females in the Western and Lagos States of Nigeria; CAFN 3, "The Achieved Small Family—Wives", "The Achieved Small Family—Husbands"; and volumes 3·1, 3·2 and 3·3; sample of 438 Yoruba females with 0–5 children by choice in Ibadan and 71 husbands; research workers include F. O. Okediji, J. C. Caldwell, Helen Ware, Pat Caldwell, Susan Soyinka, Kayode Soyinka, Bisi Adetona, I. O. Orubuloye, C. Akande, O. Adeyeye and O. Arowolo.

CAFC *Changing African Family Project—Cameroonian segment*; field work 1974; based on Pan African Institute, Douala; principal researcher, W. Vagliani.

CAFG *Changing African Family Project—Ghanaian segment*; field work, 1974–75; based on Institute of African Studies, University of Ghana, Accra; principal researcher, Christine Oppong.

CAFT *Changing African Family Project—Togolese segment*; field work, 1974–5; based on the National Institute for Scientific Research, Lomé; principal researcher, I. Sossah.

NF *Nigerian Family Study* (partly described in Caldwell and Caldwell, based on the Demography Department, Australian National University with the co-operation of the University of Ibadan; field work, 1974–75; research financed by the Australian National University; Field Directors, J. C. Caldwell and Pat Caldwell; other research workers include Kayode Soyinka, I. O. Orubuloye, O. Adeyeye and C. Akande; surveys and volumes held by the Demography Department, Australian National University, are: NF 1, "Intra-Family Flow of Money and Assistance: A Value of Children Study"; sample of 300 Yoruba households in Nigeria's Western State; NF 2, "Post-Natal Female Sexual Abstinence"; sample of 300 Yoruba females in the Western State with at least one weaned child; NF 3, "Terminal Female Sexual Abstinence"; sample of 420 Yoruba females in the Western State 40–44 years old; NF 4, NF 5, NF 6, "Biographies of Successful Men Originating in the Traditional Rural Sector", "Biographies of Successful Women in the Traditional Urban Marketing Sector", "Reports on the *Esusu*".

3

The economic rationality of high fertility: an investigation illustrated with Nigerian survey data

Few social scientists find themselves in such a perplexing predicament as is probably the lot of most demographers engaged in studying the social and economic determinants of high fertility in the developing world. Most of their reading suggests to them that the high fertility of the great majority of people among whom they are working is detrimental to the economic interests of these people. Yet any assertion to this effect is met by widespread scepticism except among some academic colleagues and officials who have often read the same books. This anomaly should be a matter for very great concern to demographers. There is a danger of their living in an unreal world of their own construction. It will be suggested here that this unreal world has been built on poor data and a misunderstanding of non-*Western* social structures.

The great majority of demographers in the field certainly accept the argument that rapid natural increase reduces the rate at which incomes per head can be raised,[1] and probably most feel that the same logic can be applied to high fertility at the individual family level. While most of the argument has been carried on at the macro-economic level, and it is quite proper to maintain that an individual family restricting its fertility prior to its neighbours behaving similarly is in a very different position from a national economy in which birth rates are declining, yet some of the macro-economic arguments can be taken to have implications at the family level. The

[1] As argued in Coale and Hoover (1958), van de Walle (1975), Enke (1966) and Ohlin (1971).

proposition that the change in age structure brought about by declining fertility means a highter ratio of producers to dependants applies equally at the family and national levels; and it can also be argued at both levels that reduced fertility permits greater labour force participation by women and even that the lower child–mother ratio would result in better maternal care and hence more productive children.[2]

Existing survey data have been employed in apparent demonstrations that children are clearly an economic liability even among rural families in Africa and Asia, while some survey responses seem to show that this fact is widely recognized in such populations. Eva Mueller carried out such an analysis, employing data from a range of sources (although only India appeared in both the production and consumption statistics), and concluded that "children have negative economic value in peasant agriculture. Up to the time when they become parents themselves, children consume more than they produce" (1975, p. 66). "The work contribution of children is not large enough to prevent them being an economic burden on peasant societies" (ibid., p. 50), and "children of either sex consume substantially more than they produce until they reach the 15–19 age bracket" (ibid., p. 42). The analysis assumes the dominant importance of cash sales and hence emphasizes the significance of the finding that "it would appear that in most LDCs children under 15 do relatively little market work" (ibid., p. 19). When it appears that children do in fact contribute to such production, it is argued that this tends to be substitute and not additional work: "Adult men may gain leisure by having large families, or women may be freed from the market place. In the limiting case, work by children may be merely a substitute for work by others in the household" (ibid., p. 32). Finally, "raising a large number of children would seem to be an expensive method of providing for the relatively minor aggregate burden of old age support" (ibid., p. 46). It is easy to secure majority assent in a survey to the assertion that educating children costs a good deal directly and indirectly (Caldwell, 1967a, Table 3, p. 226; Caldwell, 1968a, pp. 104–110), and almost as easy to assume without much further enquiry that such agreement has the same implications for desired fertility or for the impact on parents of large family size that it has in the researcher's own society.

However, the uncritical acceptance of such conclusions has major implications both in terms of fertility research as a branch of the social sciences and for the individual researcher in terms of his scientific integrity. The reason for this is that such conclusions can only be maintained by assigning a wrong order of priority to both personal experience and systematic findings in fertility field research among most of the rural population and substantial parts of the urban population, at least in Africa,

---

[2] All these arguments are put forward in Freedman (with Mueller) (1974), p. 7–8.

South Asia and considerable parts of Latin America. Two facts stand out above all others with regard to fertility in these societies. First, fertility remains high and in most is declining slowly or not at all. Secondly, there is very little evidence that large families are any worse off than small families. Few members of such families seem to feel very strongly that they are worse off; it is difficult from inspection or measurement to find any difference in living standards between large and small village families; it is difficult to show that the new elites in the towns were more likely to be drawn from small rural families than from large ones.[3]

The continuing high fertility in much of the developing world, and the lack of much concern over high levels of reproduction in many sections of the society in these countries, should have been taken as "hard" information in the very uncertain field of the economic determinants of high fertility, and as the starting point for further investigation. The failure of fertility researchers to do this has often resulted in a near-inability to communicate with anthropologists or rural economists studying the same populations. Instead, the demographers have often sought to escape the dilemma posed by the difficulty experienced in explaining the present by a kind of future orientation—an undue concentration on change and on minority groups exhibiting some differences from the majority of the population, usually employing significance tests on fertility and other differentials to do so. In the upshot they misunderstand the nature of the change and usually cannot predict the direction and rate of change because of a failure to understand the present. They frequently place too much weight on responses to certain questions about the costs of children—a weight that is frequently unjustified, because small changes in the questions can easily reverse the direction of the majority of replies.[4] More seriously, they often tend to accept the rationality of their own economic analysis by assuming that simple peasants do not understand the economic realities of their own lives, or that they are inhibited from responding rationally by inherited taboos and quasi-religious attitudes,[5] or that insufficient access to anti-natal facilities makes it impossible for them to respond rationally. It is not easy to live and carry out research in a peasant society for any sustained period and retain this outlook. Peasants, once the language barrier has been overcome, turn out to be extraordinarily hard-headed about things that affect their own interests. Nor is ignorance the essential explanation: in Nigeria, farmers

[3] Imoagene (1976) reports on the contrary that significantly higher proportions of persons joining the elite in Western Nigeria came from families of unusually large size (his respondents averaged ten surviving siblings, although admittedly this appears to have included half-siblings).

[4] Many questions in CAFN 2 (see Appendix to Chapter 2) can be paired this way, and further reference will be made to this below.

[5] See for instance Butz (1972) and the reference to "culture survival" in Olusanya (1969), p. 15.

have been shown to be only one-fifth as likely to turn contraceptive knowledge into practice as are townsmen.[6]

It is the purpose of this paper to suggest explanations for the gulf between reality and much research analysis in this area, and then to probe reality in one society by examining the situation among the Yoruba of south-west Nigeria.

Biases in Research and Analysis

Fertility research in developing countries suffers more often than not from three severe limitations: ethnocentricity, an obsession with modernization, and a restriction of the scope of the investigation to the point where the questions supply their own answers. In addition, analysis from the economic standpoint is rendered difficult by data which are often much poorer than the analyst realizes.

The type of fertility research that attempts to provide social and economic explanations for fertility levels and trends has arisen almost entirely for modern *Western* quantitative sociology and very largely from American sociology. Many of its practitioners in the Third World have had relatively short periods of residence in the countries in which they undertake research—and usually none in rural areas—and they work with nationals of these countries who were as often as not their students or colleagues in the universities from which they come. Inevitably, concepts are taken from the *West* to the culture being studied. Often the concepts are sufficiently inapplicable seriously to distort the findings.

The most harmful distortion probably relates to the nature of the family both as a social and economic unit. *Western* sociologists are capable of perceiving that the *nuclear* (or *conjugal*) family of the *West*, with an economic concentration within a group made up of husband, wife and non-adult children and usually residence restricted to the same group, is not universal—that traditionally it may have been a rarity elsewhere. But when carrying out social surveys outside the *West* they tend to treat other types of kinship as if the differences were restricted to having financial responsibilities towards a few more relatives—often assuming that these responsibilities must be more reluctantly borne than those towards members of the nuclear family—or living with a few more of them. They find it difficult to appreciate that a married man might prefer to spend his earnings on his brother rather than his wife, that he might have budgetary arrangements more in common with his father than with his wife, that he might feel that his uncle comes

[6] Caldwell (1975b), footnote 1, p. 84, employing data presented in Caldwell and Igun (1970), Table 3, p. 26.

within the circle of his immediate family of affection and preferred expenditure as much as his children. In sub-Saharan Africa, parts of Asia and undoubtedly elsewhere, the nuclear family is usually the creation of the research worker, and further economic analysis based on such a unit is quite invalid. Reuben Hill, when explaining decisions taken in planning a Puerto Rican fertility study which was to become a prototype for work in a number of other countries, wrote:

> "Of the possible units considered—the individual, the marriage pair, the nuclear family group, reference groups, communities—one met all the criteria satisfactorily, as one would expect with a family sociologist as director, the nuclear family of procreation" (1967, p. 7.)

In the World Fertility Survey's *Occasional Paper* on "Economic Modules for use in Fertility Surveys in Less Developed Countries" the costs and benefits of children are spoken of entirely in terms of *parents* and *couples* (Freedman with Mueller, 1974, pp. 16–17). The extended (or joint) family is recognized as having some financial impact, but the problem is then dealt with by identifying the economic family unit by employing a kind of "cooking-pot" definition—the extended family or common household includes those persons and their dependants who pool a significant portion (perhaps a minimum of 50%) to common or family expenses so as to make him a "sharing member" (ibid., p. 23). Inevitably, such a definition when used in field survey work would be employed as if it meant day-to-day living expenses—probably largely confined to food. The real extended family of mutual obligations which determines the extent to which large family size exerts economic pressure on parents (or brings economic benefits to them) has as little relationship to this *kitchen* family as it does to the extended family of common residence (i.e. those living in the same structure and excluding those living in the adjacent structure) which has excited the interest of historical demographers and census analysts (Laslett (1972); Hsu (1943); Colver (1963) and Burch (1967, 1970)). The economic analysis of fertility in sub-Saharan Africa is prone to error if it identifies budgetary considerations with the nuclear family, not merely because it underestimates the obligations and pleasures connected with spending money elsewhere, but because it overestimates the unity of the conjugal family's finances—most parental expenditure is not in fact on common property, and the expenditure on children and receipts from them are not felt in common or equally. In the World Fertility Survey module it is recommended that data should be obtained distinguishing the earnings of husbands and wives (Freedman (with Mueller), 1974, p. 26) but not their expenditure, obligations and budgets.

The concept of *fertility norms* has been carried over from *Western* societies, where its employment has probably brought mixed benefits, to other societies where its use has in large measure been disastrous, at least in so far as clear thinking by research workers is concerned. Most tend to identify the concept of a *fertility norm* with that of *ideal family size*, although the concept is undoubtedly supposed to be somewhat more complex than this. Freedman, in a recent bibliography of the sociology of human fertility (in which 60% of the entries in the main bibliography appear under headings including the word, *norm*), poses the important question as: "Will having particular numbers (or ranges of numbers) of children affect the ability of the reproducing unit to attain socially valued goals?" and explains that: "The assumption here is that family-size norms will tend to correspond to a number that maximizes the net utility to be derived from having children in the society or stratum" (Freedman, 1975, p. 15). The use of such a construct at least in sub-Saharan Africa tends to make the research worker ignore or regard as a rationalization such responses as imply that these are either not areas for human decision or that humans are impotent in such matters (the "up to God" responses). More seriously, such use often leads researchers to underestimate the conflicts which when resolved result in the achievement of a certain level of fertility, as well as the lack of agreement or even the existence of confrontation between the spouses in reaching that resolution. The position in sub-Saharan Africa often seems to be that there is an abhorrence of a family so small that it might mean the extinction of descendants needed to perform services for their ancestors; in traditional society nearly all parents have social and usually economic gains which increase almost indefinitely with the size of the family; fertility is at first restricted not because such gains are not there but initially to guarantee better health for children and to a lesser extent for mothers, and ultimately by the woman giving up sexual relations because she regards herself as too old or sick for further reproduction or because the family system could not stand the emotional stress of her having parallel maternal and grandmaternal responsibilities and obligations.[7] In addition, children in traditional African society belong to the lineage rather than to their parents, and there is little expectation that decisions about conception will be a personal matter between husband and wife. Such complexities can be subsumed under the concept of *norms* or of *ideal family size*, but in practice research workers seem more likely to be misled by them into oversimplifying the situation and employing survey and analytical techniques appropriate to that simpler situation.

A subtler influence on research is the belief held by most investigators that the high-fertility traditional societies must change. There is an emphasis on *threshold* studies,[8] and on elite studies, which may divert attention from

[7] These matters are explored in NF 2 and NF 3 and in Caldwell and Caldwell (1977).

[8] Some of the more important threshold studies have been: United Nations (1965), pp. 141–151, Freeman and Coombs (1974) and Oechsli and Kirk (1975).

studies of the traditional society which could probably do more to illustrate how social change will take place and why certain thresholds are important. There is such a strong belief on the part of the foreign research worker in *modernization*, that he is often incapable of distinguishing those aspects of social change which are concomitant with economic change and those which are the effect of imported *Westernization*. For instance, mass schooling, which in the *West* largely gave students a concentrated dose of the experience of their own society (admittedly with an emphasis on the experience and attitudes of their middle class), in much of the Third World results in imported values being taught with considerable impact—in Africa influential administrators, many teachers and the models for most textbooks have been of European origin and the emphasis in the schools is undoubtedly on monogamy rather polygyny, on a nuclear rather than a joint family, and on children being at school and mothers in the kitchen rather than on either labouring on the farm. Unless this is understood it is impossible to recognize and investigate changes in economic ends which derive from social changes.[9]

Finally, the economic analysis of high fertility is rendered difficult, even when there is an understanding of the economic ends of the society studied, by poor data—often rendered poorer than they need be by the respondents providing biased data meeting what they perceive to be the emotional needs of the researcher. It is difficult to establish the probable level of a peasant's income, because he has no employer and no wage scale, although the market price for staples and his area of cultivation may be a guide to receipts for staples. However, his supplementary income may be substantial, difficult to detect and almost impossible to assess. In Nigerian research, employing survey techniques which yielded plausible answers to most responses and data that were consistent with others collected independently, we have not been able to show satisfactory relationships of provable accuracy between stated income and other characteristics of respondents, such as occupation or education. McDevitt, after a long period of intensive survey work in rural Nigeria, concluded that most of the money data were of little value (McDevitt, 1975, pp. 8–10) and pointed out that the rural businessman does not make a distinction between his household and his business economy (ibid., p. 5). Taylor, working in rural Kenya, employed an unusual research strategy to show that there the likelihood of income being revealed declines as its source becomes less respectable or less derived from personal exertion and more from investment: statements of income derived from coffee-growing were more complete than on income from a

---

[9] For an example of an almost complete failure to understand the difference between *modernization* and *Westernization* in education, see Inkles and Smith (1974), pp. 15–35 and 139–143.

share in a lorry let alone a share in a bar or takings from prostitution.[10] The failure to disclose all earnings, investment and expenditure to interviewers is conventionally explained as fear of taxation authorities; yet out experience in Africa suggests that a much more potent fear is that the responses will be overheard by relatives and others who have never been certain of the amount of money dispensed by the respondent, and who have claims on his care and may have received different assistance from that given to others. This is not evidence that such persons dislike expenditures of this type and will increasingly move to reduce them; rather is it an attempt to minimize competition, jealousy and envy. Mueller attempts to circumvent the inadequacy of money data by employing an approach based on labour inputs into the growing of staples. This has two major weaknesses. First, it underestimates the complexity of peasant economies, which is particularly unfortunate in the context of her type of analysis, because a particularly high proportion of children's inputs is into work other than the production of staples and because the question of the value of children's work is likely to become a real issue in modernizing economies where diversification is taking place. Secondly, it is based upon measurements of labour inputs and consumption, which are suspect, at least in the case of the latter where none are clearly derived from adequate measurement in the developing world.[11]

The Yoruba of Nigeria

The data employed in this discussion are derived mainly from survey programmes carried out in the years 1973–75 in the Western and Lagos States of Nigeria (see Appendix to Chapter 2).[12] However, it will be argued that aspects of traditional Yoruba society have had similarities in many other cultures[13] and that the implications for fertility are much the same.

[10] Frazer Taylor (Carleton University, Ottawa, Canada), personal communication. Taylor, when interviewing, employed only English and Swahili, and did not disclose his knowledge of Kikuyu, thus enabling him to listen to the discussion in Kikuyu as to how much should be revealed to him. Our experience in Nigeria has been that even the income recorded in this way would substantially understate all income, because of an unwillingness by the respondents to reveal their total incomes to each other.

[11] Mueller (1975), pp. 10–11. Those which appear to be based on measurements from the developing world, such as Lorimer's and Epstein's turn out, when checked, to be derived measurements.

[12] The Appendix explains the nomenclature employed below for identifying sources of data. Much of the argument which follows derives from findings in CAFN 2, consisting of a probability sample of 1497 males and 1499 females over the age of 17 years taken in 1973 among the Yoruba population of the Western and Lagos States of Nigeria. The Western State was sub-divided in 1976 into Ogun, Ondo and Oyo States.

[13] All land must originally have been held communally, although freehold in Europe seems to date back in Greece to the reforms made by Solon in the sixth-century B.C. However, freehold is still rare in rural Africa and was instituted in most of rural India only in the nineteenth century. Extensive obligation to relatives outside the nuclear family is the common pattern of life in Africa and Asia, and to a lesser extent in Latin America.

The fundamental aspect of such a society has been settlements of groups of people, many related, living close together as their ancestors did for generations, farming land which is disposed of by communal decision, and owing each other all kinds of obligations and guarantees of security. These various characteristics are, of course, interrelated and in turn imply other features of the society.

Where a limited population has lived together for a long time exhibiting a complex network of of relationships by blood and marriage and where they live in small villages or even in large family compounds as do the Yoruba, it is unlikely that there will be a marked distinction between the nuclear family and the wider family. Indeed, any degree of nucleation would endanger the stability and security of the larger organization. Such nucleation is always a threat because marital sexual relations may strengthen the conjugal bond and parental (especially maternal) feelings for children may develop into an exclusive possessiveness. This is countered in sub-Saharan Africa by all kinds of cultural practices aimed at weakening the conjugal and parental bonds (Gluckman, 1955, pp. 54–80)[14] and the need for such mechanisms in societies elsewhere with joint family and land tenure systems has also been noted (Gore, 1968, pp. 2–39; Goode, 1963a, pp. 238–247).[15] In sub-Saharan Africa the conjugal bond is weakened and the concept of a simple nuclear family with common budgeting made less meaningful by the practice of polygyny—most monogamously married wives know that their marriages may become polygynous ones and safeguard themselves emotionally and financially against this. The parent–child bond is often weakened by children being brought up wholly or partly by someone else: grandparents, because parents are in the city working or because this is the tradition; siblings, because they are near educational institutions. One study in West Africa claimed that only a minority of the children studied had been brought up by their parents.[16]

The position amongst the Yoruba can be measured by survey findings, although admittedly foreigners may place a different interpretation on these data than do the members of the society themselves. In 1973, about half of all Yoruba women were in polygynous marriages (CAFN 2), which means that a considerably higher proportion would spend some of their lives in such marriages. Only one-third of wives normally slept in the same room or ate at the same table as their husband (CAFN 2) while five-sixths reported that they had no regrets about the cessation of conjugal sexual relations

[14] For a description of the weakening of the bond between a mother and her first child, see Trevor (1975) p. 240.

[15] According to Gore (pp. 22–23), in India, in contrast to Africa, the conjugal bond is weakened by emphasizing the wife's role as a mother.

[16] Clignet (1970), p. 161, where it is shown that in an Ivory Coast survey 47% of children in monogamous families and 43% of those in polygynous families were brought up by their parents.

during the long periods of post-natal sexual abstinence (NF2). When married persons with children of either sex were asked about their closest emotional bonds, fewer than three out of ten said these were with their spouses, six said they were with their children and one with their siblings.[17] The Yoruba woman, frequently expected to be the head of an at least partially independent economic sub-unit of a polygynous family, with strong ties to her own lineage, is often surprisingly independent in terms of what she does and in her finances. The majority of Yoruba women report themselves as fully employed, most being petty traders.[18] One anthropologist concluded that one could not speak of a single society but only of separate male and female societies (and economies) which exist in the same place and time but rarely intersect each other (Marshall, 1970, p. 181). These are not circumstances where one can carry out a simple analysis of the comparative costs and returns of children to parents and relate these to fertility decisions.

Joint family decisions and some degree of joint family economic interests are inevitable wherever land is not under the control (freehold, rented, leased, share-cropped, etc.) of a single nuclear family. This appears to be the case, and to have demographic implications even when the land controlled is freehold.[19] Traditionally in Yorubaland, as elsewhere in tropical Africa, land has been controlled, distributed and redistributed by communal decision, a practice which has been compatible with shifting cultivation.

Communal economic interests and residence close together of nearly all the persons to whom any single individual is related (often, in Yorubaland, in large compounds) have, in a society which has experienced multitudes of disasters, produced an intricate system of obligations and assistance which not only go far beyond the nuclear family, but do so to such an extent that the boundary of the nuclear family is almost imperceptible. Sub-Saharan African societies still experience the world's highest mortality rates and have always known disaster—epidemics, invasion, droughts, floods and crop diseases. The only protection against such scourges and the only guarantee of personal survival has in the past (and in some areas, in the present) (Caldwell, 1975d, pp. 57–58), been in numbers and in assurance of mutual help.

This has had two effects amongst the Yoruba: a great respect for the system of mutual obligations and a belief in increasing the number of persons contained by each system.

[17] Similar patterns have probably been almost universal in traditional societies. In a survey of married women in Melbourne, Australia, reported in Australian Family Formation Project (1972) it was found that agreement to the proposition that the bond between spouses was closer than that between mothers and children was agreed to by seven-tenths of the native-born and of immigrants from Northern Europe but by only four-tenths of those from Southern Europe.

[18] As reported in: Nigeria. Federal Census Office, *Population Census*, 1963; *Western Nigeria*, vol. 11, p. 125; and *Population Census*, 1963; *Lagos*, vol. 11, p. 8 (both Lagos, undated).

[19] C.f. the *zadruga*, or large extended household which held land jointly in parts of the Balkans until the present century, as described by Sklar (1974), pp. 234–236.

In an investigation by prolonged interview in depth, from which biographies were produced (NF 4 and NF 5), of persons in both rural and urban areas who had prospered, the expenditure patterns and the satisfactions derived from such spending were probed. What surprised the foreign investigators most was how frequently the spending on relatives, often quite distant ones, and even on non-relatives was put as the most marked increase in expenditure, and how frequently this was the "consumption good" which gave most pleasure.[20] Again and again, interviewers explained their pleasure at the increased or new respect and love these expenditures had brought them. It might be noted that these largely unstructured interviews brought out the relative importance in producing satisfactions of this kind of expenditure in a way in which exhaustive formal questionnaires employing expenditure questions did not (CAFN 2). In the past, such expenditures, made earlier than necessitated by personal need or community disaster, certainly strengthened the efficacy of the whole system from the standpoint of the persons undertaking the expenditure and incurring the obligations. A Nigerian, undertaking a study of the elite, also expressed his surprise at the lack of hostility among this group at the massive and continued help that nearly all (98%) gave to poorer relatives in response to innumerable and incessant demands, "Help was an accepted way of life"; almost all consider aid to both parents as unavoidable; and two-thirds are perfectly happy at receiving gratification and do not grumble at all (Imoagene, 1976, pp. 144–146).

Such networks can be increased in size by having children who in time marry into other families. Survey questions (CAFN 2) elicited the information that nearly all Yorubas approved of the role of children in linking their families with others (96%) and five-sixths felt that they could ask these new relatives by marriage for assistance to an extent that they could not ask non-relatives.

Certainly, Yoruba society is changing. The main vehicle of change in the rural areas has been cocoa, introduced around the beginning of the century, dominant since the 1920s, and now requiring the purchase of expensive spraying equipment to suppress diseases attacking the trees. Tree crops have, as elsewhere in tropical Africa, upset the traditional system for the control and redistribution of land both because it rendered access to land competitive and because it placed a valuable individual or family possession indefinitely upon a specific area of land. Consequently there has been a move towards individual claim—although not freehold title—upon land and, in some places, a marked shortage of new land for planting (Vanden

---

[20] M. H. Peil (personal communication) reports that, in her previous surveys in Nigeria, the proportion of respondents reporting helping kin as the preferred use of money has been in the range 3–28%.

Driesen, 1971). By 1963, two-fifths of the population lived in urban areas, while by 1975 the proportion may have been closer to one-half with over one-fifth in two centres, Lagos and Ibadan, with around two and three-quarters of a million inhabitants respectively.[21] By 1963, fewer than half the members of the male labour force described themselves in the census as farmers, while most women returned themselves as full-time traders. Education had spread dramatically, so that by 1973 almost half the population over 17 years of age had had some schooling, with the proportion reaching seven-tenths for persons in their twenties (CAFN 2). About three-quarters as many women had been to school as had men. Few reported themselves as belonging to the traditional African religion, although that should not lead to an underestimate of its continuing influence on attitudes and ideas; instead, the society was split statistically, but not seriously socially, between Christians and Moslems with the former slightly predominating. The civil war in the late 1960s, with its recruitment of young men, catalysed social change, while oil revenues over the last decade have accelerated economic change and the move from the rural areas into the towns.

In some ways the family was responding to this change. There had apparently been a slow decline in the incidence of polygyny (Vanden Driesen, 1972, pp. 49–53) probably arising largely from the reluctance of more educated women to have co-wives.[22] Most town families were living well away from their traditional home areas, and husband and wives, although frequently living with relatives beyond the nuclear family, were less likely to be living close to adult siblings or parents with whom decisions would have to be shared. Indeed, the elite families often turned in on themselves to the extent that they seemed to have an almost obsessive interest in their children's education (Lloyd, 1966).

However, there was as yet no certain evidence of fertility decline in any part of the society. The evidence from the 1973–75 survey programme was that the adjusted total fertility ratio for all surveyed women was 7·4 (CAFN 2 corrected by the Brass technique) and that there was no statistically significant fertility differential between women of completed fertility by size of centre of residence or by other socio-economic characteristic. However, the average number of children borne by women 17–19 years of age in the two cities was only two-thirds of the level in villages with fewer than 20 000 inhabitants, although the difference fell to only 5% for women aged 30–39.

[21] All 1963 statistics are from Nigeria Federal Census Office, *Population Census*, 1963: *Western Nigeria*, vols I and II; and *Population Census*, 1963: *Lagos*, vols I and II (both Lagos, undated). Estimates for 1975 are pro-rated from 1973 estimates obtained by CAFN 1 and CAFN 2.

[22] In CAFN 2, 7% of polygynously married women and 35% of monogamously married women had received some secondary education.

The explanation lies partly in a higher proportion of very young women in the city, partly in later marriages there, and probably partly because unmarried or childless young women were more likely to leave the village for the city; but the explanations do not seem to cover the whole gap and it is possible that the beginning of fertility decline, at least in the city, is now being observed. Evidence from a larger sample drawn entirely from the city of Ibadan (CAFN 1) reveals that the average number of children borne by women over 45 years of age declines by one child from women with only primary school education, through those who did not proceed beyond secondary schooling to the relatively small number with tertiary education.[23] No other socio-economic characteristic yields an indisputable differential or one that is unlikely to be explained by the educational differential.

Little attempt is made to control fertility, and the major constraints upon it are very substantial periods of sexual abstinence by women after birth and a high frequency of female terminal abstinence which probably begins in many cases before the menopause. These controls are rarely explained in terms of the economic difficulties resulting from high fertility, but the former is almost always justified in terms of preserving the infant's health (NF 2) and the latter for personal reasons such as being too old for the worry of raising more children (NF 3) (Caldwell and Caldwell, 1977). But those women who have at any stage attempted any anti-natal practice except continence numbered only 16% by 1973–75 in the city of Ibadan (CAFN 1), 4% in the villages of Ibadan's rural hinterland and 2% in the villages of the less urbanized Ekiti Division (Orubuloye, 1975 and 1981), figures which were nevertheless higher than those recorded from four to six years earlier.[24] Nevertheless, there is very little evidence that family planning is securing a rural toehold: further investigation of the few women practising contraception in villages around Ibadan or in Ekiti showed that they were mostly the wives of school teachers or of men with white collar jobs in the distant towns (Orubuloye, 1975 and 1981).

In 1973 (the following analysis is entirely from CAFN 2), the proportion of all women in the Western and Lagos States who had ever used any anti-natal method other than sexual abstinence was 11%, which was

[23] However, women with no education recorded lower fertility in Ibadan than women with primary education (CAFN 1). David Lucas has reported the same finding from his survey in Lagos (1976), Table 9.6, p. 218. It is possible that illiterate women may be more affected by sterilizing disease (some of them are probably prostitutes, but the ramifications of ill-health are undoubtedly much wider than this); they may also be more likely to adhere strictly to long periods of post-natal sexual abstinence. However, it is also probable that they report a lower proportion of deceased children, while undoubtedly experiencing a higher level of mortality among their children.

[24] Caldwell and Igun (1970), recording a survey carried out in March–April 1969, when levels in Ibadan were 8% and in the rural areas 1%. Levels of rural contraception as low, or usually lower, are the rule in tropical Africa (see Caldwell, 1975, p. 87).

sub-divided into 5% currently using modern contraceptives (apparently largely pills, condoms and IUDs, in that order), 5% who had used such contraceptives in the past and 1% employing rhythm or withdrawal.[25] The use of contraception rose steeply with education and occupation and was markedly higher in the larger urban centres and amongst younger adults. Women with education exceeding three years secondary schooling and with husbands in white-collar occupations,[26] made up only 11% of the sample but 55% of the current users of modern contraception; such women living in Lagos or Ibadan formed only three per cent of the sample but 35% of current users.

There was thus no significant reaction in the society as a whole to having reached a fairly high level of education, non-agricultural employment or urban residence, even though urban residents exhibited levels higher than that of many low-fertility countries.[27] Nor is it a simple case of still being below the threshold or not realizing the new economic conditions.

It will be the theme of this paper, to be explored through the accumulated survey data, that such high fertility levels do not show any misunderstanding of the nature of the contemporary Yoruba economy. Rather are they a rational response to the social economic ends of the society. In fact, given those ends, the parent of a large number of children can prosper relatively to the parent of a small number even more in the modern economy than in the traditional one.

Fertility will certainly decline in the future, but it will not do so because of more rational economic analysis by parents. It will do so because the economic calculus will change with the crumbling of the old social and economic ends of the society—those based on mutual obligations and formed in a society of large family compounds and communal access to land.

Nor will the old order crumble as a direct or sole reaction to economic modernization. If economic change were to be halted now, the crumbling would continue, although doubtless more slowly, and fertility would fall. This will happen because continued change in family structure has attained a momentum that would be difficult to reduce, especially in the new conditions of towns, cash-cropping, office jobs and so on which offer no

[25] CAFN 2. The separate questions of past use of various methods, and other evidence from the survey programme, suggest that current use of rhythm and withdrawal is probably understated and these probably amount to at least 2% and 1% respectively.

[26] White-collar occupations are defined here as all professional, administrative, clerical and other indoor occupations which are non-manual and necessitate literacy. They include military and police officers and even government messengers (partly because these people will otherwise misstate the nature of their job to interviewers). Most of these people do not in fact work in white collars.

[27] By proportion of population in urban centres of each size class the Western and Lagos States combined are close to the median levels of urbanization of those industrialized countries and of European countries reported in the United Nations (1974b), pp. 388–394.

obstacles to the new type of family. But it is not this lack of obstacle which causes the change—on the contrary, it is mostly imported cultural innovation.

The basic change will be family nucleation, not in residence patterns but in the concentration of expenditure and obligation. It will be marked by (and caused by) a movement towards monogamy, a strengthening of the conjugal bond over all others, a strengthening of the parent–child bond over all relationships external to the nuclear family, and ultimately an emphasis on what parents owe children rather than what children owe parents.

These are not necessarily rational changes even in terms of fitting in with an industrial economic system. Far more are they imported *Westernization*, for much of this behaviour was characteristic of Europe long before most of its population lived in towns or worked in factories. Such *Westernization* began during the last century with the arrival of missionaries who almost invariably identified the Christian family with the European family. But it has reached flood tide with mass schooling and with an increasingly literate population being exposed to the mass media. Schools, newspapers, magazines, television programmes, and even radio broadcasts, draw almost exclusively on material from the *West* and the material is presented by people most affected by that culture. In primary school, children are taught about a family unit consisting of a father, mother and children, the parents being primarily devoted to rearing the children. However, the most damaging thrust at the traditional system probably comes from the enormous coverage of sex in the newspapers and magazines, which in Nigeria compete with the more sex-oriented publications in Europe and North America and, indeed, draw heavily upon them. At present much of the impact of the emphasis on the importance of sex is contained outside marriage—by girls in bars and nightclubs, by prostitutes in brothels and by extra-marital relations—but inevitably husbands are increasingly likely to think that the message also refers to marital relations, especially when the wife is educated and particularly when she too, receives and heeds the message.[28] The joint family has always appreciated that its greatest danger lies in the strengthening of the conjugal link through an increasing enjoyment of marital sexual relations.

Such changes will not reduce fertility markedly in the near future. One reason is that they take time to percolate through the whole society and are only partly accepted at first. There is very considerable cultural resistance. A woman may be a wife, but she and her husband know that she should also be a good daughter, sister and mother. The elite may concentrate more on their children, but they still have firm ideas about not spoiling them, which continues to keep a ceiling on the cost of children. Most children know that

[28] C.f. for Sierra Leone, Harrell-Bond (1975), pp. 488–489.

their consumption patterns are based on the relatively meagre consumption patterns of their peers; the fact that a father might eat better or own something or make a journey somewhere does not mean that his dependent son can aspire to do likewise.

The main reason why social changes will not produce rapidly declining fertility in the near future is that the present system of mutual obligations actually works, and will continue to do so until a sufficient number of people opt out of it to topple the whole system—rather like breaking a *chain letter*, except that the mutual obligations system is, when intact, a stable system with none of the tendency of the *chain letter* to destroy itself by uncontrollable expansion. As long as children ungrudgingly share their earnings with their parents, it will pay to have a large family and to educate them. As long as children are helped by their older siblings, by grandparents, uncles and cousins, and, indeed, by the other parent when that parent has a separate income and budget, the parent will not bear the full cost of the large family, and will not escape expenditure on other children by limiting his or her fertility. It is better still if the system generates a good deal of heart-warming gratitude as it undoubtedly does in Yoruba society. There are, of course, other sanctions preserving the system. The most important is that a person, who can meet obligations and provide assistance but refuses to do so, no longer has access to communal property. He has no right to land in his place of origin; he cannot build a house there: his very presence will probably be unwelcome; he is thus cut off from his ancestors. Modernization has in some ways strengthened the system of mutual obligations; the two most common financial crises associated with a deadline for payment and necessitating appeals for assistance arise from taxes and school fees. While the system works economically it also works socially; high fertility brings with it honour and prestige; indeed, children are themselves identified with wealth.

Thus, high fertility is still economically advantageous in Yorubaland. There is no threshold as measured by socio-economic indices. If the mutual obligation system had been dismantled long ago, and if the conjugal family had nucleated its relationships—as apparently happened well back in European history—then high fertility would have been impoverishing for most urban families, and certainly those in the middle class, decades ago, at the threshold levels of those times. By now fertility would be falling and there would be a greater and more insistent demand for contraception. If some kind of nationalist cultural revolution had succeeded in blocking all contact with the *West* except trade and the import of machines, and had enshrined African cultural values, then modernization probably could have continued until well into the next century without affecting fertility.[29] As it

[29] Nkrumah's Ghana emphasized the need for cultural nationalism until 1966 but favoured many *Western* familial values; China exhibits the reduced contact but has created social and economic organizations which substitute for the extended family.

is, the family system, and through it the system of mutual obligations, is under assault. When significant sections of the society foreswear major obligations outside the nuclear family, and invent a rationale for doing so which can be used by others to justify their own actions, then the whole system could decay fairly rapidly. One of the first measurable indications of this may be fertility decline among some sections of the population. Probably the process will begin in the cities in the near future and will have penetrated the society deeply by the end of the century.

Some aspects of the existing system, and the inroads already made into it, will now be examined in more detail.

Desires, Needs and Wants

Perhaps the weakest aspect of fertility and KAP survey work has been to ask questions about ideal family size and desired number of children without attempting to discover anything about other ideals and desires. It is almost unbelievable that debate should have raged around the meaning of "up to God" responses without anyone knowing whether other questions about hopes and aspirations elicited similar replies. Accordingly, we have endeavoured during the Nigerian research programme in recent years to probe a wider range of desires and expectations (especially in CAFN 2 which is the main source of the findings quoted below, although non-directed responses from NF 4 and NF 5 are also quoted).

Questions about plans and hopes, about the expenditure of small sums likely to come their way and about larger windfall gains that are most unlikely to do so, and about both probable and improbable choices, yield a surprisingly clear pattern.

Yoruba society is strongly commercial and most people have a very clear idea of choices and costs. In spite of a widespread conviction amongst development planners that pre-industrial societies are essentially non-quantitatively oriented and innumerate (and amongst demographers when explaining bad age data), the awareness exhibited by respondents of just how far even large amounts of money would go was comparable with that of the only industrial society the writer has studied in similar depth, Australia.

Two points stand out. The first is that Yorubas want extra money in the very great majority of cases to make investments, to make the future more secure with the help of today's good fortune. They wish to start up businesses, buy stock for existing small businesses (mostly trade stalls), improve housing[30] and educate children or themselves. Consumption goods

[30] M. H. Peil (personal communication) reports that housing is a good investment for those who have ancestral rights to urban land and so are in a monopolistic position with regard to building houses and renting accommodation to strangers.

very much take second place, although clothes are a partial exception here. This is especially true in the more traditional society for two reasons. One is that the villagers have not yet felt the full impact of the acquisitive society: salesmen and advertisers do not try to tempt them with new goods; such goods are not easily obtained or repaired in rural areas; and many consumer durables would be impracticable because of the lack of electricity, the shortage of kerosene or the expense of both. A more important reason, however, is that there are limits on individual conspicuous consumption in a traditional society. Not only is it decidedly bad taste to flaunt too many belongings that other villagers do not have or that no one has ever found necessary, but expenditure on such things advertises the fact that one could do more to assist others. Many African societies have mechanisms for removing the surplus wealth from individuals; Ibo society does it through a ladder of honoured positions, where accumulated wealth indicates that the possessor should be raised a rung but where the cost of the elevation consumes most of the surplus wealth. Certainly, there is a growing village demand for transistor radios, bicycles and small kerosene stoves, and a real need for cocoa tree spraying equipment, but such things are often better brought as presents on visits by educated children working far away in the modern sector of the economy. Similarly, the male head of a household is more likely to buy his family cloth for clothing in the form of a necessary expenditure or even presents for an important family occasion or village festival than to do it as a matter of routine. The fact that a villager who appears to be relieved of one kind of expense (perhaps school costs because he has few children) may find it difficult to resist additional calls for assistance, and that it is in better taste to acquire possessions above the conventional necessities as a present from an adult child than by purchase have obvious implications for the rationality of high fertility. It should also be emphasized that the giving of presents in the society demonstrably generates additional pleasure over and above that received from the utility of the object.

The second point is that respondents just do not think of children as a competitive form of expenditure—as drawing on money which would otherwise be available for alternative expenditure or investment. When we asked 3000 people to discuss what they could do if they unexpectedly acquired some more money, no one said that it would now be possible to have a baby or to increase the family by an extra child. When we forced the point by providing a list of acquisitions to be placed in preferential order according to what they could afford, and included "another child", an astonishing and quite unprecedented 29% of all respondents queried the structure of the question itself by pointing to the anomaly that the list of alternative ways of disposing of additional income included opting for another child. Obviously, most of the remainder thought so too but did not think that it was up to them to judge the nature of the questions. One in ten actually chose the child but interviewers often had the impression that they were expressing their strong desire for another child rather than understanding that the question was really about the allocation of resources.

Three-quarters of the women agreed, often with some puzzlement, that they would defer having a baby for three years if offered a good job which they could only take up by postponing the birth. This may some day be part of the mechanism of fertility decline; but, at present, the question is an excellent example of getting out of questions answers that are structured into them because of experience in very different societies. The truth is that the problem does not yet arise in acute form; employers and relatives know that working women usually have a lot of children and will have to make arrangements—and those arrangements are usually fairly easily made because of the assumption of extended family and sibling responsibilities and because poor and young relatives often with little education or others from the home village are only too pleased to be nursemaid for little more than their keep especially if it means moving to the city.[31]

What does stand out clearly is the strong desire to have children and to educate them.

Only 1% of respondents describe ideal family size as being less than four children and only one-third as being less than six. Half of all respondents still agree that "A man with 12 children is blessed", while nine-tenths of both men and women hold that "Bearing children is the most important thing a woman can do", and subscribe to the statement "I love children—nearly all children".[32] Certainly, three-quarters of respondents agree with the Yoruba saying, "Lots of children, lots of misery", but the median estimate of the number of living children that there would have to be before the onset of this misery is eleven or higher in all but one of 54 sub-groups of the population defined by sex, educational, occupational and urban-rural residence criteria. The exception is women with husbands in white-collar occupations who are nearly all educated themselves and who mostly live in the cities and larger towns. The fear of the extinction of the family cannot be underestimated—a fear that may rationally grip the parent of a three- or four-child family in a society where mortality levels are still high in considerable sections of the population (Orubuloye and Caldwell, 1975) and where there may well be an association between the chances of siblings dying because of common environmental or child-care conditions. Amongst respondents of each sex, 98% believes that "A man lives on through his

[31] Reported by Arawolo (n.d.) to be still the case in Ibadan, although some shortages are developing in the supply of suitable nursemaids in Accra (Oppong, 1975c).

[32] The statements chosen were proverbs or other everyday sayings in the Yoruba language. See Caldwell (1974) especially pp. 16–19.

sons", 92% that "The real dead are those who die without descendants", and 85% that "Children are still needed to perform services for the ancestors". The latter assertion is now open to some questioning, but amongst white-collar workers in Lagos with extended secondary or tertiary education assent did not fall below 81%, even amongst men under 30 years of age.

The desire is not only to have children but to educate them for jobs and ways of life other than peasant farming (even when it is dominated by cocoa growing as it is in the Western State). All but one-sixth of respondents would be unhappy if their children remained peasant farmers, and the proportion did not fall below one-third amongst illiterate farmers (NF 1, which was addressed only to male household heads). With regard to education, only 8% would be satisfied with anything less than secondary education and 54% with less than tertiary.

When asked about occupational aspirations (without any attempt by interviewers to suggest jobs), farmers and both urban unskilled and skilled workers wanted to be successful business men or women, while white-collar workers aimed at the professions, clerical jobs or successful businesses according to the level of their education. Hardly anyone desired to be a farmer, but most knew accurately enough the limits that their education imposed. But for children who had yet to complete their education the position was very different: 85% wanted their sons to be professional or white-collar workers—almost half specified doctors; while 82% wanted similar jobs for their daughters—almost half nominated nursing.

The outline of how and why high fertility successfully operates in a society in transition from peasant agriculture to a more urbanized society, with most people working in commerce, administration and to a lesser extent small factories, is now beginning to emerge. The essential factor in the system is the retention of the traditional system of assistance and of the direction in which that assistance flows, a system which developed in huge rural compounds where four generations of the lineage often lived together. A Nigerian research worker contrasted, with some surprise at the extent of the difference, his survey sample of the new elite in Nigeria's Western State, where 97% of employed children with living parents assisted their parents financially, irrespective of the level of the parents' income or health, with a study of an American New England population where a similar proportion of parents emphasized that they would not accept help from children even though most had spent massively on the children up until the time of their employment.[33] An important subsidiary factor is a considerable urban–rural income gap and a massive differential in income by education. The latter is taken for granted by nearly everyone; it originated at a time when missionaries highly valued their few literate assistants and was sustained by a

---

[33] Imoagene (1976), comparing his findings with those of Sussman (1953).

continuing shortage of educated Nigerians for work in the colonial administration and with European firms, and ultimately in the massive extension of education preceding and following Independence. The new world of excitement and honour, of "big men" and important undertakings, of consumer goods and sufficient money is the world of the large towns and of jobs within them that require educational qualifications. Yorubas honour their traditional ways more than most West Africans, but they know where contemporary rewards are to be found: only 1% of respondents of either sex hoped that their children would secure chieftaincies or other positions of traditional honour as their main occupation, and all dream of their families securing beach-heads in the urban middle classes. There are immediate benefits in having children so placed, quite apart from the remittance of money. Successful children will visit the village often (Adepoju, 1974, pp. 385–387) and will invariably bring presents with them; their presence will honour their parents and they will be consulted by both their families and by other villagers; they will be noticed at ceremonies and festivals and will contribute substantially to the cost of them. A parent will proudly display a luxury good presented to him in this way with none of the explanations that would be necessary for a personal purchase. Successful children will often plan and pay for improvements that their village relatives would not have brought themselves to think about: house wells, latrines, improved drying areas for cocoa and so on. In one study, all improvements in water supply and sanitation in the village had been provided by children working elsewhere (Orubuloye and Caldwell, 1975). The children will improve the house itself on successive visits, perhaps first the room in which they stay, but possibly later the outside walls will be strengthened with concrete, or additional windows will be added. Eventually, the village may be honoured by the building of a separate house as splendid as those found in the city and felt to contribute to the progress of the centre even if it is mostly untenanted. Educated, elite children will contribute from afar—often with the assistance or compulsion of an association formed by city dwellers from their town or village of origin—to the creation of community facilities in their home place: a school or an additional school room, a community hall or meeting place, new farming equipment and the like. They may also use their influence or the power of their arguments on government to try to secure teachers, roads, electricity, a water supply and so on. There are other benefits in having successful children living in the town. A parent can enjoy a visit to the town and be welcomed into comparatively luxurious conditions; he can meet his children's important friends; he can make purchases in the town at leisure. He can also arrange for another child to come and stay while being educated.

The path to all this is well known. The parent with little or no education can improve his lot only by establishing a successful business—perhaps a small shop selling food or a larger one with building materials, or even a saw mill or a lorry or a wholesaling supply service of perhaps cloth from a Lagos mill. It takes ability and self-confidence and a deftness with money and even accounts. It also takes luck, the advice of wise relatives, a benevolent providence and perhaps a monopoly of supplies from a certain producer arranged by friends or relatives. These are the invariable ingredients of success in the autobiographies collected from such men and women (NF 4 and NF 5). But to gain further benefits from the modern world one usually needs to educate a child to break into its heartland. The trouble is that not all children can do this in spite of encouragement (which often takes the form of incessant nagging and an obsessive interest in school results). There are two essential elements in maximizing the chance of success. One is a kind of "lucky-dip" principle or the backing of many horses: with a large number of children there is a good chance that at least one will do well, and one elite salary will outweigh the earnings of a string of children working in traditional or poor urban occupations and will make up for expenditure on several educations. The other is the value of a sibling chain of assistance. The child who breaks through first into extended education and the jobs that this secures almost invariably helps his siblings (usually, but not always, younger ones). He can provide money for fees and usually accommodation in a large centre near a secondary school or some tertiary institution. He can also serve as a model and a guide: he knows this new world and what one should aim at; his conversation and even his books assist the young student brother to change into the type of person the school will encourage; his house and his possessions are something worth striving for. Both elements depend on high fertility. This may be less true when there is a modification of the present system, in which great numbers struggle to stay in the educational system which almost capriciously throws off many at every stage; luck certainly plays a role in keeping on the ladder.

This description may seem to apply only to rural families or at least to poor ones. Surprisingly the evidence seems to be that the urban elite as yet prosper more than any others. Most of their children continue to spend on their parents and relatives, and most have high incomes, for the urban elite understand the system, can afford the fees, know the headmasters and assist each other in placing their children in suitable positions.

The rest of this paper will fill out this outline with evidence from existing data, investigate the balance of costs and returns in high fertility, and look at high fertility as a preferred investment.

Children: Activities, Costs and Returns

The Yoruba do not perceive themselves as being disadvantaged by high fertility (evidence in this section is from CAFN 2 except where otherwise noted). Fewer than one-fifth believed that, if they were to have an extra child in the year following the interview, they would be poorer in the future. A majority believe that one needs a *very large* number of children (and many more merely believe that one needs a large number) to ensure first that some will grow up, secondly that some will be willing and able to help their parents once they are employed, and thirdly, so that they will have this ability, that some will be bright enough to win the educational qualifications that will secure them a job with a high income. There is almost unanimity in agreement about the need for this assistance in the parents' old age, a view held so strongly that it often obscures the profitability of such help at earlier times.

Probably the key error in the analysis of the economic support for high fertility is to focus only on this return from adult children and then to assume that the support given during their rearing must be of the nature of an investment. It is only one further step to suggest that there are cheaper ways than high fertility of achieving the same return, especially if the apparatus of the State can be used.

The problem is that nowhere, except possibly amongst limited numbers of the urban elites, can one ever secure much strongly felt agreement in Yorubaland or elsewhere in tropical Africa that even dependent children are particularly burdensome. The fact that differentials in family size do not appear to impose equal differentials in financial loads upon parents obviously may be related to extended family flows of money and assistance. But this is not the whole answer. One reason for the lack of disquiet is that there seems to be fairly general agreement that more hands grow more food. This is related to the ability of larger families to farm larger areas, and, where land is limited, to farm existing areas more intensively.[34] Admittedly, very young children can contribute little labour, but a condition where no children can contribute to food growing is found only for the first two or three children and is found in the cases of both small and large families.

However, the failure of economic analysis to show why large families feel no worse off than small families even before the returns from employed adult children begin to flow is almost certainly a failure to understand the consumption as well as the production side of the partially-subsistence household and a failure to take into account market activities other than the sale of staples. It is a failure to understand societies where the distinctions are much less clear than in advanced industrial societies between producers and consumers and between the hours of the week devoted to production and those devoted to consumption.

In societies like that of the Yoruba a much larger proportion of wants are

[34] See Galletti *et al.* (1956), pp. 307–334, where production is shown to increase with the labour input into a specific area.

satisfied within the household by human activities than by machinery. The technical aider in the Third World, finding that he keeps his household together only by using the services of a large number of people (including those who merely call with goods or messages), is apt to think that this is very largely the result of demanding a different way of life, standard of living and pattern of consumption from that of the local population. The very fact that this is partly true may prevent him from observing just how much very humble households depend on human services.

In the West an ever larger proportion of the possessions in the home do not supply aesthetic pleasure in themselves and cannot be consumed for direct satisfaction, but instead supply services. Telephones bring messages into the house and the family car brings purchases, the vacuum cleaner dusts the floor, the washing machine cleans the clothes and the washing-up machine the dishes, the refrigerator and freezer keep food so that fresh food has to be brought into the house less frequently, the mixer breaks up and mixes food while its grinding attachment grinds, the hot water system heats water and takes it to where it is needed, the electricity system brings fuel into the house, the incinerator removes waste and so on. In rural Yorubaland most of the consumer durables and other gadgets which provide these services cannot be afforded or even easily purchased or adequately serviced even where money is available; nor is electricity usually available, and, where it is, the cost is enormously high compared with that of human labour. But every one of these things can be done by human activity. Most involve carrying, picking up or pounding, all of which can be done by children. Indeed, in a traditional society they are done as a matter of course by children with little complaint. Nine out of every ten of our respondents agreed that "small children save adults from menial tasks", and that "children are important because of the help they give in the home". Even outside the home such tasks abound. The Western observer often makes the mistake at first of assuming that most rural activity is clearing, digging, planting and harvesting, and that the great reductions in labour can be made by the introduction of tractors, saws, ploughs, mechanical cultivators and the like. In fact, more energy is probably consumed in the course of a year by carrying water, fuel, products for sale in the market and purchases from the market, and by walking to and from the nearest road or distant fields. Eventually, much of this activity will be reduced by the multiplication of feeder roads and vehicles, by the digging of wells closer to the village and even by the reticulation of water and electricity and the sedentarization of agriculture. In the meantime, there is much for children, even small children, to do. In a partly-subsistence economy, children are not only producers for the market and for household consumption; they also provide subsistence services and make life for adults pleasanter and more gracious than it would otherwise be. In a different sense from that in which the term has previously been used, children are, indeed, "consumer durables".[35]

We have attempted to measure children's activities and to analyse them by sub-divisions of sex, age, education and size of centre of residence (CAFN 2). Children (and their parents as well) assume that children (at an early age) will do most of the things that adults of the same sex do. Around the age of five, imitative play seems to give way to activities that relieve others of some work.[36] Amongst the very young there is little division by sex, and work is fairly evenly divided between doing housework and carrying things or messages outside the house. These are heterogeneous categories and an analysis based on them hides the changes in the balance of tasks that takes place with age: in the former a change from sweeping and light tasks to washing up or washing clothes to cooking and ironing among the older girls, and splitting wood among the boys, while in the latter the progression is from carrying messages and water to bearing heavier objects like firewood or fuel or to errands where responsibility is required such as when making purchases. Minding younger siblings depends more on birth order than age. In the traditional society (and still in rural areas amongst children who have not attended school), farming became an increasing proportion of all boys' work as they grew older, although there was a change in emphasis from tasks like weeding to such heavier labour as clearing and making yam mounds, and, amongst girls, marketing became more important although it by no means replaced housework. Schooling reduces the numbers undertaking such traditional work as farming and marketing, and urbanization has a similar impact in reducing the number of boys engaging in farming (although not the number of girls marketing). It is not the time in school that prevents educated boys from farming; it is a different attitude to life which is accepted, although often with misgivings, by their parents (Galletti et al., pp. 78–79; S. A. Aluko, personal communication).

Children from quite young ages help with market-oriented activities: the production of cocoa and foods eaten locally; the processing and preparation of foods derived from the oil palm, cassava and maize; spinning, weaving and dyeing; plaiting hair and so on. Children can also earn money on neighbouring farms during peak agricultural activity, and can collect firewood and wild plantain (the non-sweet banana) from the forest—in fact it appears that the possible earnings from the latter activity determine the minimum wage which can be paid for casual agricultural labour.[37]

[35] Blake (1968) examined whether having a child is an alternative economic choice to purchasing a consumer durable and whether the child yields a psychic utility, but not whether it yields services of the same type as those from the consumer durables.

[36] For almost identical descriptions, see, on Ghana, Oppong (1973), p. 51 and, on the Philippines, Nurge (1956), pp. 7–11.

[37] Personal communication from I. H. Vanden Driesen referring to the findings from his field research in the Ife Division of the Western State during 1968–69.

The attempt to measure parents' feelings about the balance of cost and return on children has been made in both Ghana (GRH and GA) and Nigeria. The results are unsatisfactory because many parents inevitably think of the question in terms of cash returns either from individual earnings or the expansion of the household's capacity for market production. There is little point in pressing the question whether the extra services in or outside the house make up for the extra costs and disadvantages of children, because most respondents state that additional children at no time result in additional costs or disadvantage. In terms of the current money balance of costs and returns, most respondents say that children who are not at school bring in more than the cost they impose by the time that they are about 15 years of age, while those still at school never do so. In terms of the cumulative return on children, most respondents over 50 years of age say that they have received back more than they spent. Indeed, 97% of respondents felt that: "The best investment is in the education of one's children (or relatives)."

An attempt was made to trace all money flows in each direction between parents and children in 300 families (NF 1). The investigation showed quite clearly that the present system of parent–child financial relationships—a system which does not penalize high fertility—depends for its working on the concept of extended family and communal help: those who can help usually do so. Most parents who did not give any assistance were unable to do so and were not blamed for their failure. At least they were not blamed sufficiently for it to result in any restriction of subsequent assistance from their children—if anything their greater need provoked a little more assistance. Similarly, those children who do not help are mostly those who can least afford to do so—the predicted revolt of the educated in favour of a Western type of system of obligations has not yet occurred on any significant scale. Investment in children is probably an investment in the real sense of the term. But this does not come about because there is any correlation between giving assistance to a specific child and receiving help back from that child. It comes about because greater financial help to capable children—and this qualification is clearly understood by the parents—may allow them to reach the urban white-collar occupations, and perhaps even the professions, with high and regular incomes. If they reach such heights they will in most cases return more money and remit it more regularly.

Children on average are reported to remit money to parents amounting to ten per cent, or a little more, of both fathers' incomes and household incomes; among those who remit at all the reported proportion is around 15%. For perhaps half of all parents the number of remitters may eventually be three or more, thus increasing parental income by half. Such an analysis is illuminating but misleading. It hides much of the return on the investment.

First, the monetary return is probably understated. Secondly, the non-monetary returns may well outweigh the monetary ones (speaking only in terms of goods and not of other gratifications). Thirdly, the successful investment buys security; the main aim is that the child should obtain employment with guaranteed tenure and regular salary that will permit help to be given to parents no matter what disaster should strike them—blighted cocoa crops, drought, flood, cholera, urban unemployment, a succession of funerals, or many other domestic or village crises.

There are, in fact, few other competitive sources of investment for rural populations. Peasant farming offers few outlets for extra money in contrast to extra labour; spraying equipment costs money but its acquisition is no longer thought of as optional. Usury is practised by some farmers but is more the speciality of the businessman.[38] Money is safely invested in a small business only if that business is run by a trusted and competent relative. More land can be acquired with money now that communal tenure has been modified, but it can only be profitably used if farmed by near relatives, usually children or a wife (Vanden Driesen, 1972, p. 53). These are not restrictions which favour low fertility.

One type of activity—once universal but now practised only by those grown-up children who remain in the village—has not been mentioned and does not appear on the kind of balance sheet just discussed. Sons tend to help their fathers on the farms throughout their fathers' lives. In fact, the most comfortably-off old man will be he who has some non-migrant children helping him locally and other migrant ones channelling the new forms of wealth from afar.

A Society Subject to Rational Economic Analysis

The ethnocentric Western economist is tempted to conclude that the society has not yet reached a level of economic rationality with regard to fertility; in that he feels that children should either involve a net loss, in which case the family should be small, or a net gain, in which case fertility should never be restricted. He is likely to feel justified in this attitude when the same survey (CAFN 2) secures agreement from five-sixths of respondents to assertions that "a brother who has four children and is able to study and travel is wiser than his brother who has eight children and has to work all the time", and "a rich man with a few children is more important than a poor man with many children" while at the same time finding the following distribution of answers in a forced choice between four statements: "Children are better

[38] M. H. Peil (personal communication) on farmers; I. H. Vanden Driesen (personal communication) on businessmen.

than wealth"—25%; "Children are wealth"—54%; "Children are almost as good as wealth"—10%; "Children use up wealth"—11%. However, subsequent discussion with respondents easily brings to light the fact that most believe that a man is more likely to be helped towards riches than hindered, and even more likely to be helped towards international travel, by a large number of children than by fewer. If the investigator sets the rules of the game then the respondents will abide by those rules—of course one chooses the options that offer wealth or travel!

For most of the society the position seems to be that a minimum number of children (usually a fairly high minimum given the mortality levels) is needed to ensure prosperity, security and even immortality. Beyond that number, there is some eventual increase in prosperity with each child. But there may also be some increase in difficulties in organizing the larger family especially in terms of meeting schooling costs, and ultimately, for women, physical or social problems in continuing to reproduce. There is then a non-economic upper bound to female reproduction (eventually got around by most men by the practice of polygyny), which no more forbids the application of Western economic analysis below that limit than such analysis is prevented in the West by the existence of a non-economically determined two-child floor to family fertility in most populations.

The Inevitability of Change

Changes in the economy and society following the massive intrusion of the *West* over the last century have lessened the need for the extended family system by weakening communal tenure of land and common residence. In addition, many forms of insecurity have been reduced by a host of changes stretching from modern health measures to a smaller chance of being destroyed by local disasters because of better communications, greater commercialization and a strong central government.

Such a reduction in the need for the extended family has not led to its being an inefficient unit for profiting from economic opportunities. In fact, it has proved surprisingly efficient in selecting and financing children to climb the educational ladder to high salaries. It has also proved more efficient than the nuclear family would have done in exporting prosperity from the towns to the countryside.

However, the import of the new economy has been accompanied by the import and teaching of different cultural values. It is now inevitable that nuclear family values will spread in the decades ahead. There is admittedly considerable cultural resistance to an uncritical conversion to *Western* familial practices—again and again West Africans deplore in conversation and in the press the failure of *Western* families to take in uncomplainingly their aged parents. The break-up of the large families has been assisted by rural–urban migration, but this alone would not have shattered extended family emotional and economic priorities.

The nucleation of the family will not of itself make high fertility unprofitable. That requires the adoption of a system in which the lifetime net flow of money is from parent to child rather than in the opposite direction and a rise in children's costs which makes a large number of them prohibitively expensive. The former change has hardly begun—there is no particular economic reason why it should as long as the system remains intact. If the system were to crumble significantly, there may then be a landslide to the new values. But it is most unlikely that one aspect of a culture can be imported without the rest, especially when so much of the balance is to do with children and seems to be taught by the educational system. At present, the community draws on both traditional values and those of an austerer Christianity—that of nineteenth century Europe which lingered long in the sometimes humble missionary centres of West Africa—to justify the failure to offer children the range of goods or expensive pleasures their parents might have. It seems probable that, with the example of *Western* culture which is continually being pressed upon them by the media and the schooling system, the very children who demand more from their parents, and thus change the parent–child relationship, will be the ones who return least. This change will be assisted by the transition from a society where most honour is earned by activities and generosity within the local community to one where the proudest achievements are those performed in the wider community and are marked by examination results, appointments to new occupational positions, the achievement of high salaries, reporting of doings in the national press and so on. Eventually the State may intervene, charging "corruption", to make it less easy for families to assist each other in achieving such appointments. Eventually, too, wives will be more likely to question husbands for spending money on their brothers' education while their children or household are in need. Certainly, the economic calculus of fertility is already changing. Whilst only six per cent of farming families agreed that "children use up wealth", 25% of white-collar workers in the larger urban areas did so.

None of our Nigerian or Ghanaian research has ever detected much evidence of cultural lags in the sense of behaviour that is irrational in terms of the contemporary social and economic ends of the society but was rational in terms of the ends of an earlier time. What is clear is that there is no economic behaviour distinct from social ends. Rational economic behaviour exists only in terms of the structure of the society. Even by *Western* economic reasoning Yoruba behaviour and fertility is rational given certain aspects of the society: an extended family in both emotional and financial terms; a system of mutual help which assumes very substantial assistance by adult, and even married, children to parents whether the latter are still working and in good health or not; a condition where very substantial residential and educational change is still both possible and probable so that the differentials between generations in rural–urban residence and educational qualifications are great and where such differentials are reflected in parallel income differentials; the retention of a loyalty to a traditional home town where esteem and security are still important and can still be obtained to some extent by expenditure; and a respect, at least in this centre, for leisure and, even more, for ceremony as an alternative to plaudits being given solely for achievement in occupational advance and expenditure on personal ends (as distinct from expenditure on community activities).

Certainly, this system will change but not because most of its aspects are incompatible with economic modernization and industrialization—clearly in contemporary Lagos they are not. It will change because educational and literacy levels are rising and because the message being absorbed from the media and school lessons points the way to a different society. If there are thresholds for demographic transition they are likely to be levels of education, literacy, urbanization or occupation which, with a certain level of exposure to an imported culture, hasten familial change and lead to a different economic calculus with regard to fertility. The time it takes to bring about familial change will depend very much on the original nature of the family and the rate at which the new culture is being imported. It seems unlikely, therefore, that such threshold measures can be related directly to fertility change; any appearance of this will probably be accidental in view of the lag necessary for decisive family change—the real threshold will have occurred earlier and the threshold values implying the inevitability of change will have been lower than the analysis suggested. Certainly, relating such threshold values to those of the *Western* transition, which started with lower fertility and a different family structure, will be unwise. It may yet be proved that family and social changes were a prelude to the increasing postponement of marriage and the presumable downward drift in fertility paralleling it in Europe of the late middle ages. Indeed, change in European family relationships may have been a continuing phenomenon—may, indeed, still be occurring in terms of conjugal relationships—and such change may explain different periods of fertility decline.

The Yoruba evidence would suggest that fertility decline is a product primarily of social rather than of economic change and that the economic rationality of high fertility depends largely on social relationships and the economic behaviour expected in such relationships.

C

The Construction of
a Theory

4

Toward a restatement of demographic transition theory

Our interpretation of past population movements and our expectations about future trends rest primarily on a body of observations and explanations known as "demographic transition theory." The conventional wisdom of this theory has had a deep impact and guides the work programmes of international organizations, technical assistance decisions by governments, and popular analyses in the media.

The theory has changed little in the last 20 years. Indeed the period has seen a plethora of analyses of differentials in fertility, especially those found in contemporary American society, which have tended to obscure the all-important distinction between the origins of fertility decline and the subsequent demographic history of societies experiencing such decline.[1] This failure to update the theory is curious because the last two decades have provided researchers with far more experience of pretransitional and early transitional societies than they had previously been able to obtain.

It is also unfortunate because it has led to unnecessary misunderstandings, misinterpretations and frustrations. It will be argued here that an inadequate understanding of the way in which birth levels first begin to fall has led both to premature gloom about the success of family planning programmes and unnecessary hysteria about the likely long-term size of the human race, as well as to antagonisms at such forums as the Bucharest World Population Conference between countries at different stages of demographic transition.

Development and Testing of the Theory

The thrust of this chapter is that there are only two types of fertility regime, with the exception of the situation at the time of transition: one where there is

---

[1] See Leibenstein (1974), 457–479 for a survey of primarily economic theory that brings out the lack of concern of that theory with the onset of fertility decline.

no economic gain to individuals from restricting fertility; and the second where there is often or eventually economic gain from such restriction. In both situations behaviour is not only rational but economically rational. Another corollary is that there is not a whole range of economically rational levels of fertility in different societies, but instead only two situations, the first where the economically rational response is an indefinitely large number of children and the second where it is to be childless. It is admitted that in many societies at different times there is not a steep economic gradient between different levels of fertility; however, maximum and minimum family sizes in these societies are determined by personal, social, and physiological reasons, not economic ones. Further, it will be posited that the movement from a society characterized by economically unrestricted fertility to a society characterized by economically restricted fertility is essentially the product of social, rather than economic, change, although with economic implications. It will also be argued that the forces sustaining economically unrestricted fertility are frequently strengthened by economic modernization unaccompanied by specific types of social change and that this is the explanation for sustained high fertility in a situation in which "modernization"—urbanization, increase in the proportion of nonagricultural production, and so on—is demonstrably occurring. The social revolution—one of familial relationships and particularly of the direction of intrafamilial flows of wealth dictated by familial obligations—need not by its nature accompany economic modernization. However, it almost inevitably will occur either simultaneously with, or to a considerable degree preceding and perhaps hastening, economic modernization in the contemporary world. This is due largely to the phenomenon of Westernization, an essentially social process with a range of mechanisms for its spread (which have depended on economic advance in the West and to a more limited extent elsewhere, but which have not been dictated or formed by economic growth).[2]

The discussion will cover three types of society: (1) primitive society where food gatherers, nomadic pastoralists or agriculturalists live in largely self-sufficient communities feeling little or no impact from a national state or a world religion; (2) traditional societies, predominantly agrarian, where the apparatus of a state government or the attitudes, and often the structure, of an organized religion make an impact on both community and individuals, especially in giving guarantee of safety or assistance; (3) transitional societies where rapid change in way of life towards that followed

[2] Although many European countries remained in a state of transition for a long period, such conditions are not likely to recur, partly because of the existence of mass schooling. In contemporary transitional societies, families tend to be clearly in one fertility situation or the other, and hence fertility differentials appear; even whole societies are likely to move rather rapidly through the transition as the social and economic calculus changes.

by people in lands with a "modern" economy usually in recent times has been catalysed by outside contacts. It will be maintained that, at least in the contemporary world, the supports for unlimited fertility finally crumble in the transitional society, and that the analysis of this crumbling and of its preconditions is largely unrelated to the analysis of the frequently slow and sometimes vicissitudinous reduction in family size that subsequently occurs in transitional and modern societies. Much of the argument draws primarily on African examples, both because of my experience in Africa, and because all three types of society are well represented on the continent.

Demographic Transition Theory

By the end of the nineteenth century it was common knowledge that fertility levels were falling in many Western countries and there was a presumption that birth rates would stabilize at lower levels (although there was no agreement about what the new levels would mean in terms of natural increase). An attempt was made by Warren Thompson[3] (1929) to divide this transition into three phases and by C. P. Blacker[4] (1947) to distinguish five phases. Neither could be said to be the father of demographic transition theory in that neither suggested an explanation for fertility change.

Modern demographic transition theory was born almost in mature form in a paper written by Frank Notestein in 1945. Notestein offered a twofold explanation for why fertility had begun to decline. Fertility in premodern countries had been kept, if not artificially high, then high only by the maintenance of a whole series of props: "religious doctrines, moral codes, laws, education, community customs, marriage habits and family organizations . . . all focused towards maintaining high fertility" (p. 39). High fertility was necessary for survival because otherwise the very high mortality rate would have led to population decline and extinction. But eventually in country after country mortality began to decline, and the props were no longer needed or were not needed at their original strength. One could leave the explanation here and argue that the props would inevitably wither, as social adjustments were made in response to other changes. However, Notestein put forward the view that, in the West at least, more positive forces (arising out of the same process of modernization that had brought the death rates down) were at work destroying the props. Fundamental was "the growth of huge and mobile city populations," which tended to dissolve the largely corporate, family based way of life of traditional society,

[3] In his 1946 publication, Thompson largely supported the view put forward by Notestein in 1945.

[4] The term "demographic transition" is first employed on p. 41 of this article, after reference has been made to "demographic evolution" and "transitional growth."

replacing it with individualism marked above all by growing personal aspirations. Large families became

"a progressively difficult undertaking; expensive and difficult for a population increasingly freed from older taboos and increasingly willing to solve its problems rather than accept them." (1945, pp. 40–41).

Again in 1953 Notestein pointed to the "urban industrial society" as the crucible of demographic transition and stated, "It is difficult to avoid the conclusion that the development of technology lies at the root of the matter." Once again he placed emphasis on the erosion of the traditional family, "particularly the extended family," and on the growth of individualism, but he also drew attention to other important social movements: "the development of a rational and secular point of view; the growing awareness of the world and modern techniques through popular education; improved health; and the appearance of alternatives to early marriage and childbearing as a means of livelihood and prestige for women." However, this time the description of pretransitional society was not drawn largely from the experience of the West but was generalized to include the developing world:

"The economic organization of relatively self-sufficient agrarian communities turns almost wholly upon the family, and the perpetuation of the family is the main guarantee of support and elemental security. When death rates are high the individual's life is relatively insecure and unimportant. The individual's status in life tends to be that to which he was born. There is, therefore, rather little striving for advancement. Education is brief, and children begin their economic contributions early in life. In such societies, moreover, there is scant opportunity for women to achieve either economic support or personal prestige outside the roles of wife and mother, and women's economic functions are organized in ways that are compatible with continuous childbearing" pp. 15–18).

The mainstream arguments of the theory are that fertility is high in poor, traditional societies because of high mortality, the lack of opportunities for individual advancement, and the economic value of children. All these things change with modernization or urban industrialism, and individuals, once their viewpoints become reoriented to the changes that have taken place, can make use of the new opportunities.[5]

The argument appears at first clear and convincing, but it has elements and implications that are more complex or debatable and that have had an enormous effect on our way of looking at demographic change. The most fundamental issue is whether the theory actually deals with reactions and accommodations to material circumstances. There is a persistent strain in

[5] Some social scientists emphasized isolated parts of the argument: Stycos (1964) emphasized the possibility of advancement in life. Ogburn and Nimkoff (1955) stressed the great departure in the city from rural household economy. And Carlsson (1966) wrote of the new life style of the urban industrial society and the export of that style. Others, notably Hauser and Duncan (1959), p. 94, complained that too many explanations had been given, and that some of the supposed causes were material changes, while others were ones of ideas.

demographic transition theory writings that claims that rationality comes only with industrial, urban society, and a related strain that regards traditional agrarian societies as essentially brutish and superstitious. This arises in two distinct ways.

The first is from the references to pre-demographic-transition society. The concept of the brutishness of the poor, and their inability and unwillingness to help themselves, is a fundamental proposition of Malthus. But the origin of the view in modern demographic transition theory is the argument that, in spite of the high mortality, insecurity, and lack of cost of children in pre-demographic-transition societies, all kinds of religious and social institutions and preserves were needed to keep fertility high. This is why demographic transition literature is full of references not to the behaviour or reactions of such people but to *attitudes*, *beliefs*, *traditions*, and *irrationality*. Kingsley Davis wrote of the contrast between traditional societies and "the growing rationalism of modern life" (1949, pp. 599–600) and, again, describing sex and reproduction in the former, that "towards this aspect of life the woman has mainly a nonrational approach—religious, superstitious and incurious" (1955, p. 37); George Stolnitz described "a shift in attitudes from the traditional fatalism of peasant societies" (1964, pp. 33–34); Eva Mueller observed that, "it is difficult to influence deep-seated attitudes" (1972, p. 383); William Rich believed that "large-scale fertility declines cannot be expected until the living conditions of the majority of the population improve enough so that they no longer *consider* large families necessary for economic reasons" (1973, p. 2)[6]; Stephen Enke deduced that, "many simple peoples understand very little about why reproduction occurs and how it can be prevented" (1966, p. 54); Michael Endres has written recently, "people directed by tradition resist rational intervention and choice between behavioral patterns," and "to urge upon a traditional people a rational technical means of birth control is to challenge the tenacious hold of a hard-won culture to which choice and change are the enemy" (1975, p. 74); while G. T. Trewartha indicted the irrationality of premodern society for causing not only high fertility but also maldistribution of settlement: "Indeed, much of the distribution does not appear to be particularly rational . . . Tradition, which is unusually strong among the tribal peoples of Negro Africa, plays a more than ordinary role" (1972, pp. 182–183).

The second respect in which an implicit assumption of pretransition irrationality enters into the theory is through references to cultural lags in making fertility adjustments to the arrival of the new urban, industrial conditions. Such references are plausible in a way because a period of change is under consideration instead of an extended stable situation.

[6] Emphasis added.

Several of the quotations above do refer also to such lags, but the concept is both implicit and explicit in Notestein's 1945 paper. There he argued that the supports for high fertility "change only gradually and in response to the strongest stimulation" and described "a population increasingly freed from older taboos and increasingly willing to solve its problems rather than accept them," (pp. 39–41).

That the central tradition of demographic transition theory is still very much that of Notestein's 1945 and 1953 formulations and that the belief in increasing rationality with modernization is still an integral element has been demonstrated vividly by the publication of the most recent United Nations *Population Studies*, which justifies the latest United Nations population projections. The argument is worth quoting at some length:

"The entire process of economic and social development . . . itself changes people's outlooks from traditions and fatalism towards modern concepts and rationalism. . . . The past record in the more developed countries demonstrates . . . that it (fertility decline) can . . . be expected to occur in the normal course of the modern development process . . . the deliberate regulation of fertility defies age-old custom . . . A high frequency of childbirth . . . was necessary for the continuation and security of families and this found emphatically strong support in the prevailing values and customs. In many cultures it has also been considered that children provide a much needed insurance against destitution in old age. Associated with such cultural norms has been the regard for women in their seemingly principal function as bearers and rearers of children, limiting thereby their participation in economic and social roles held to be mainly the prerogative of men. Interwoven with such attitudes there can also be a fatalistic refusal, or even an abhorrence, to contemplate any regulatory interference with the reproductive process. It is not to be wondered at that such a traditional outlook on life can be highly resistant to change. But as shown by the earlier experience of the more developed regions . . . change is possible or eventually to be expected" (1974a, pp. 2, 17 and 14).

Much of the argument for demographic transition concepts as they are now widely held turns on the definition of rational. The term "economically rational" is frequently substituted so as to avoid having to judge "social rationality" with the possibility of having to agree that a certain mode of behaviour was rational in a given setting in that it met the ends of religious beliefs or of community obligations. Even so, the criteria employed are highly ethnocentric and are laden with Western values. It is assumed that it is rational for a man or a couple to maximize the expenditure on the individuals in his or their nuclear family; but there are any number of non-Western societies in which there is greater pleasure in spending on some relatives outside the nuclear family (adult brothers for instance) than on some within it, and in which children are happier to spend on parents than are parents on children. Obviously the fundamental choices are social ones and economic behaviour is rational only insofar as it is rational within the framework established by social ends. What demographic transition theory has always regarded as rational are primarily Western social ends with economically logical steps to maximize satisfactions given those ends.

The underlying assumption of this study is that all societies are economically rational. The point is a simple one, but its acceptance is absolutely necessary if we are to arrive at an adequate theory of demographic transition, if we are to understand the contemporary population changes, and if we are going to make adequate predictions for planning purposes. It is, in fact, difficult to have a rigorous analysis on any other assumption. Social ends differ but can be largely explained on a rational basis—usually even in economic terms. Furthermore, change in social ends can often be observed, measured, explained, and predicted. The view that the fertility behaviour of the Third World arises largely from ignorance and should be combatted with education and guidance is held strongly by many family-planning movements and leads to friction and even confrontation; the same reaction arising out of much the same origins was witnessed writ a little larger at the Bucharest Conference. Indeed the view that peasants are usually mistaken in evaluating the effect of their fertility on their own economic well-being has recently been seriously argued in a paper by Mueller (1976).

A second implication of demographic transition theory, at least as originally conceived by Notestein, is that industrialization and concomitant urbanization are preconditions to development. Notestein placed stress on "urban industrial living" (in 1945) and later on "urban industrial society" (in 1953), as the context in which the social changes leading to fertility decline occur. Similarly Thompson (in 1946) referred to "industrialization" as the necessary condition. In the last 20 years such terms have largely been replaced by "modernization" or near synonyms like "the modern development process" as it became clear that great numbers of people in the Third World were unlikely to be living in industrial cities for generations. The demographic transition theory did allow for the possibility that the new way of life and the consequent new fertility behaviour might be generated in the urban industrial setting and then be exported to nonurban and nonindustrial populations either by exporting some of its institutions (such as schools, women's rights legislation or a full market economy) or by simply exporting its attitudes or ideas. This tenet received historical support from the decline in fertility among rural populations in the West. The theory did not specify whether the urban industrial melting pot from which the changes were derived had to be in the same society or whether a global economy and society was beginning to operate that could export the necessary ideas and institutions from the economically developed countries to the commercial cities of Asia and Africa and on to the rural hinterlands. (Demonstrably this has long been happening with regard to governmental institutions and more recently in terms of schools and political ideology.) In any case the link with the emphasis on the props for high fertility is clear. If high fertility in developing countries were a wholly rational response to economic circumstances, then the small family pattern could never be exported; but, if the large family were to a considerable extent the product of beliefs and attitudes sustained largely by religion and shibboleth in order to compete with high mortality rather than to meet the needs of the economic system, then export was quite possible. Those who doubted the validity of a theory based only on the transmission of ideas but who were prepared to accept the possibility that the spread of small families could be achieved by the spread of institutions made little progress in identifying those institutions that were minimally necessary for fertility transition—schools? nonagricultural employment?

A third problem lurked in demographic transition theory but was not specifically identified. Was it primarily modernization that was being exported? Is there a specific form of social modernization that is a necessary adjunct to economic modernization? Or is the export Westernization, which by historical accident has been tailored to fit the world's first economic modernization and which is easily exportable partly because of the West's economic strength (clearly visible in its earlier ability to colonize) and partly because this tailoring makes it easily adaptable to modernizing economies? Notestein wrestled with problem areas in his 1953 paper and the whole question of Westernization almost arose: why had fertility fallen steeply between World Wars I and II in almost wholly agricultural Bulgaria while failing to do so during the 1950s in the larger urban areas of Egypt and the Far East? (pp. 17–18).

Suggested Modifications to the Theory

Without actually saying as much, Davis argued in 1955 and again, with Judith Blake, in 1956 that the props were not needed. High fertility was a perfectly rational response to socioeconomic conditions in a traditional agrarian society: the extended family means that the cost and care of children are shared; children, once past infancy, may in fact pay for their costs, especially in conditions of cottage industry, but more generally in any farming situation; both husbands' and wives' families of origin may help establish the newly married couple, often on a farm of their own; large families may bring economic strength through political strength in the local decision-making organizations.[7]

---

[7] The relationship of fertility to kinship was stressed a year earlier by Lorimer, but he retained the religious and cultural props (See Lorimer, 1954).

Recently this aspect of the demographic transition debate has been summarized and evaluated by Thomas Burch and Murray Gendell (1971), who demonstrated that research findings from India and Taiwan fail to show the predicted fertility contrasts between families residing as nuclear families and those living together in larger agglomerations of relatives. The point is an important one, and, in order to clear the way for the subsequent argument in this paper, should be dealt with here. The research in India and Taiwan is almost certainly irrelevant for three reasons, of which the second is most important. The first is that survey or census data do not accurately measure even residential family size. The building materials, mud and stone in contrast to bamboo and thatch for instance, often determine whether considerable numbers of people can be housed in a single structure or alternatively in several smaller structures adjacent or close by. The second (a point to be elaborated later) is that family residence arrangements have little or nothing to do with the true extended family of mutual obligations, at least as long as residence outside the traditional community is not specified. It is the size and ramifications of this family of obligations that may well help to determine fertility. The third is that family residential patterns are often a function of the life cycle; in some societies nuclear residence is most likely to be found immediately after husband and wife (often with children of their own by this time) first move away from their parents to a farm or business of their own. What demographers should really be interested in are the families of this type who are unlikely to subsequently attract or retain many other relatives (except perhaps aged parents or nephews and nieces undergoing education) often because they have moved to a city or have been fairly highly educated and so have opted for a different way of life from their relatives.

Family sociologists added some riders to the picture. William Goode decided that the nuclear family's fundamental demographic characteristic was not that it leaned toward small size but that it was more flexible than the extended family in reacting to economic conditions favouring high or low fertility; thus at much the same time (eighteenth and early nineteenth centuries) European populations had chosen high fertility in frontier North America and moderate fertility in their homelands in Europe (1963b, p. 240).[8] This had, of course, been a major contention of Malthus. Some, Colin Clark, for example, went further and identified nuclear families with advanced economies and extended families with nonindustrial societies—probably, as will be argued later, a fundamental mistake at least in terms of European history (1967, pp. 186–187).[9] Another attack on the props came from David Heer and Dean Smith

[8] It is possible to argue, at least in the Australian context, that they opted not for high fertility but for early female marriage in frontier conditions where women were scarce, but had an important role to play and that high fertility was the unplanned consequence (Ruzicka and Caldwell, 1977).

[9] It is true, however, that some preindustrial peoples appear to have a family structure nucleated not only in residence, but in closeness of relationships; but nevertheless they shared food and animal skins for clothing on a basis going beyond even distant relatives at the same camp. See Graburn (1971), pp. 107–111. For the argument that the true extended family is largely a product of agrarian societies, see Blumberg and Winch (1972).

(1967) who argued that the props had at every stage been wholly rational because of high mortality and had withered as the death rates fell.

Recent Ideas

An important contribution in the 1950s was that of the economists, especially Ansley Coale and Edgar Hoover in 1958 with a major analysis of India, together with Mexico. What is apt to be overlooked is that Coale and Hoover accepted as their starting point the existing demographic transition theory (1958, pp. 11–12)[10], and that most of the subsequent economic analysis is independent of theories about when and if fertility is likely to fall. Coale and Hoover spelled out the economic implications of transition theory but they did not test its basic assumptions. Their analyses were essentially those of macroscopic data, and their main conclusion was that national economic growth is impaired if fertility levels too greatly exceed mortality levels. However, most nonspecialists received the message that they had shown convincingly that high fertility is economically disadvantageous for every size of population unit, and the view that high-fertility agrarian families were behaving irrationally was given a powerful boost.

It is possible to extrapolate part of the argument from national populations to individual families: to suggest that lower fertility will produce a family age structure with a higher ratio of potential adult producers to child consumers than will high fertility and that fewer children will allow mothers to participate more in economic activity (Freedman, with Mueller, 1974, pp. 7–8). For reasons analysed below all these arguments ring somewhat hollowly in an actual agrarian society: children work at young ages; often the peasant's analysis is dynamic in contrast to the demographer's static one in that the peasant is thinking less of the present and more of safeguarding the future; and, in many societies, the peasant's wife already works long hours (freed from minding the product of her recent fertility by the child care being practiced by the product of her earlier fertility).

Two years before Coale and Hoover's study appeared, R. Nelson had produced his "low-level equilibrium trap model" (1956). Subsequently Harvey Liebenstein made the model more specifically demographic, suggesting that in "backward areas" people are merely caught by circumstances: they lack the inducement to save or invest and are unlikely to make quantum jumps in technology; as a result, per capita income remains static, mortality does not decline, and, hence, population does not grow (1957, pp. 170–173). The model does imply at least short-term rationality, although it could also be taken to mean that the society as a whole was incapable of planning its course to a better future. A more important limitation is that the model seems to have no real significance for social

[10] Their summary is essentially based on Notestein (1953).

theory (except for historical studies) in a world where societies are no longer isolated from each other and where imported health technology means that population is growing increasingly fast, even in many societies with largely subsistence economies.

In 1974 Julian Simon summarized and assessed much of the research evidence available on fertility and stage of economic development, concluding that "fertility is everywhere subject to much rational control." He largely avoided the question of why—within this framework of rational decision—fertility decline sets in, contenting himself with pragmatically observing that "we may rely on the fact that, as education rises, fertility will fall" and that "if one wishes to reduce fertility, one should think about raising educational levels as well as aiding birth control" (p. 130 and 163–164).

Since the 1950s, sociologists have contributed powerfully—not always intentionally—to the thesis of irrationality by apparently showing a substantial gap between desired and achieved fertility in the Third World (together with a smaller gap in developed economies). The origin of this formulation dated from the beginning of fertility studies, when the Indianapolis Survey of 1941 asked American respondents what they considered the ideal family size. The concept of "norms" had been one of the basic planks of modern sociology, and in the early 1960s Ronald Freedman applied it to fertility studies in a way that seemed to have implications not only for behavioural rationality but for behavioural economic rationality: "family size norms will tend to correspond to a number which maximizes the net utility to be derived from having children in the society or stratum." In developing countries, he concluded, "there may be a delicate balance of pressures towards higher fertility to ensure at least a certain minimum number of children and counter pressures to minimize or eliminate an intolerable surplus of children under difficult subsistence conditions" (1961–62, pp. 40 and 48).

During the mid 1960s, knowledge, attitude, and practice (KAP) surveys were used to measure desired or "ideal family size" in the developing world using questions about the "best" or "ideal" number of children or the family size that would be desired if the respondent were to start her reproductive history all over again. Comparisons made in 1965 between "desired" and "actual" fertility promoted W. Parker Mauldin to state, "although it is not yet true that people in the developing areas share the small family ideal, it is true that most of them no longer want very large families" (1965, p. 6), and Bernard Berelson to calculate that, while ideal family size in the United States was 97% of the achieved size, it ranged in a number of developing countries between 60 and 92% (1966, p. 658).

The whole question of ideal family size is of the utmost importance for the discussion of demographic transition theory in this paper. It is not necessary to regard the gap between ideal and achieved size as evidence of irrational behaviour; indeed Berelson regarded it as arising from "lack of information, services and supplies" and this was the most common position taken during the 1960s by technical aid organizations in the family planning field. Indeed the significant gap—that created by the props, according to demographic transition theory—is essentially that between the family size which would be dictated by economically rational behaviour and ideal family size. In fact there is little relationship between the demographic transition concern with the attainment of economic rationality and the KAP study attention to ideal family size; KAP studies essentially attempt to measure potential consumer demand, and in this they ignore the issue of rationality except to the extent that it seems reasonable for a person to do what he wants to do. Some researchers appear to take it for granted, however, that a movement in ideals is almost inevitably a movement toward rationality and, hence, evidence of the decay of the props.

There are three fundamental questions. The first is whether there are "norms" at all in the high-fertility situation. It will be argued here that economically there is no ceiling in primitive and traditional societies to the number of children who would be economically beneficial; the actual number is kept down because physiological and social problems arise from too frequent childbirth and the failure to cease childbearing at a certain stage. Achieved fertility is a product of this conflict and can hardly be described as approximating a norm.[11]

The second question is whether fertility behaviour must be regarded as mainly economically motivated, or whether social motivations are also important or even dominant—whether norms, if they exist, and fertility behaviour can be taken as an approximate measure of the individual's reaction to economic circumstances. Simon argues that fertility can be taken to be primarily economically motivated and justifies "an important omission [from his study] . . . , social norms and values. The reason . . . is that in the context of long-run analysis, culture and values do *not* have independent lives of their own." (1974, p. 105).[12] This, it will be noted, is a direct assault

[11] This view is also at odds with Lorimer's attempt to produce a more sophisticated interpretation of fertility levels, kind of "plural society" way of looking at the world, when he argued that there is not a simple contrast between the low fertility of developed countries and the high fertility of developing countries but that the latter exhibit a wide range of fertility levels reflecting their social and economic structures and presumably their norms. See Lorimer (1954). Carr-Saunders had earlier argued that societies might be able to sustain different levels of fertility and that "the evidence . . . shows that the mechanism whereby numbers may be kept near to the desirable level is everywhere present" (1922), p. 230.

[12] He buttresses this by deciding that fertility behaviour is rational, largely on the basis of the Princeton Office of Population Research demonstration that fertility is nearly everywhere substantially lower than it would be if presumably largely uncontrolled Hutterite fertility behaviour were prevalent (see, e.g., p. 11).

on the props. The proposition differs from that put forward in this paper in that the argument here is that fertility is economically rational only between certain limits that are set by noneconomic factors; that there are two types of society, one in which it is economically rational for fertility to be even lower, but in which a floor is interposed by noneconomic considerations, and the other, in which it is rational for it to be ever higher, restrained only by a noneconomic ceiling.

The third question is whether fertility can be used as a measure of desired behaviour. The apparent demonstration by the KAP surveys that there is a wide gulf between what Third World people want to do and what they succeed in doing introduced a large element of chance (and not random chance at that) into the whole matter. It is perhaps impossible to study the motivation behind fertility decline if the populations of the Third World habitually exhibit fertility well above what both economic rationality and the attitudes moulded by the props dictate. I suggest that this apparent gap is partly the product of the present unusual circumstances, but largely an artifact of the method of investigation. Change is at present so rapid in many societies that there is a fast increase in the number of people who will economically benefit from lower fertility. However, the "ideal family" questions ultimately fail to measure likely fertility behaviour even under conditions of adequate access to contraception because they are imported almost undigested from Western society and contain a range of assumptions about non-Western societies that will not bear up under examination. The fundamental problem is the questioning of a woman about the "best" number of children, as if the chief cultural thrust were optimization of family size instead of a range of other concerns such as meeting the expectations of husband and other relatives, conforming with peer group behaviour, and so on. In many surveys most respondents probably do not fully understand the question. They know what the words mean, but they also know that they are being asked to define "best" in a modernizing sense by interviewers (and, behind them, some institution) who interpret "best" in a futuristic sense or in the sense of the elites. The "politeness response" is only a small part of the reaction (Jones, 1963). The "ideal family" question was shaped by Western, middle-class researchers, living in conjugal families in which husbands and wives consult each other over matters of reproduction and sex, and it achieves its greatest reliability among such people. In this chapter it will be taken that achieved fertility everywhere comes close to being a rational response to the circumstances of the society.

In 1965 the publication of a United Nations study directed the attention of researchers to the prime importance of the changing conditions that lead to fertility decline at a point identified as the "threshold." The analysis distinguished six levels of fertility, in what was essentially a cross-sectional and not an historical analysis, but for further analysis combined the levels into two groups, one in which relatively low fertility had been achieved and the other in which it had not. Every Asian and African population, except Japan, was in the high-fertility group, while, with the exception of Albania, every European population in Europe, North America, and Oceania was in the low-fertility group. In Latin America, only Argentina and Uruguay were among the low-fertility countries. The United Nations recognized that it was "perhaps no coincidence that most of the countries where fertility is low . . . are in Europe and European-settled regions," concluding that "fertility levels might . . . be due . . . at least partly to culturally determined circumstances affecting the interactions between fertility and economic and social changes" (p. 143). This dichotomy had the disadvantage that the nations identified as being beyond the threshold had in many cases passed it long ago; and neither the nature of the actual threshold nor the changes sufficient to ensure movement across it were actually detected.[13]

Other attempts to apply or develop threshold analysis have been made. Etienne van de Walle and John Knodel failed to find it a usable tool when analysing fertility decline in France and Germany (1967). Dudley Kirk proclaimed the value of such an approach in 1971, and in 1975, together with Frank Oechsli, applied it to Latin America, calculating a "Development Index" and relating it to declines in both mortality and fertility. But Oechsli and Kirk's data unmistakably evidence a cultural dichotomy: most of the countries with reduced fertility either are areas of almost purely European settlement in the extreme south or are Caribbean Islands with very mixed cultures and population origins. Island nations have been conspicuous in recent fertility declines, and the United Nations has identified ten and attempted to explain the change in terms of their small size and hence the easy penetration of ideas and health measures (1974a). Yet seven of the island nations were settled entirely by immigrant populations while under European control: Réunion, Jamaica, Mauritius, Trinidad and Tobago, Guadeloupe, Martinique and Puerto Rico; one has been entirely Christian-ized: American Samoa; one is a mixture of an immigrant and a fully Christianized indigenous one: Fiji; and one has achieved universal Western-style education: Sri Lanka.

In contrast to the approach of the thresholders, there has recently been renewed interest in the innovational explanation. (In the late nineteenth and early twentieth centuries, governments and other institutions almost

[13] Among Western European countries, the first declines in fertility paralleled the beginning of marriage postponement perhaps as early as the seventeenth century (see Hajnal, 1965) and even the restriction of fertility within marriage began a century ago. Therefore, at the threshold itself, many of the post-threshold societies identified in the study exhibited different index values (a range of socioeconomic and demographic indices was calculated) than their current ones—most, indeed, were then within the range of the contemporary pre-threshold societies. (This assumes that the UN studies mean the threshold to be between Groups 3 and 4. There is some tendency to alternate between the concept of a threshold and that of a continuum.)

invariably explained fertility control innovationally, as the spread of pernicious ideas.) Much of this has arisen from the Princeton Office of Population Research European fertility project and its demonstration that fertility declines spread fairly rapidly through linguistic or religious units only to be halted at their borders (Coale, 1973, pp. 62–63).

The threshold and innovational approaches share a common problem in explaining the onset of fertility decline. Their data are usually for considerable aggregates of population, and, hence, it is difficult to determine whether the measured drop in fertility is attributable to a single socioeconomic group or not. If it is, then the threshold explanation holds up (provided that the threshold indices are meant to apply to subsections of a society), but the spread of innovation is shown to have an impact only on groups that have already reached some potential state of receptivity as measured by socioeconomic indices and not by attitudinal changes; if it is not, then the threshold indices can be discarded as measures of the sufficient conditions that must be met for demographic change to occur. In any case both approaches have failed as yet to specify the kinds of changes necessary for individuals or couples to alter their fertility behaviour and why such alterations take place.

Attempts have of course been made to investigate these changes around the beginning of transition, the most ambitious to date for developing countries being the East–West Population Institute's Value of Children Study.[14] So far the published national reports (on the Philippines and Hawaii) have had a strong social psychological orientation toward beliefs and values—stronger even than the questionnaires upon which they are based. The approach is clearly an aspect of innovational theory and has a good deal in common with explanations that rely heavily on the props; and, although it does not spell it out, the Philippines report could be described as an analysis of the import and diffusion of nonindigenous cultural values. So far, the project had insufficiently investigated the changing material aspects of life and the extent to which changing values could be said to be rationally moving parallel to economic realities.

New Experience

Increasingly massive family planning programmes in Asia and parts of Africa, Latin America and Oceania over the last quarter of a century have presented an enormous increase in opportunities to watch and measure fertility transition and to identify the innovators. This should have allowed

[14] The only two national survey reports published at the time of writing were Bulatao (1975) and Arnold and Fawcett (1975). The emphasis on a psychological approach is set out in Arnold et al. (1975), pp. 5–6. The report on the orginal workshop is also available but it is more economically oriented than the subsequent project (Fawcett, 1972). There have been separate Value of Children projects, such as the survey carried out as part of the 1973 Nigerian segment of the Changing African Family Project to be described later in this paper.

demographic transition theory to be rewritten with the sureness that arises from large-scale field experiments. This has not happened, and one of the keys to the whole problem may be why it has not happened.

An important reason is undoubtedly described by the well-known precept in other areas of endeavour: applied science has increasingly limited returns, unless based on continuing fundamental research. Too much of the research has taken as its starting point and framework the preexisting conclusions of demographic transition theory. Too many frustrated family planning fieldworkers and administrators have been only too willing to blame the props for the failure to achieve programme targets. Most indigenous and all expatriate administrators and advisors are in circumstances in which they economically benefit from controlling their own fertility, and they find it hard to understand why this should not be so for everyone else—irrationality is an easy answer especially when it can be demonstrated that education and demand for the family planning services are highly positively correlated. Probably too much of the research has been programme-based instead of concentrating on the mechanisms of change in the society as a whole. Yet this is not the whole explanation. The operational research has permitted the identification of large numbers of innovators— at least in terms of using contraception, if not always in terms of deciding to restrict family size—but research has not clearly established the basic changes that have affected these people. On the face of it this seems hard to believe, and yet it is true for a number of reasons. One (as will be seen below) is that the innovators do not really know themselves; they differ in various ways from their parents and these differences make fertility control rational, but they usually cannot identify the essential differences. Another reason for the failure to identify preconditions is that comparison of the characteristics of family planning acceptors and nonacceptors shows that the former are much more likely to exhibit not merely one "modern" characteristic but a whole interrelated set (more education, nonagricultural employment, higher incomes, and so on), so that there is a chicken-and-egg problem. There has also been a research failure: failure to investigate in detail the way of life and circumstances of individual acceptors parallel to similar studies of the population as a whole.

In relation to the last point it might be noted that there has been over the last half century a considerable advance in economic anthropology, which has been almost entirely ignored by demographers.[15] Fierce debate has

[15] The origins of economic anthropology lie, appropriately for the demographic transition theorist, in premodern European history and economic history, but its genesis as a separate field is to be found in German ethnographic studies of the second half of the nineteenth and the first quarter of the twentieth centuries and French studies of the 1920s. In English a literature also began to develop from the 1920s with the work of Malinowski and Firth, leading to the attempt by Herskovits at the end of the 1930s to compile and synthesize what was known. Controversy and new studies have found a renewed vitality in recent years. For a good review of the field, see Firth (1967), with references to the syntheses of Wilhelm Koppers in 1915–16 and Max Schmidt in 1920–21 and the later work by Richard Thurnwald. And on more recent studies, see also, for instance, Dalton (1971), Sahlins (1972) and Epstein (1967).

raged in economic anthropology between the Formalists and the Substantivists, the former claiming that Western economic analysis can be applied unchanged to all economic life and the latter maintaining that economics serves social ends and that every culture has its own economic theory. The Formalists narrowly define the subject of modern economics as allocation of scarce resources between either unlimited or numerous ends, while the Substantivists contend that rational economic behaviour is rational only within a given social context and that these contexts are diverse and often startlingly different from those of the modern West. The Substantivists have also established that, even where money and market exist, these may embrace only part of a society, and, more importantly, only part of the life of much of the population. The rest of the society, and perhaps the bulk of the life of most of its citizens, falls in the more traditional sector, where it is not rational, and usually not possible, to act out the life of market-economy man. The implications for demographic transition theory are that transition is made possible only by profound changes in the social structures of such societies, and that analyses of the economic rationality of high fertility reach different conclusions in different social structures.

Fundamental Problems of Research

Part of the failure to advance demographic transition theory can undoubtedly be blamed on inadequate research. The basic problem has not been inadequate methodology but rather poor application, especially of methods in cultures other than those for which they were developed. The problems will only be summarized here as they have been treated more adequately elsewhere. The general failing, and one that encompasses the others, has been ethnocentricity. Too much research has been done too quickly and on too large a scale with research instruments, and often researchers, brought directly from contemporary Western society. Too often, the representatives of the non-Western society in the research have been completely inculcated with Western research approaches and conclusions in Western universities. As a result, the research approach often predetermines the range of findings and asks questions that provide the appropriate answers almost by an echo effect.[16] What prevents the researcher from worrying about the extent to

[16] For example, in the Nigerian Segment of the Changing African Family Project, respondents were asked, "If someone offered you a good job for three years, but you could only take it if you put off having a baby for that time, would you be prepared to try to stop having a baby for three years?" Only one-quarter of both women and men replied "No" and that response was not much higher even in remote villages. Very few Nigerians would be offered a good job (defined by most as meaning one in the modern, white-collar sector) and fewer still with a guaranteed period of employment. In practically no case would a woman have to agree not to have a child (and never in the case of men). Should such an extraordinary offer ever be made, of course many might opt for the good job. The fundamental fact about developing economies is that choices of this kind do not exist and, therefore, a question of this kind is not appropriate.

which the pattern of responses fails to represent the society is the magnitude and flow-chart nature of modern social scientific research: the large sample, the hierarchy of command, the precoded questionnaire, the responses as invisible magnetic recordings on a computer tape, computer editing, the computer print-outs of marginals and cross-tabulations that necessarily balance to the last unit, the written report in a predetermined pattern, and finally the cross-cultural international comparison with other research using similar or even identical instruments.

Four pitfalls of current research have particularly contributed to misunderstanding of the nature of demographic transition.

1. The magnitude and direction of wealth (money, goods, services, guarantees) flows and potential flows are areas of research that are often neglected or misunderstood. Such research is difficult. In premodern societies much of the wealth is still outside the monetized economy. Often money-equivalents are not visualized; services usually have an element of obligation; investments in future security may be discounted in the opposite direction to that to which Western economics is accustomed (discussed further below); the details about wealth have often not been disclosed even to immediate relatives (who exert competing demands and from whom details must often be hidden, more to prevent resentment and to allow equity to prevail, than to deprive people of their just deserts); and there is sometimes also a fear about tax officials and other authorities knowing about earnings. In these circumstances, small-scale, painstakingly thorough research is needed by investigators with a thorough knowledge of the society. Hardly any good research has yet been done. There is a temptation to quote inadequate or incomplete research, with highly misleading results. There would be less danger if the errors were random, but, without question, there is a great understatement of all flows of wealth and potential wealth.

2. The "family" of the fertility survey is often an artifact of the survey. Women are asked about their own reactions and their husbands' reactions, and of course, the women answer in these terms. No one describes the role in decision-making of the husbands' and wives' lineages; no one explains that the husband regards his brother as a nearer relation than his wife in the sense of that close inner circle where one no longer regards expenditure as depriving one personally of wealth; no one explains the intricate system of decision-making and obligations that may far exceed the nuclear family or residential group and in which the nuclear family may not even be a recognizable subunit.

3. The nature of family formation and of related decisions in developing countries is frequently misunderstood. Family size decisions are usually out of the respondents' hands for several reasons: both the physiological side of reproduction and the obeying of cultural practices may seem (sensibly enough) to them to be something they cannot control and hence there is an element of fatalism; family size is often the product of decisions taken for family reasons not primarily aimed at determining fertility; and, where there are decisions to be made, they may not be primarily decisions of the "couple". All these factors must be taken into account when interpreting "Up to God" and "Don't know" responses, which may be closer to the truth than the numerical ones. In these circumstances the value of any "ideal family" type of question is debatable, and the employment of the concept of "norms" misleading.

4. While fertility transition research is essentially a study of change, such investigations have been impeded by too much emphasis on modernization. Change can be understood only if emphasis is given to studying the fundamental nature of the society that is being subjected to new forces. Too many survey questions are focused on the modernizing features, and too many of them have a built-in assumption that everyone is reaching for such change. Demographers have been far too rarely concerned with familiarizing themselves with the knowledge other social scientists have already accumulated about the society being examined. Perhaps even more serious is the fact that modernization has been accorded such respect (by all development researches, but specifically by population researchers, in that they regard modernization as being the chief mechanism for reducing fertility and hence eventually containing global population growth) that its components have usually not been analysed and the all-important distinction has not been made between Westernization, which may proceed at a rate unrelated to economic change, and residual modernization, which must go hand in hand with economic change because it is either a necessary condition or a necessary product.

What we obtain from research that is vitiated by these weaknesses is a reflection of the way a poorer version of our own society might be expected to behave if set down in a Third World context. We fail to appreciate significantly different social and economic structures and the extent to which these yield rewards to the highly fertile.

A Society Experiencing Change

The observations in this section are primarily of Nigerian Yoruba society. The Yoruba are the indigenous inhabitants of Nigeria's Western State (recently subdivided into Ogun, Ondo, and Oyo States) and Lagos State, as well as considerable parts of Kwara State in Nigeria and Southern Benin, or Dahomey. The Western and Lagos States are believed to have contained about 8·5 million people in 1962 (Okonjo, 1968) and contain perhaps 13 million now, of whom over 11 million are Yoruba, out of a total of 13 million Yoruba in Nigeria and Benin. The Yoruba of the Western and Lagos States have been the focus of the largest segment of the Changing African Family Project and of the Nigerian Family Study, and many of the data used here are drawn from that study.[17] The area is well suited to this kind of investigation, because a primitive society (as defined here) existed over most of it until the latter part of the nineteenth century (and aspects of it can still be studied in any rural area); the traditional society is now paramount; and some of the population—largely the urban population and especially the middle classes of the cities (Lagos probably has over 2 million

[17] The argument will not repeat that of the various research papers from that work but will draw on them: Chapters 1 and 2 of this volume, Caldwell and Caldwell (1976, 1977 and 1978), Caldwell and Ware (1977), Okediji et al. (1976) and Imoagene (1976).

inhabitants and Ibadan 750 000)—are part of transitional society.

The Primitive Society

A primitive society is one in which the largest organizational institution is the tribe, the clan, or the village. No overall responsibility is taken by the larger apparatus of State or Church, which means that security within the groupings that exist is not augmented or guaranteed by an outside entity. Indeed, security outside the group is minimal; nearly everyone continues to live among their people of orgin; and the size of that group is often the measure of safety.

Several aspects of such a society are of prime importance for understanding all pre-demographic-transition societies.

Perhaps the foremost is that the society or economy (for they cannot be separated) of the group is a single system in which the participants have time-honoured roles and duties. There is usually communal land (which is essential in nomadic, food-gathering, and most shifting-cultivation systems); residence in propinquity to large numbers of people—mostly relatives—with whom one has lived all one's life; government by these same people; and a simple economy where much cooperation is needed for the larger tasks. The absolute right of individual ownership is unknown. In fact economic relations and social relationships intermingle. Edward Evans-Pritchard wrote of the Sudan, "One cannot treat Nuer economic relations by themselves, for they form part of direct social relationships of a general kind," (1940, p. 90) and C. K. Meek of Nigeria, "One of the main distinctions between Native systems of holding land and those of Western societies is that the former are largely dominated by personal relationships, whereas the latter are subject to the impersonal legal conception of 'contract'." (1949, p. 16) Marshall Sahlins summarized the position as, "A material transaction is usually a momentary episode in a continuous social relation. (1972, pp. 185–186)[18] Transactions and gifts are not in fact markedly differentiated, especially as the latter are almost invariably also the cause of two-way flows of wealth.

Gifts of goods or services and later reciprocation allow the creation of a security system of mutual obligations (which will be dealt with in this review of the primitive society, even though such systems are of fundamental economic and demographic importance in traditional and transitional societies and survive even into modern society).[19] In all primitive and most traditional societies the maximization of profit or other ends in good times is of small importance compared with the minimization of risks (which often

[18] See also Mauss (1969), especially pp. 37–41.
[19] See Lomnitz (1971) for a description of the extensive system of reciprocity still existing among the Chilean middle class.

means ensuring survival) in bad times. Describing the Fulbe (or Fulani) of northern Nigeria, C. Edward Hopen reported that they "have an almost pathological concern (and often fear) for the future. Their conversation abounds with expressions as 'tojaango' (what of tomorrow) and 'gam jaango' (because of tomorrow). . . . The prospect of a secure and relatively care-free old age under the care of their sons will often restrain young women from deserting or divorcing their husbands. Both men and women in many respects show a remarkable disposition to forego present convenience (or pleasure) in the interests of future benefit" (1958, pp. 113–114).[20] Such attitudes are universally reported by field researchers, even among the businessmen of Ghana's capital, Accra (Garlick, 1971, pp. 110–118).

The fertility implications are obvious. It is in such conditions, where one lives with almost all one's relations and possibly with families whose ancestors have dwelt near one's own for generations, and where one has no other social environment and no other source of cooperation, and where social organization tends towards gerontocracy, that it is inconceivable that the nuclear family should crystallize out and that such a unit should attempt to gain economic advantage over other units.[21]

It is the survival of the extended family system as economic change occurs that helps to sustain high fertility. This survival is rendered more likely by a system of mechanisms that retain the full rigour of the extended family system even through the primitive and traditional societies. After the observations above, it might seem unlikely that primitive society would need such mechanisms, yet they exist throughout sub-Saharan Africa (Gluckman, 1955).[22] The reason is society's awareness that conjugal sexual relations can intensify conjugal emotional relationships, and that parent–child emotions can also become of overriding importance. Therefore,

[20] For examples from other cultures, see, for instance, Wharton (1971) and Johnson (1971).

[21] Although this conclusion seems obvious, misinterpretations on this issue abound. Thus, one economist/demographer, Julian Simon, arrived at the right conclusion by making the unfounded assumption that in high-risk situations one cannot afford to worry abut the future and, hence, is irresponsibly fertile. George Peter Murdock's analysis of family types from the Yale cross-cultural survey file in *Social Structure* (New York: Macmillan, 1949) confused the whole position by placing emphasis on such simple characteristics as residence units and groupings during movement, so that his successors began to draw parallels between independent, nucleated families found on the one hand among food gatherers and herders and on the other in industrial societies, and to contrast these with the extended family of settled agriculturists. (See, for example Nimkoff and Middleton, 1960.) Nothing, as we will see, could be less illuminating. The inward-turning nuclear family where obligations exist largely between spouses and toward their nonadult children is a very recent phenomenon almost everywhere except in the West. In spite of Murdock's followers' attempts to show resemblances between Eskimo and Western families, the former in fact have traditionally shared all the food they caught, and it is hardly possible that a nuclear family could improve its diet at the expense of others (see Graburn, 1971).

[22] See also Trevor (1975) on the breaking of the emotional bond between a mother and her first-born in Hausa-Fulani society of northern Nigeria.

African cultures successfully weaken both types of relationship, because communal residence and occupational cooperation would be endangered if men listened to what their wives said was in their mutual interest rather than what their brothers or fathers said, while matrilineal societies would disintegrate if preference were to be shown for sons and daughters over nephews and nieces. In fact (and this is important in terms of demographic transition), relationships between spouses, even in monogamous marriages, are not very strong in traditional Yoruba society and parents do not exclusively focus their attention on their biological children. Even in 1973 only one-third of Yoruba spouses slept in the same room or ever ate together (admittedly indexes of affection regarded as less significant by Yorubas than by outsiders), and fewer still identified the person to whom they felt closest as their spouse, while children were commonly brought up by a number of kinsmen.[23] This should be seen in the context of traditional Yoruba residence in extended family compounds, which persisted even in Ibadan until only a few years ago.

Networks of relatives are important in the primitive society and remain so in the traditional society. They increase the size of the security system and of the cooperating group in less serious situations; they increase the number of close allies in the political contest in the traditional political system in which success is due to the ability to tap more or better communal resources; they increase the number of relatives who can attend family ceremonies and hence magnify one's social importance and sheer consumption pleasure. In rural Yoruba society it is still taken as one of the immutable facts of existence that family numbers, political strength, and affluence are not only interrelated but are one and the same thing. Furthermore, such a base still forms an excellent springboard to success for young aspirants in the modern sector of the economy.[24] There are only two ways of increasing the size of one's network of relatives and they are interrelated: by reproduction and by the marriage of one's children. Data from the second survey in the Nigerian segment of the Changing African Family Project show that 80% of all Yoruba still hold that children are either better than wealth or are wealth, while those who maintain that on balance they consume wealth fall to 6% in rural areas; 96% agree that increasing the number of relatives by means of marriage is a good thing and 83% that they can ask relatives by marriage for help with material things or services to a greater extent than they can ask nonrelatives.

[23] Data from CAFN 2 (see Appendix to Chapter 2). On the traditional upbringing of children by a number of kinsmen, see Mair (1953), p. 2, and, for survey figures showing fewer than half of children in the Ivory Coast to be with their parents, see Clignet (1970), p. 171.

[24] The new elite are more likely to have come from larger rural families than from smaller rural families even when allowance is made for the anticipated differential between the two in the number of children supplied to the succeeding generation (see Imoagene, 1976).

But, if this is the way to wealth and power, why do extra children not press more on resources, especially on the supply of food? The question seems to have no meaning in most primitive societies and in traditional society among the Yoruba, even in densely settled rural areas or among urban populations. Part of the answer is that each new pair of hands helps to feed the extra mouth (to paraphrase the kind of proverb that seems to be found widely in Africa and Asia). Part is the nature of the communal economy, where "a man does not acquire more objects than he can use; were he to do so he could only dispose of them by giving them away" (Evans-Pritchard, 1940, p. 91). Indeed, in such an economy underuse of resources may be far more common than pressure upon them, a situation generalized in Sahlins' rephrasing of Chayanov's rule: "the intensity of labour varies inversely to the relative working capacity of the producing unit (i.e. the household or family)" (1971).[25] Lorimer constructed a model for agrarian societies, which apparently showed that, even if belt-tightening was caused in some families by the birth of extra children, it was only to a small extent while the children were young (1967). Less than one-fifth of Yoruba respondents in the second survey of the Nigerian segment of the Changing African Family Project believed that the birth of an extra child would have even an immediate impoverishing effect.

African children certainly work (except perhaps in the transitional society), beginning at age 5–7 years, as they imitate ever more what their elders of the same sex do. It is often difficult, even among adults, to distinguish work completely from way of life. Nevertheless, the traditional patriarch appreciated that work had to be done, that it was often onerous, and that more could be done and others could perhaps take a larger share of the burden if the family were large. C. Edward Hopen (1958, p. 124, fn. 1) relates that he discussed with a Fulani of northern Nigeria whether the Fulani, who supposedly are filled with joy by fathering large families, would have many children in the happy Moslem Heaven that they describe, only to be told: "No, why will we want children? All the work will be done by the servants of Allah." Pierre de Schlippe (1956, p. 235), reporting on the Zande of south-west Sudan states that, "The prestige of extensive fields and full granaries was to a great extent achieved by family despotism," including "cruel punishments inflicted on wives and children." This is not now the case among either the Zande or the Yoruba, but in rural areas, wives and children obey male instructions to work (see below on the question of schoolchildren). Yoruba children work as they have always done helping to provide nonmarket goods and services, as well as helping with market production.

---

[25] Reyna (1975b) argues that, even in primitive society, the unit with greater working capacity is able to diversify its activities, thus making use of windfall gains and distant economic opportunities and raising its per capita income.

That a man benefits economically in such a society by polygyny is now widely affirmed[26] (Boserup, 1970, pp. 27–52); it is a small step from this to recognizing that he also gains if he has a large number of children.

Traditional Society

In Yoruba society the difference between primitive and traditional society is hardly worth making when analysing demographic trends; but the establishment of the latter was undoubtedly the necessary precursor for fertility-change in the transitional society. However, this has not been the case in all traditional societies, many of which evolved slowly over a long period, and indeed the beginning of fertility transition can almost certainly be found in Europe at a time when it was still very largely premodern. State and Church, long before the advent of the Welfare State, were able to provide some assurance that they would intervene to try to prevent unnecessary deaths at times of community disaster—in Europe, with intermissions, since the time of the Ancient World, and over considerable parts of China over the centuries. This may well have weakened the need for the extended family in that the family was no longer the ultimate guarantor of survival. This was probably particularly the case where the authority of the State impinged most strongly and for the longest periods: for instance, in the Ancient World, in Metropolitan Rome, and, especially, in the City of Rome. It is difficult to examine Augustus's marriage laws without concluding both that the extended family at least was under pressure and that a subsequently reversed fertility decline was under way. Rome, as Gibbon so eloquently related, never really died away in Europe: the Church inherited the marriage laws and the attitudes that framed them, as well as responsibility for those in critical circumstances; the manor guaranteed employment and set conditions on access to land, which not only implied that family nucleation (in the economic sense of responsibilities) was well advanced but also reinforced that nucleation (and possibly held fertility in check by preventing early marriage) (Russell, 1949, pp. 103–107).

Traditional societies with their greater overall organization either introduced or increased the use of money. This, together with their greater guarantees of security to the traveller, expanded trade. With their national legal systems, they were more likely to move toward freehold tenure of land, although the demographic transition theorist should note how recently communal tenure has been important in non-European parts of the world. In fact, in most of sub-Saharan Africa freehold land still exists on only a very limited scale. All these changes had implications for the family.

[26] An analysis of the startlingly rapid change that occurred in another southern Nigerian society (the Ibos) with the imposition of colonial government found massive development in trading and other economic adaptations, but nothing worth reporting on the family and reproduction. See Ottenberg (1959).

Wealth Flows in Primitive and Traditional Societies[27]

As analysed by an outsider from a modern society, children have demonstrable values of several different types in primitive and traditional societies. They do a great deal of work for or with their parents not only when young but usually during adulthood as well; they accept responsibility for the care of parents in old age; they eventually bolster the family's political power and hence give it economic advantages; they ensure the survival of the lineage or family name and in many societies undertake the necessary religious services for the ancestors.

This list, like much value of children research, obscures two very important points.

The first is that such disaggregation is a product of external observation or, even more significantly, of hindsight. In relatively unchanging societies no one sees these separate bonuses conferred by fertility. The society is made of a seamless cloth: children fit into a non-introspective society where they behave as their parents behaved and where their role is to work when young and to care for the old. This is why they may have great trouble in listing any good things (or bad things) about large families when asked by the researcher. Indeed, the respondents' ability to see clearly the separate aspects of children's roles are not as certain as before. These roles, then, become important in what is now the transitional society and help to explain the options and decisions of such a society.

The second point is that the value of children to the lineage and ancestors is not really a prop with a strength of its own. Rather, this aspect of the role of children reflects the fact that the other aspects conducive to high fertility are positive as well. When the other props begin to deteriorate in the transitional society, so does the concern for ancestors (often with the help of imported religions, or new interpretations of existing religions, or the spread of secularism).

Nevertheless it is important for the analyst of a society moving toward transition (and this is true of most developing countries) to identify the nature and magnitude of the intergenerational wealth flows in the society. In pretransitional and essentially rural societies, at least six different economic advantages of children to one or both parents can be distinguished: (1) Situational gain is of particular importance to patriarchal males. The obsession with per capita analysis has obscured this type of gain. In Yoruba society there is nothing approaching an equal division of wealth or consumption within the family: there are inequalities by sex, age, and family

[27] Strictly speaking, economists describe these "wealth flows" as "income flows", retaining the word "wealth" for a stock rather than a flow. However, most social scientists assume that "income" excludes the giving of a helping hand in the house and many other items included in this discussion. Hence, it seemed necessary to use a new term.

status. As the number of children beyond infancy grows, and, indeed, as the number of wives and ultimately the number of children-in-law increases, it is inevitable that the person on top of the pyramid controls more resources and has access to more services (as well as enjoying more obvious power), even if per capita income remains static. (2) Children work in the household and on the farm not only producing goods but providing a range of services that adults regard as wholly or partly children's work and that they are loath to do themselves: carrying fuel, water, messages, and goods; sweeping; looking after younger siblings; caring for the animals; weeding the crops; and so on. (3) Adult children usually assist their parents, especially with labour inputs into farms (which frequently increase as the parents age) and with gifts, to a much greater extent than the older generation readily admits or than is spontaneously reported to survey-interviewers by either parents or children. (4) Adult children provide particular assistance in making up the family contributions to community festivities and to such family ceremonies as marriages, funerals, and celebrations connected with births. (5) The care of aged parents, who may insist on having their farms, businesses and households propped up as if they were still running them, can be a major undertaking. (6) Parents can invest in training or education of children so as to increase their ability to make returns (although the motive is usually only partly economic and is much more complex than is baldly stated here).

The key issue here, and, I will argue, the fundamental issue in demographic transition, is the *direction and magnitude of intergenerational wealth flows* or the net balance of the two flows—one from parents to children and the other from children to parents—over the period from when people become parents until they die. In premodern society much of the flow is indirect, because of the existence of extended families, clans, and even villages that share in these flows, and because the child's contribution to the parent may be largely by the augmentation of political strength to allow the tapping of a larger share of the communal wealth. The concept of a net balance is still valid, however, even if difficult to measure. It may even be closer to the truth in the older traditional village to speak of the flow being from the younger to the older in the community as a whole with the parent–child relationships in each family playing only a secondary role.

In all primitive societies and nearly all traditional societies the net flow is from child to parent. This is often partly obscured (especially in recent times) from the researcher by the very mechanisms that help to keep it working and to some degree determine the magnitude of the flow. Parents continually point out to children how much they have done for them and how much the children owe (not specifically as money or goods, but more as duty, which in the end means much the same thing). Such protestations may not have been needed in primitive society; to a large extent they help to provide guarantees in a changing and increasingly uncertain society. Three points should be noted. First, such protests are heard most in societies where the wealth flow is still from child to parent; they are much less a feature of a society where the flow has been firmly established toward the child. Second, the protests are not likely to bear much relation to the size of the family and hence to the size or reality of the outlay. Third, the researcher is likely, on hearing the protests and recording them as responses in his questionnaire, to take them as evidence of the economic disadvantages or even irrationality of high fertility. The protests are likely to be supported by details of actual expenditure, without equal concern for details of the returns, and these the researcher may regard as quantified data. There is evidence from one study of a region adjacent to Nigeria that the work of single, adult sons is so important to fathers that they deliberately use their control of bride wealth and marriage ceremonies to space out and postpone sons' marriages so as to organize an even flow of the labour first of unmarried sons and eventually of grandchildren (Reyna, 1975a).

There is then a great divide, a point where the compass hesitatingly swings around 180°, separating the earlier situation in which the net flow of wealth is toward parents and in which hence high fertility is rational and the later situation in which the flow is toward children and in which hence no fertility is rational. Why the divide is where it is, and why the compass swings, will be our major concern when investigating the transitional society.[28]

What this means is that before the divide economic rationality dictates unlimitedly high fertility. On the whole, discussion and even survey work in African primitive and traditional society seem to support this. Fertility is limited for all kinds of noneconomic reasons (some of which, however, like child survival, have economic implications). In Yoruba society, the Nigerian segment of the Changing African Family Project found that easily the most important reason is the spacing of births so as to contain infant and early childhood mortality and, hence, to maximize the number of living children. The second most important reason (at least in the past, because it has now been displaced in importance by delayed marriage) has been the cessation of sexual relations by a woman on the birth of the first grandchild so as to avoid the social and psychological tension arising from competing maternal and grandmaternal obligations. Other reasons have been the cessation of sexual relations in some cases when the husband takes another wife or when he moves elsewhere to work or because the woman feels increasingly old or battered by reproduction. Increasingly, fertility is being held in check by postponed age at marriage, which in the case of females already averages several years past puberty; this postponement arises out of competition with education or job opportunities and holds fertility in check because it is

[28] This is discussed at greater length in later chapters in this volume, and in Caldwell (1977a).

accompanied by continence, less sexual activity than in marriage, contraception, or abortion. When the numbers of children become really large, they raise problems of control, noise, and emotional deprivation even in rural societies. The list of noneconomic reasons is quite formidable and is incontrovertible evidence that economic rationality alone is unlikely to determine fertility in any society.

Similarly, after the economic divide, economic rationality dictates zero fertility. This does not happen, and fertility often falls slowly and even irregularly, again for social and psychological reasons—the extent to which alternative roles are available to women, the degree to which child-centredness renders children relatively expensive, the climate of opinion, and so on.[29] Fertility does not reach zero for reasons that are entirely psychological and social.

It is then necessary to attempt to measure intergenerational wealth flows, an endeavour that is rendered difficult in pretransitional society by a host of problems: much of the flow is not direct but is derived from the extra political power exerted by a man with many children, especially grown-up sons and daughters married into other families; much of the flow is not money but goods and services; some of the flow forms part of family contributions to meet community obligations and does not reach the parents at all; most people have good reason for diffidence about revealing the total flow of wealth, or at least that received. All of these difficulties except the last diminish as the economy becomes more monetized and society more urbanized, and hence transitional society allows easier measurement. Attempts to measure the near-lifetime return on investment in children as well as the outflow from older children were made in Ghana in 1963, and a more comprehensive attempt to examine intergenerational money flows was made in Nigeria's Western State in 1974–75. Both showed clearly that returns from children are substantial.[30]

It is essential to emphasize that the divide is not mechanistically determined by economic conditions. On the contrary it is almost entirely a social phenomenon (except that parent–child net flows of wealth, with the exception of labour and other services such as care for the very young and very old, are hardly possible in subsistence conditions or in the primitive society), and can be reached only when the economy of the nuclear family has been largely isolated from that of the extended family and when a subsequent change of balance has occurred within the nuclear family. The necessity for economic nucleation arises in several ways: the change of economic balance inside the nuclear family is essentially one of emotion and

---

[29] This problem was examined toward the end of fertility transition in Australia (Ruzicka and Caldwell, 1977). Reported child-centredness in this population is noted in Caldwell (1973).

[30] See Caldwell, 1965 and 1966 and, especially, pages 65 to 69 of this volume.

sentiment, which requires emotional nucleation (and other changes of emotional balance within the family) that is incompatible with the extended family economic system, which also needs a parallel system of emotional obligations to work; the change of economic balance in the nuclear family really means that the parents of the family are wholly in charge of their own family economy.

Even if the divide would probably eventually be reached in any urban-industrial society, attitudes and social organization could long delay its advent. Alternatively, a different set of circumstances could bring it on early, even, in fact, before the creation of the modern economy. This seems to be what happened in Western Europe.[31] The feudal system, built on the inherited ruins of the urbanized civilizations of the ancient world, went far toward making a nuclear family economically viable. Doubtless, economic obligations existed to more distant relatives. But these obligations were supported by moral forces and were susceptible to the weakening or reversal of those forces. This seems to have happened with the rise of Protestantism, which put much store on self-sufficiency of all types and on moderation in expenditure and desires. It allowed a man to tell his relatives that they should be more careful in their expenditures, more frugal in their wants, and more foresighted in planning for times of need. More importantly, it allowed him to do this and cautiously refuse to give any (or much) assistance, while retaining his pride and even preaching his practice. Given that the divide had been reached, fertility could be increasingly controlled, even if, at first, mostly by postponed marriage.

In Africa, substantial support for the thesis that emotional nucleation precedes economic nucleation comes from a study in Ghana where Oppong showed among male undergraduates at two universities a significant correlation between the kind of family and kinship obligations the students believed in and the number of children they wanted, and an earlier study by the writer that presented evidence on the extent to which urban elite families were emotionally turning in upon themselves (Oppong, 1974; Caldwell, 1968a).

The Transitional Society

An increasing proportion of the Third World population lives in transitional societies that are laboratories for the study of demographic change and lack of change and for determining the origins of demographic transition.

---

[31] It is doubtful if this happened in the traditional stage of any other society, although in Japan families did exhibit "rapid segmentation in each generation," partly because of a kind of primogeniture system, and because fertility levels were probably moderate. (See Vogel, 1967, pp. 91–92; and Taueber, 1958, pp. 52–53.) Extended family help was the rule in India and China (Lang, 1946, p. 169), while in northern Nigeria it could be institutionalized into the *gandu* (Hill, 1972).

"Transitional" here refers to rapid changes in the way of life, especially changes in the impact of children and in the possibilities available to parents for limiting the number of their children.

Nigeria's second largest city, Ibadan, is such a laboratory.[32] Its population is almost 750 000. Although agricultural links are still strong, only one-sixteenth of males report farming as their main occupation; one-third work in nonmanual occupations and another one-third work as soldiers, policemen, or craftsmen, or in similar jobs requiring a degree of training or imported skills and often with an orientation toward the nontraditional world. One-twelfth of women work in nonmanual occupations; but a similar proportion is employed in skilled occupations and over one-half in marketing, often of a somewhat different order from similar employment in rural areas. Three-quarters of the men and one-half the women have been to school; of the latter, one-quarter have experienced some secondary education and almost one-eighth have completed secondary school. More importantly, in terms of the strains on families frequently depicted by demographers, nearly all their children are now receiving some formal education and the majority are proceeding on to secondary schooling. It is rapidly becoming easier to limit fertility if that is the aim. Sexual abstinence has long been widely known as an approved method of avoiding pregnancy. Modern contraceptives are now available from several clinics, a large number of pharmacies, and other retail outlets; in 1973 one-sixth of all women aged 15–59 years had used modern contraception and one-ninth were currently doing so, while the doubling time for the levels of each category of behaviour (i.e. the time taken for the proportions behaving in this way to double) had for many years been only four years.

However, fertility (and "ideal family size") appear to have changed little. Significant differentials exist neither between Ibadan and Yoruba rural areas nor within Ibadan society (except that the small group of very highly educated women exhibit lower fertility at younger ages). Nor were contraceptors less fertile than noncontraceptors within Ibadan (Caldwell and Ware, 1977).[33] The conventional answer in terms of accepted demographic transition theory would be that attitudinal lags prevented parents from fully assessing the new economic situation, that innovation is not fully accepted and implemented at once because the props do not disintegrate at once, and that insufficiently motivated contraceptors are inefficient. None of these propositions appears to hold good in Ibadan, nor are they likely to elsewhere: the parents' assessment of the economic situation appears to be realistic with no time-lag involved; the innovators (as

[32] Data from the Changing African Family Project, mostly from the first survey in the Nigerian segment.

[33] Comparisons were made by age at given parities and changes in parity, and age-specific birth rates were also estimated.

discussed in the section below) do not seem to be aware of their courage in disregarding the props; the contraceptors are mostly doing precisely what they meant to do with the contraceptives.

High fertility remains rational in nonagricultural urban conditions as long as the flow of wealth is predominantly from the younger to the older generation.[34] This is still overwhelmingly the case in Ibadan. The 1974–75 Survey of the Intra-Family Flow of Money and Assistance in Nigeria's Western State surprised us by showing that the return from investment in children is greater for urban than rural residents and is the greatest of all among the city white-collar and professional class. Yet the reason is not far to seek. The urban population working in the modernized economy have both the means and the understanding of the system to keep their children moving up the educational ladder to the top positions in the modern society—positions with high salaries and fringe benefits, as well as control of the levers of power and hence access to opportunities for more wealth, some, but not all, fraudulently obtained. The parents can provide a background suited to continued study, and they know the headmasters and the people who allocate jobs. Perhaps more unexpectedly, the younger generation do not resent the system because they expect to receive wealth in turn from their own, even more successful, children. In fact, as Adepoju has shown, it is the more successful children who would feel most guilt about not sharing their wealth and who visit their parents most often to share it (1974, pp. 385–387). Furthermore, as the Nigerian Family Study's biographies of the successful clearly demonstrated, a major joy (perhaps the single most important consumption good for the successful) is meeting all family obligations in a more than generous way—in (as they repeatedly said) seeing distant relatives and even non-relatives recognize the donor's success and generosity.

This picture of the success of the urban middle class is but a segment of a wider picture of a whole modernizing society existing in a situation where wealth flows predominantly from the young to the old and where there are marked differentials in earning powers by rural–urban division and by education. The route from the rural area to the job in the modern sector of the economy is almost solely by extended education. Most parents can no longer manage to travel this way, but their children can. To get children far up the educational ladder and into the high-salary positions three stratagems are necessary: relatives outside the nuclear family must be encouraged to help with school fees or with accommodation and subsistence at centres where the right educational institutions exist; older children must help the

---

[34] This is a different argument from that put forward in Davis (1955), p. 4, where it is argued that the growth of cities at first reinforces high fertility in rural areas by providing greater outlets for agricultural produce.

younger ones in the same way (the sibling chain of educational assistance); and priority must be given to channeling the most assistance, at least early in the establishment of the sibling chain, to the children with the most chance of success—usually the brightest but occasionally those with unusual application, although the distinction is not often made. The first and second stratagems depend on the retention of the system of mutual obligations; the second and third work best with high fertility. The society, like many others in the Third World, believes that the birth of bright and potentially successful children is a matter of capricious fate to which some kind of probability can be assigned (the lucky dip, or lottery, principle) and that large families are likely to have one or more of such children whose existence far outweighs any disadvantages arising from a larger number of less successful siblings. Poor people have limited investment opportunities in such societies, and economic and political caprice can upset what appears to exist, so educational investment in children is thought to be the best investment in both Nigeria and Ghana, and doubtless in many similar societies. The child who has broken through to a job in the modern economy can assist the parents through flows of wealth (sent regularly and at times of crisis, brought on visits, or spent on visiting parents and siblings) or through influencing authorities and manipulating power; the child can bring honour to the parents by visiting them; and can give them access to the joys of the modern world during their visits or final retirement to the child's house. Children in urban areas are usually needed to bring earnings into the household, in circumstances where the total income of a poor household is often the sum of many small parts.[35]

Contraception may in the future be used largely to limit family size, but for the time being there is a substantial and increasing demand for contraceptives in Ibadan for other, more pressing reasons: to substitute for female sexual abstinence after birth (in a world where the message of the enjoyment of sexual relations is increasingly being heard); to permit sexual relations during the increasingly long period before marriage in a situation in which pregnancy might destroy the investment in education or dictate a marriage regarded as less than desirable by the family; or to allow safe extramarital sexual relations in a society in which long periods of abstinence, substantial age gaps between spouses, and late marriage of males have meant that discreet relations of this kind have been to a large measure condoned.

More work needs to be done on individuals and families in dire poverty in both traditional and transitional societies. We have investigated a considerable number of cases in West Africa and one point seems clear: they are

[35] On the economic impact of rural–urban migrant children in Ghana, see Caldwell (1969); for a discussion of the role of children in the family economy in India, see Mamdani (1972); for a description of the situation in a cloth-weaving town in south India, see Pethe (1964), p. 112.

most likely to be products of an atypically inadequate family structure—often one that has been greatly eroded by mortality and that was vulnerably small in the first place because of accident or subfertility.

Identification of the Primary Forces of Change

The transitional nature of Ibadan society also allows the identification of the extent, nature, and cause of fertility transition. This is best done by identifying the innovators. Two methods were employed in the Changing African Family Project. The first was the isolation of all those women in Ibadan (together with their husbands where the marriage was a first, monogamous one with the husband still present) who had indubitably succeeded in demographic innovation: women already over age 40 years with fewer than six live births achieved by intention and any method of restricting fertility.[36] The second was the examination of all women in the three 1973 Nigerian surveys who, regardless of age at the time, had had fewer than six live births, but desired no more and were at the time employing modern contraception to try to ensure this.

The first point established was that there are still very few demographic innovators. Ibadan contains about 62 500 women over age 40 years, but only 438 or 0·7% had intentionally and successfully restricted fertility to less than six births.[37] Women of all ages with fewer than six live births and using modern contraception to avoid further pregnancies numbered less than 2000 in Ibadan, out of about 153 000 women aged 15–49 (or 1·3%) or about 128 000 aged 20–44 (about 1·5%). The size of this demographically innovating group (i.e. under 2000) can be compared with the number of so-called family planning innovators, for in 1973 the number of Ibadan women practicing modern contraception was over 17 000 or almost nine times as many. In the whole of the Western and Lagos States (which include rural areas but which also contain Lagos with its 2 million people and rapidly changing society as well as many other towns), only 0·5% of women are currently demographic innovators according to the first Nigerian survey. The 1·5% of demographic innovators in Ibadan can also be compared with the number of socioeconomic innovators: 46% of women have had schooling, and 15% have experienced at least some secondary education; most have their children of school age in full-time education; one-tenth are employed in the modern sector of the economy; one-third of the husbands work in

[36] CAFN 3, Changing African Family Project: Nigerian Segment, Survey 3. The latitude allowed with regard to contraception, namely the use of any method, including abstinence, to achieve the small family was necessary because the survey was restricted to older women who had relatively little access to modern contraception.

[37] This is a very conservative definition of fertility innovation; however, even some of these women might have achieved this fertility by chance and then have rationalized the position. See Lesthaeghe and Page (1976).

nonmanual occupations, while no more than one-fourth could be said to be employed in the traditional sector of the economy. Clearly, continuing high fertility is not explained by lack of access to or even use of contraception, or by only limited modernization, or by children still maintaining the occupational roles they filled in traditional rural society.

The problem is, then, to study the demographic innovators in depth and to find out how and when they separated themselves from the rest of the community. The quest should be easy. One might infer from demographic transition theory that the decision to do without the props might well be traumatic, and some demographers have wished that they could talk to the eighteenth-century French couples who first daringly decided to innovate. In fact, at first the most frustrating and then the most illuminating discovery was that the demographic innovators are for the most part unaware that they have done anything unusual. After all, contracepting is no longer unusual, particularly in the educational and social groups to which most belong. The use of such contraception to limit family growth just seemed an obvious thing to do in their economic circumstances.

The fundamental question is then: What were the economic circumstances of this group and how did they differ from others who were supporting children at school? The first hint is given by some of their characteristics: demographic innovators compared with non-innovators are 1·6 times as likely to have been to school and 2·7 times as likely to have been to secondary school; they are 2·0 times as likely to have husbands in nonmanual occupations, 4·5 times as likely to have had fathers in such occupations; they are 6·5 times as likely to have all these characteristics—to have fathers and husbands in nonmanual occupations and to be in such occupations themselves and to have had secondary education. Background and education are more important than current occupational experience or indeed any other contemporary circumstance or experience.

These findings could be said to be consonant with the knocking away of the props. However, the Nigerian segment of the Changing African Family Project contained a battery of questions and propositions of a psychosocial kind, relating to phrases taken from Yoruba proverb or song and of a type that could be made in a semi-philosophical way in everyday conversation. The responses showed clearly that what distinguished the demographic innovators from others was not their lack of superstition or their rationalism but their attitudes toward family and children. They have emotionally nucleated their families; they are less concerned with ancestors and extended family relatives than they are with their children, their children's future, and even the future of their children's children. They are more likely to have been "spoilt" themselves in the sense that their parents gave them more emotion and wealth than they expected back, and this is the way they tend, although usually to a greater extent, to treat their own children.[38]

What causes this emotional nucleation of the family whereby parents spend increasingly on their children, while demanding—and receiving—very little in return? Not the urban-industrial society, at least to the extent that it has developed in Ibadan. The majority of the society, even among the elite, is still one where net wealth flows over a lifetime from child to parent. Nor is that majority system buffeted by the institutional requirements of the modern economy; on the contrary it can adapt not only well but profitably to such a society. It might well be able to continue and improve the adaptation for decades, or perhaps generations, except for the factor that has already brought about change among the small minority of demographic innovators.

That factor is undoubtedly the import of a different culture; it is Westernization. Just as Western ethnocentricity has bedeviled Third World research and introduced wholly inappropriate attitudes, assumptions and methods, it has in a perversely negative way upset the whole study of "modernization" (i.e. the social changes that seem to precede, accompany, or follow economic development). Western researchers have all too frequently decided to become "objective" or at least "non-self-centred" by achieving the almost incredible feat of omitting transmitted European cultural traditions from the study of modernization; it is like leaving Hellenization out of an examination of social change in fifth century B.C. Macedonia or leaving Roman social influences out of a treatise on Britain in the second century A.D. This may sound like hyperbole, but it is not. In one of the major texts on social change in the Third World, Alex Inkeles and David Smith fleetingly recognized that the difference in their division of the world into that which was modernized and that which was not was almost entirely a contrast between the West and the rest: "With the exception of Japan . . . all the major nations which we can consider modernized are part of the European tradition" (1974, pp. 17–18). Rather than pursue this theme, they decided not to be "arrogant" and instead broke up the Western tradition into components that could be used for measuring not "Westernization" but "modernization".[39] Throughout William Goode's important

[38] There has been previous evidence pointing this way from studies in Ghana. The author, drawing on a 1962–64 research programme, emphasized that the family–building practices and attitudes of the new urban elite could be understood only in terms of relationships restructured in terms of a fusion of an existing culture with an imported one (1968a, especially pp. 52–73 and 183–188). Oppong (1974) has shown how presumably rational decisions about desired family size among younger members of this elite reflect the type of family situation they desire and will probably try to construct.

[39] Their index lists "European influence" only to suggest "See Western bias," and, on following this into the text, we find them preparing a defence because "some of our critics would be prepared to argue that the use of the O. M. [Overall Modernity] scale borders on being a social science form of cultural colonialism" (p. 297). Their scale is of little use for the demographer trying to relate modernization to family and fertility change, for two of its important components are "kinship obligations" and "family size" (both measured negatively) (pp. 25–27 and 34).

study, *World Revolution and Family Patterns* (1963), with its investigation of recent family changes in the Arab, sub-Saharan African, Indian and Chinese worlds, "revolution," except in the discussion of slower growth over a long period in the West, is a synonym for "Westernization".

Curiously, it is only the well-trained, over-sensitive Western researcher who does not see and hear the obvious. In West Africa, survey respondents (as well as the conversationalist met in the street, the villager in the compound, and the Lagos newspaper) speak continually of adopting European ways—often, in fact, embarrassing the researcher in rural areas by going on to summarize this as "becoming civilized".

How, then, is the European concept of family relationships and obligations imported? The answer is that the import has been on such a massive scale that the slow erosion of traditional family structures is a measure of cultural durability.

Sailors, traders, and slavers may have disrupted some families, but they preached little and few took their examples as a model. However, in the mid-nineteenth century British colonial administration reached Lagos (less than 160 kilometers from Ibadan) and missionaries arrived at Ibadan itself. According to the Changing African Family Project, by 1973 nearly one-half the population of Ibadan were Christian and only 0·5% still described themselves as adhering to traditional African beliefs; two-thirds of those who had achieved small families were Christian. Missionaries and their successors have for over a century preached the Western family as the Christian family: monogamy as God's way instead of polygyny; husbands and wives looking after *their* children.[40] Administrators tended to take the same viewpoint, and nearly all Europeans in the developing colonial society advertised the Western family by example and viewpoint.

The mass infusion of European manners, however, has been relatively recent and it has had two interrelated vehicles: mass education and the mass media. Schooling for a very small minority, mostly male, dates back in Ibadan for over a century, but the movement toward some schooling for most children got under way in Yorubaland only in the 1950s. "The family," as taught by the school, is almost entirely the Western family. Textbooks either come from England or are local products modelled on English prototypes. Readers, used in the first years of schooling, are very much concerned with the family and generally tell of a house with a father who goes out to work, a mother who stays home and looks after the children, and the children themselves, who are good and who can expect help and gifts to rain upon them from their two parents. School teachers, even when their

---

[40] There has been some revolt against the identification of Christianity with the West, and the African pentecostal churches, which do not preach Western values, have attracted about one-quarter of Ibadan's Christians (CAFN 1).

own family lives are not fully Westernized, are unlikely to offer non-Western family precepts to their pupils.[41] Researchers have sometimes tried to relate fertility change to the Westernized context of the syllabus (Loewenthal and David, 1972, p. 42), while activists have introduced a "population awareness" ingredient into existing syllabuses; almost certainly such formal ingredients are trivial compared with the inbuilt assumptions of the system and its teachers. Education systems are not easily changed, and are much more likely to be imported intact. In much of the Third World they are essentially a reflection of the modern West, both in their origins and messages, and rarely mirror life in a largely communal and subsistence village. By the mid-1980s many of the women who flooded as youngsters in the late 1950s into the new primary schools may well be faced with the question of calling a halt to family size rather than continuing to reproduce. Then we will discover what impact their schooling had on their families' social and economic structure and what impact this has for their fertility.

Mass media in Nigeria have only had a marked impact since Independence in 1960. Only the newspapers and magazines require the literacy that comes from schooling, but education is likely to lead to the higher income that facilitates the purchase of a radio or a television set or a cinema ticket and to the interest in the nontraditional world that makes these purchases more profitable. All cinema films, most television films that portray family life, much of the magazine content, and a considerable proportion of the newspaper feature content are imported, and the models on which they are based are wholly imported from the West. The same message of nuclear family structure is relayed as is imparted by the schools. But another message is also presented in Nigeria: the great importance of sexual relations. This is luridly presented in newspaper and magazine features, news stories, and question and answer sections. Taking a single important example, the emphasis on sex in the widely read *Lagos Weekend* must boost the market for contraceptives, because until recently the main interpretation has been on the excitement of relations outside marriage. But, with the increase in the proportion of educated (and partly Westernized) wives, it is inevitable that the message will be increasingly interpreted to mean also sexual relations within marriage. Such a change, certainly already well under way among the elite, cannot fail to affect the traditional system of family relationships (as has always been recognized in the society) and by strengthening the conjugal emotional bond will tend to nucleate the family, at first emotionally and ultimately economically.

---

[41] A comprehensive study of teachers, their family lives and problems, their attitudes and their fertility will be available when Christine Oppong analyses the Ghanaian Segment of the Changing African Family Project.

Transition Theory Restated

In general, in societies of every type and stage of development, fertility behaviour is rational, and fertility is high or low as a result of economic benefit to individuals, couples, or families in its being so. Whether high or low fertility is economically rational is determined by social conditions: primarily by the direction of the intergenerational wealth flow. This flow has been from younger to older generations in all traditional societies; and it is apparently impossible (or at least, examples are unknown) for a reversal of flow—at the great divide—to occur before the family is largely nucleated both emotionally and economically. A fair degree of emotional nucleation is needed for economic nucleation; and considerable amounts of both are required before parents are free to indulge in ever greater expenditures on their children.

Pre-divide populations do not aim at females conceiving as frequently as possible during the full reproductive span, and post-divide populations do not favour childlessness. The reasons are not basically economic; they are social, psychological, and physiological. It is possible, however, that the marginal economic advantage of each additional child in pre-divide society and disadvantage in post-divide society in some circumstances modifies the impact of the noneconomic determinants. Nevertheless, economic analysis on its own can do nothing to predict the timing of the divide and very little to explain the levels of fertility on either side of it—probably the course of fertility in the twentieth century West owes less to the economics of each additional child born than it does to the extent to which parental emotional and expenditure patterns have become focused on the children and the degree to which their society renders such focusing expensive in terms of alternative uses for money, emotion, and time. Similarly, demographic evidence of fertility change may be valueless in terms of deducing movement toward the divide or estimating the probable timing of the reversal of the intergenerational wealth flow; the fertility change may well respect an adjustment of changing social, psychological, or physiological circumstances.[42]

Extreme external factors may influence this pattern. Pre-divide fertility may be restricted in the Kalahari Desert or on Tikopia because of very finite resources; and post-divide fertility was temporarily very high on the American frontier, where the wealth flow to children was relatively insignificant and where there were few alternative sources of labour and even company. The analysis carried out here has been largely based on Africa where access to land has been fairly unrestricted. The position may

[42] See, for example, past fertility declines reported in William Brass et al. (1968), pp. 178, 181, 346–347, 512–513.

be somewhat more like Tikopia in densely settled agrarian areas in Asia. However, the little available evidence suggests that it is not, and that even there farming families do not on the whole see the extra birth as impoverishing and do not tighten their belts as the child grows. The explanation may be partly that we are deceived by a static analysis and see the household or family too little in terms of the coming and going of people over time; partly that the extra child does in due course add sufficiently to production; and partly that in the contemporary world the existence of urban employment takes sufficient strain off the need for providing more land.

For reasons that lie deep in its history, the family was increasingly economically nucleated in Western Europe centuries ago; indeed some social groups may have crossed the divide reversing the intergenerational wealth flow as early as the seventeenth century (Henry, 1956; Peller, 1965). This phenomenon had two demographic effects: a direct one, namely that Europe's population growth rate was lower than it would otherwise have been once mortality began to decline; an indirect one, in that European culture accepted the nuclear family as the basic unit of society and included a range of values associated with it among exports to other parts of the world.

An emphasis must be placed here on the export of the European social system as well as its economic system. It is as absurd to deny that this is the central feature of our times as to deny the significance of the Hellenization of southwest Asia, the Romanization of the Mediterranean and western Europe, and the Sinoization of much of southeast and central Asia in other periods. The issue is not whether Western social structure is better or even whether it is more suited to modernization; it is merely that the West has been able to export it because of the overwhelming economic strength it derived from the industrial revolution.

From the demographic viewpoint, the most important social exports have been the concept of the predominance of the nuclear family with its strong conjugal tie and the concept of concentrating concern and expenditure on one's children. The latter does not automatically follow from the former, although it is likely to follow continuing Westernization; but the latter must be preceded by the former. There probably is no close relationship in timing between economic modernization and fertility—and, if true, this may be the most important generalization of our time. If another culture had brought economic development, a culture with a much less nucleated family system, industrialization might well have proceeded far beyond its present level in the Third World without reversing the intergenerational flow of wealth. Conversely, in the present situation, family nucleation and the reversal of the intergenerational wealth flow are likely to penetrate deeply into the Third World in the next half century, almost independently of the success of industrialization, and, almost inevitably, they will guarantee slower global population growth.

Several subsidiary points about the export of the Western economic and social systems should be made. First, this export has made both mortality and fertility declines possible in the Third World. Public health measures were acceptable deep in traditional society, and this has been taken as evidence of the reality of the props, which were so constructed as to encourage the desire for low mortality and high fertility. The props are in fact needless: in pre-divide society economic prosperity increased with the number of surviving children—the noneconomic restraints on fertility were more on the number of pregnancies and on the time-span of reproduction than on numbers of survivors. Second, the whole system of extended family obligations and the flow of wealth from younger to older generations may be disrupted by political means (China is the clearest example) with exactly the same effect in reducing fertility (although net wealth flows in a commune are probably relatively low, they are almost certainly from the old to the young). Third, the imminence of the reversal of the wealth flow and of declining fertility is usually hidden because of the increased economic benefits from high fertility in the modernizing economy of pre-divide transitional society. And fourth, the attempts to slow associations over time between mortality decline and various economic development indices on one hand and fertility decline on the other are probably valueless; even where there are direct relationships they usually cannot be proved because of the tendency for so many economic and social changes to move together.

A final note should perhaps be added on the more theoretical aspect of population growth in primitive societies. It can be argued that mortality is determined by environment, way of life, and technology, and varies widely among primitive and traditional societies. Yet, demonstrably, population growth rates over long periods have been very low, thus establishing that fertility levels must have approximated mortality levels. One can go further and maintain that this means that mortality levels determined fertility levels, an argument that not only supports the concepts of props but implies that they were subject to strengthening or relaxing until the right level was reached. A more plausible reading of the African tribal situation, however, is that fertility levels were established independently. Where they were above mortality levels, population grew, and the tribe expanded its area through warfare with its neighbours. When expansion was successfully opposed, mortality rates climbed to meet fertility rates: first, because of increasingly unsuccessful warfare and, subsequently, because of growing pressure on limited resources. Where fertility levels were below mortality levels, the tribe died out.

Research Implications

If the society is at every stage rational, and economically rational at that, then it can be studied employing economic tools, as long as it is understood that the researchers must accept the society's own ends. Those ends can be researched only by students of society, and their techniques alone—and not those of economic inquiry—can attempt to predict the approach to the divide where the wealth flow reverses.

First-class fieldwork on wealth flows in pre-divide societies is urgently needed, and that research must start with the identification of all possible types of mobile wealth and the development of methods for detecting flows. A good study of a single village would be worth a great deal; defective work on a nation could be dangerously misleading. Cross-sectional studies have some value, but it will be necessary to build up life-cycle models. Specialized investigations might attempt to discover why children do not seem to press on resources in agrarian areas even when these areas are densely settled.

Sociological and anthropological work is needed to define the extent of the true extended families of obligation and to measure the internal wealth flows. It will also be necessary to measure the strength of each obligation bond—the circumstances (and the likelihood of those circumstances occurring) that will bring it into play and the probable volume of the wealth flow under given conditions. The study of the changing family and the measurement of movement toward the social, emotional, and economic nucleation of the conjugal family are important.

A combined social science assault will probably be needed on the circumstances and conditions of the reversal of the wealth flow—and on the time taken for the flow from the older to the younger generation to grow to such an extent that it exerts a real impact on fertility control decisions.

We also need studies that can easily be done in association with family planning action programmes. We must find out the real reasons people want contraceptives and the extent to which contraception has anything to do with restricting fertility. Subtle and sympathetic studies in depth of both demographic innovators and contraceptive innovators are essential for action programmes.

Finally, we need to know a lot more about the effect on the family of the lessons learned from the media and in school. Much effort has gone into distinguishing the population content of high school lessons but little study has been done on the family structure almost inadvertently taught in the elementary school.

The major implication of this analysis is that fertility decline in the Third World is not dependent on the spread of industrialization or even on the rate of economic development. It will of course be affected by such development in that modernization produces more money for schools, for newspapers, and so on; indeed the whole question of family nucleation cannot arise in the nonmonetized economy. But fertility decline is more likely to precede industrialization and to help bring it about than to follow it.

This chapter was reprinted with the permission of The Population Council from "Toward a restatement of demographic transition theory," *Population and Development Review* 2, nos. 3 and 4 (September and December 1976): 321–366.

5

A theory of fertility: from high plateau to destabilization

If the object is to understand and predict the onset of fertility transition, then study should be focused on the conditions of stable high fertility and on the nature of destabilization. In earlier papers I advanced a series of propositions in order to elucidate the nature of demographic transition from high to low fertility.[1] The fundamental theses is that fertility behaviour in both pretransitional and post-transitional societies is economically rational within the context of socially determined economic goals and within bounds largely set by biological and psychological factors. Two types of society can be distinguished: one of stable high fertility, where there would be no net economic gain accruing to the family (or to those dominant within it) from lower fertility levels, and the other in which economic rationality alone would dictate zero reproduction. The former is characterized by "net wealth flows" from younger to older generations, and the latter by flows in the opposite direction. These flows are defined to embrace all economic benefits both present and anticipated over a lifetime.[2]

I have also argued that the conditions of stable high fertility, and of subsequent destabilization, lie largely in the nature of economic relations within the family. The family that determines economic advantage and demographic decision is not synonymous with the coresidential family usually identified imperfectly in census and surveys and often subsequently analysed with scant regard for the definitions employed in data collection. Rather it encompasses those groups of close relatives who share economic

[1] Chapters 2, 3, and 4 of this volume. See also the collected papers and comparative findings of other researchers in Caldwell (1976 and 1977a) and Ruzicka (1977).

[2] Including goods and money, labour and services, protection and guarantees, and social and political support. Despite problems in measuring the totality of these flows in each direction and their components, it is possible to secure reasonably good evidence of the recent direction of wealth flows in individual societies (e.g. in Nigeria in 1977 and Bangladesh in 1978).

activities and obligations. Within this larger and demographically more significant entity, the locus of economic and fertility decision-making is of prime importance, but has not yet been adequately investigated.

These premises suggested the need for investigation of the family both in historical situations of high fertility immediately before fertility decline and in contemporary situations of high fertility in which indexes of economic and social change suggested that the family structure and the high-fertility system might be under strong pressure. Accordingly, my recent research has been directed largely at study of a western society, namely Australia, in the nineteenth century, immediately before the onset of fertility decline (see Chapter 6; Ruzicka and Caldwell, 1977); and more sustained study of the agrarian extended family of the high-fertility belt extending from Morocco to Bangladesh.[3] The emphasis here is on the latter, and particularly on the Islamic groups studied, since they do not present the complexities of caste and of the nature of work and lifestyle implied by caste in Indian society. This research is supplemented by some further work on sub-Saharan Africa (Caldwell, 1977b).

General Propositions

The following propositions arise from the study of the family—particularly the traditional, rural, extended family—of North Africa and Southwest and South Asia, an area containing over a quarter of the population of the world, one-third that of the developing world, and half that marked by continuing high fertility. The region is characterized by some of the world's highest and most stable fertility.[4]

Six propositions are advanced as a basis for describing the relations between economic and reproductive behaviour in this region.

1. The traditional peasant economy is a familial-based economy, fundamentally different from the non-familial-based capitalist economy. The major difference between the distinct economies of the world lies in the organization of production, or the mode of production.[5] Each mode of production has its own economic, and dependent demographic, laws.

[3] Islamic and Indian components of this study are being reported separately. See Caldwell and Caldwell (1980); P. Caldwell (1977); and a paper on India is in preparation.

[4] The peasant economy observed in these societies also obtained in China until mid-century. See for example Fei (1939), Yang (1948) and Fei and Chang (1949).

[5] *Modes of production* and *relations of production* were terms first employed by Karl Marx and are suited to the analysis in that they are used in the sense that "the relations of production define a specific mode" (Hindess and Hirst, 1975, p. 9), although such relations were not equated by Marx, and have rarely been equated by Marxists, with family relations in precapitalist production, as they are in this paper. Capitalist economy is used here to describe any economy in which there is a market for labour beyond kinship or other traditional obligations to work; the industrial economy is treated as a recent manifestation of this economy.

2. Familial modes of production are characterized by relations of production between kin that give the more powerful or the decision-makers material advantage. The struggle of the decision-makers to maintain their advantage is normally seen as the assertion of natural rights and as proper behaviour; nevertheless, family economic relationships are exploitative and there is potential for conflict and change.

3. High fertility is advantageous to the peasant family as a whole and to its most powerful members. As long as the internal relations of the familial mode of production remain intact, marital fertility will not be restricted for the purposes of limiting family size.

4. Although the familial mode of production is typically found in circumstances of subsistence production, it can adapt for at least a time to urban life and to the market economy without fully succumbing to the rules of the market and, indeed, while allowing that market to operate in a highly specialized way. Thus, the economic and demographic structure of the familial mode of production may dominate in a society with a limited market economy.

5. In general, modes of production in a society do not change quickly from one to another but may exist in parallel for long periods, and families may participate in more than one mode of production. Familial modes of production other than the peasant economy include hunting and gathering, shifting cultivation, nomadic herding, and feudal.

6. A familial mode of production has long persisted within the capitalist mode of production, as an (at least temporarily) more efficient method of producing part of the family's needs, while giving material advantage to the male head of household as the dominant decision-maker. Post-transitional fertility decline arises from the continuing disintegration of this submode and its reproductive relationships, as capitalist production successfully competes with domestic production and as social change transforms the relations of production.

These proportions will be examined roughly in the order in which they are listed, focusing first on the conditions of stable high fertility and then on the nature of destabilization.

Familial Modes of Production

In familial modes of production, different family members enjoy different advantages according to their position in the family structure. Such situational advantage is characterized by both material advantage and advantage in terms of power, but even the latter is significant largely in its potential for securing material advantage. Material advantage, broadly defined, includes advantages in type and amount of labour activity, in services rendered, in security, in guarantees, and so on. The direction and magnitude of the net wealth flow determine the recipients of material advantage. There are nonintergenerational flows, such as that from wife to husband, but the intergenerational flow is of most importance in assessing the utility of fertility. As will be seen, potential conflict, antagonism, and opposed interests are inherent in the relations of production, but this does not mean that such conflict is necessarily apparent to those involved. Rather it means that there are inherent tensions (or antagonisms) that may be a vehicle for change and that indicate the direction change is likely to take.

An important aspect of material advantage is relative work inputs. Work traditionally has largely been a matter of *drudgery* (Thorner's term for Chayanov's Russian version (1966, passim.), (1966a, p. 6)[6], and human beings have always been oppressed by the long hours of toil involved in farming and primitive domestic work.[7] In these circumstances, a significant factor in material advantage lies in the nature and amount of work undertaken. A comparison of work inputs of different family members is difficult, however, for a number of reasons. The peasant family of North Africa and South Asia still produces largely for subsistence, and the growing of food in the field, the processing of it in the yard, and the cooking of it in the house cannot be assigned varying productivity values (indeed, processing and cooking cannot always be distinguished). The distinction frequently made between "productive work" and "household work" tends to obscure the value of some forms of work. Indeed, the whole subject of peasant labour inputs is so obscured by conventional wisdoms, convenient to the powerful, that it is difficult to interpret research or to discount the prejudices of researchers. The following are merely selected examples, but each is an important consideration in comparing the real value of different kinds of work.

First, there is a mystique of the plough. This is so pervasive that peasants equate ploughing, done by men, with work and thus contend that men do the real work. In reality, ploughing requires the sudden use of strength, especially on turns, but it is more pleasant and requires less constant effort than the use of digging sticks. Yet almost everywhere cultivation seems to

[6] The term drudgery is preferred by the editors over labouriousness or irksomeness for Chayanov's Russian term, *tyagostnos*.

[7] Accordingly, the Sahelian cultivators face the risk of starvation every few years rather than increase the annual level of their drudgery in order to create food buffer stocks. See Caldwell (1975d) p. 74. Chayanov argued that the Russian peasantry consciously and necessarily indulged in "self-exploitation" until reaching an equilibrium between drudgery and consumption, beyond which "continuing to work becomes pointless, as further labour expenditure becomes harder . . . to endure than is foregoing its economic effects" (see Chayanov, 1966a, p. 6).

have changed from a female to a male prerogative with conversion from digging stick to plough.

Second, there is a continuous downgrading of the value of women's work that misrepresents its significance. Those peasant households with insufficient female inputs are in just as reduced a condition as those with insufficient male imputs. The downgrading serves to keep women submissive, even grateful, and, when wage labour is employed, to keep their pay far below that of males. There is an incongruity about the whole situation: daughters are less important than sons, as any patriarch will aver, because, at an early age, they marry out into another family; yet the most hardworking labour input within the family (which largely determines living comfort) comes from daughters-in-law, brought in from other families who have conditioned them to be a submissive and hence valuable and economical labour force, precisely because of their undervaluation. Social scientists are likely to accept the obvious preference for sons as evidence that male labour must be more valuable than female. Much work done by women and children such as the collection of water, fuel, and manure, is thought of by men as menial, and, in truth they are loath to do it, although describing it as comparatively easy work. (Similarly, in capitalist production, many men who work outside the home, in occupations that do not involve real drudgery, are loath to share the woman's work within the house.)

Third, nonphysical occupations, especially white-collar and professional ones, are everywhere honoured above physical or manual pursuits, in spite of being pleasanter and much less onerous. In developing countries, such occupations are often little more than graceful role playing, and are in no way as productive as the almost dishonoured drudgery going on all around.

Another important point is that the peasant household, like those in all modes of production, is not an unguided vehicle moving with frictionless momentum along straight rails provided by societal norms. Decision-making mechanisms operate in both economic and demographic areas; and their investigation, which has hardly been attempted, is absolutely necessary for a complete understanding of fertility transition.

Power in economic decision-making usually means power in demographic decision-making. Fertility may be influenced by decisions in such areas as the practice of premarital sex, the practice of premarital contraception, whether marriage takes place, the age at marriage, the frequency of sexual relations during marriage, the practice of contraception during marriage, and the practice of abortion before or after marriage. In peasant societies none of these decisions is totally within the province of the conjugal pair, and some of them are largely or almost wholly decided by other persons. The older generation (father alone, parents, parents plus others) usually decide upon marriage and upon the age at which it will occur; they are probably the dominant influence, except in transitional economic and social circumstances, in deciding whether fertility will be controlled; and they often influence the level of sexual activity. This influence on reproductive behaviour tends to be obscured by its negative nature, which may be interpreted, usually wrongly, as *laissez faire*. Most residents of this region know of the availability of contraception, and most could practice some form of fertility control if the family wished it. Probably the great majority of adults in extended families see no gain in restricting fertility. Certainly, in three-generational joint families the older decision-makers correctly see no personal advantage from fertility restriction by their children and children-in-law. When this younger generation perceives advantage and acts upon it, the relationships that constituted the peasant mode of production are already dissolving.

The Traditional Extended Family

In the rural areas of the region the great majority of people still live in extended families, in that they live either with or in close proximity to relatives and share land, budgetary arrangements, or at least mutual obligations and guarantees against disaster.[8] There is no absolute distinction between living close to each other and living as a joint family in the same residence, although co-residence probably makes it less likely that the authority of the older generation will be eroded and that the younger (or intermediate) generation will form sufficiently strong conjugal links to encourage them to attempt to share in economic and demographic decision-making. The families of the Middle East have been described as "extended, patrilineal, patrilocal, patriarchal, endogamous and occasionally polygynous," (Patai, 1971, p. 84), a description that, with the exception of endogamy, fits well enough from Morocco to Bangladesh and even, until recently at least, across China. These characteristics go far to explain how the economy of the family works and why its fertility remains high.

The extended family is the dominant economic and security unit in this region. Help is usually unobtainable (except among minority groups) from such larger units as the clan, lineage, village, or tribe, all of which are important in sub-Saharan Africa and exist to a greater or lesser extent throughout the region. The explanation probably lies in fixed land areas

---

[8] Throughout this paper, groups of close relatives living in close proximity with mutual obligations and economic interests are described as extended families. Co-resident families containing not only husband, wife, and their children but also additional relatives are described as joint families. Thus a joint family is one type of extended family, distinguished by residence in the same household. This usage is in keeping with that set out in Smith (1968).

with family tenure and a long history of state power, which reduced the level of local physical conflict.

A key question is whether the type of family moulded by the peasant mode of production is merely one of the types of family found in the region or whether it is culturally dominant. After all, there have been considerable urban populations for millennia, and for an equally long time there have been landlords as well as peasants, wage earners as well as family helpers, and marketed as well as subsistence food.[9] Nevertheless, subsistence production is still the norm; probably two-thirds of India's food is eaten by its producers (Thorner and Thorner, 1962, p. 206). Moreover, the pyramidal family, hallowed by time and enthusiastically sanctioned by religion, prevails even in conditions other than subsistence farming. Except among the modernized urban middle class, it has managed to keep its structure largely intact. Merchant and artisan families, even in cities, retain the agrarian household organization with its unified budgetary and authority structures. Wage earning is most frequently regarded not as an alternative economy to the familial one, nor as a path to liberation from family authority, nor even as a means of accumulating individual property, but as a method for supplementing total family income or wealth. Indeed, Meillassoux (1972, p. 102) argues that capitalism has frequently contributed to this end, paying wages too small for the worker to set up a nuclear family but only enough for him to supplement the income of an extended family. And Wolf (1966, pp. 55–67) maintains that increasing outside opportunities have reinforced the residential joint family and contributed to its survival. This indices of urbanization, or even of the proportion of produce reaching the market, are not good measures of change in the familial economy or of the approach to demographic transition thresholds.

It is the internal economy and the relations of production of the peasant family that are dominant in terms of production and central in terms of demographic decision-making. The economic and social structure of the peasant family is focused on the control of familial labour and consumption. Its demography can be fully and satisfactorily explained in these terms. Why, then, have the economists and anthropologists told us so much that is marginal, while ignoring the essentials?

The major reason seems to be the sanctity of the family. Marx and his successors pointed to the existence of different modes of production, and indeed described capitalism as the last of a series of modes characterized by antagonistic relations of production and by the exploitation of man by man. Yet, Marxists preferred to recognize the peasantry either as a class exploited by landlords and rulers or as incipient capitalists. Even when actual, as well as potential, antagonisms within the Russian peasant families were

[9] For the argument that peasants are a minority, see Béteille (1974).

documented in the 1920s, these were employed merely as political evidence against the continued existence of this way of life (Kubanin, 1931). Chayanov (1966a), also employing data on the Russian peasantry, argued that there was a distinct peasant economy that could not be analysed in terms of the classical factors of production, but he always referred to the family and its labour as a unit. Sahlins, who concluded that "a material transaction is usually a momentary episode in a continuous social relation", (1972, pp. 185–186), described the domestic economy as a setting in which "decisions are taken primarily with a view toward domestic contentment. Production is geared to the family's customary requirements. Production is for the benefit of the producers" (1972, p. 77). Elsewhere, the importance of family relationships in "primitive" economies has been taken to demonstrate the dominance of social goals rather than the essence of the organization of production. Herskovits (1952) examined the family without analysing its internal forces; Polanyi concluded that "man's economy is submerged in his social relationships . . . the economic system will be run on non-economic motives" (1968, p. 7); the Thorners identified the noncapitalist nature of peasant farming but left the family as an atomistic unit: "Peasant farming . . . is inextricably woven into the fabric of peasant family life. To rip cultivation out of its family context and pretend that it is a family business, is to distort rural reality" (1962, p. 206); the women's movement also puts a gloss on the agrarian family, as shown by Mitchell: "The peasant family works together for itself—it is one. The family and production are homogeneous. . . . Under capitalism, each member of the family is supposed to be an 'individual.' . . . No wonder there are tensions" (1971, p. 157).

Redfield and Wolf, the leading anthropologists of the peasantry, exhibit somewhat contrasting approaches. The former (1960) makes few references to economic activities, and none to production. The latter, essentially economic in his approach, nevertheless equates exploitation solely with the removal of the peasant surplus production by the politically powerful, and decides that "economic relations of coercion and exploitation and the corresponding social relations of dependence and mastery are not created in the system of production" (1966, p. 3). There is a real aversion to even considering the nature of intrafamilial economic relations. Schultz treads carefully even when analysing the modern American family: "I anticipate that many sensitive, thoughtful people will be offended by these studies of fertility because they may see them as debasing family and motherhood. These highly personal activities and purposes of parents may seem to be far beyond the realm of economic calculus" (1973, pp. S2–S3).[10]

[10] See also Schultz (1974), p. 4.

The all-important internal economics of familial production has been almost entirely ignored, while great (and demographically misleading) emphasis has been placed on the marketable surplus, on the marginal production being exchanged, and on nonfamilial economic relationships (Firth, 1967; Dalton, 1971; Epstein, 1962). One can speculate that this emphasis arose because these less important economic relationships were closer to those of capitalist society; therefore they were easily recognizable, could be analysed with the techniques developed by economists to explain the capitalist economy, and gave reassuring promise that development toward a "modern" economy was inevitable. Production hardly seemed to fit into the picture, so it was conveniently forgotten, leaving economic anthropologists to concentrate largely on exchange. Another reason was that the surplus was commonly identified as the origin of civilization itself in that it supported non-farming populations (e.g. Childe, 1964, pp. 30–31).

We are not likely to be able to understand stable high fertility in agrarian societies, however, unless we analyse the peasant family in terms of the material advantages arising from production and reproduction.[11]

The Relations of Production in the Peasant Family

Many, often subtle differences in material advantage favour the old and the male in the extended family. They include consumption: the kind and amount of food eaten, precedence in feeding, the clothing customarily worn, use of house space and facilities, and access to transport. They include power and access to services: who can tell whom to do what; the right to be pampered and have the little services performed that make life graceful; the guarantee of support in argument, danger, or a bid for social or political power; and the right to make unchallenged decisions. They include labour: the amount of work done, the kind of work done, the right to control one's own working time, and access to leisure or to activities (such as bargaining) that give real pleasure.

Except when the society and economy are undergoing fundamental change, these differences in privileges and rights are accepted with little or no bitterness. This does not mean, however, that they are not recognized as conferring distinct levels of material advantage and are not valued as such.

[11] The necessity for analysing the relations of production in precapitalist societies has been pointed out by Meillassoux (1972 and 1973) but he, rather curiously, did not analyse relative advantage and the role played by the relations of production in maintaining such relativity. Instead he emphasized the priority of reproduction and of the role of male dominance in organizing female marriage and childbearing, and produced a tortuous argument explaining the power of the aged in peasant society in terms of the need of the young cultivator to be sustained through his initial season until he reaped his harvest. This may have been the influence of Lévi-Strauss. See Lévi-Strauss, (1971). Firth (1967), p. 6, confirmed precapitalist awareness of economic advantage, but identified it solely in terms of interfamilial relations, usually of the exchange type.

This is proved by the tenacity with which such rights are held and by the animosity with which the privileged react to any threats of change.

So entrenched is the system that it is difficult to find researchers from within it to evaluate the real distinctions. The usual reaction is that expressed by an observer, trained in the British school of anthropology, of a Chinese village in the 1940s: "If the father or mother eats better food, it is not because he or she has the privilege of claiming it but because the children want to favour the parent in this way. . . . It is true that women, especially young women, usually have less choice food than their men have, but the difference is by no means significant, and the women usually take it for granted" (Yang, 1948, p. 77.). Much the same description is repeatedly given in rural Bangladesh; yet these privileges, usually taken for granted, are almost certainly the major factor in raising female mortality to almost 50% above that of males for the first three decades of life (Ruzicka and Chowdhury, 1977–78). Consumption privileges begin early: in the Middle East boys are frequently weaned at twice the age of girls. It is difficult in the North Africa–South Asia region to find field workers who will agree that female household processing or preparation of food involves labour inputs comparable to those of the men in selling the surplus, let alone in ploughing the field. Usually only direct observation,[12] not report, reveals that middle-aged men spend much of their time managing or talking or drinking in the coffee shop while their sons take over the heavier field work, or that the effort mothers-in-law put into direction and management is decreasingly onerous and usually pointless since their daughters-in-law can hardly err in carrying out the usual repetitive tasks.[13] Islam, it should be noted, enjoins the young to take over the harder labour.

The task of measuring labour inputs (as well as relative consumption) should be attempted, although the results will always be unsatisfactory and debatable. Chayanov (1966b, p. 180) calculated that Russian peasant women and girls worked 1·21 times as many hours as men and boys, respectively, while Fei and Chang (1949, p. 33) calculated a similar ratio in terms of the sex division of labour inputs per acre, although the former seems to have underestimated household labour and the latter to have ignored it. Societies in which women are largely secluded or confined to the household almost invariably appear to arrange tasks so that a high proportion are undertaken in or around the house. In such societies children have two additional values: to deliver the messages and do the carrying and marketing that their mothers cannot do; and, in the case of sons, to help their fathers in the field from a very early age because the woman cannot do field work.

[12] Direct observation has been attempted in Bangladesh by several researchers: Cain (1977), Khuda (1978), Jalaluddin (in preparation) and Caldwell *et al.* (1981a).

[13] Similar work has also been undertaken in Indonesia by White and in Nepal by Peet; see Nag, Peet and White (1977).

It is probable that larger peasant families would generally be more prosperous than smaller ones even if the individuals shared production and consumption alike. Where, as is usual, the advantage lies with the old and the male, the material advantages of these decision-makers would tend to be undermined by limited fertility resulting in smaller families with a less broadbased pyramidal structure. Large families facilitate division of labour, permitting specialization and enabling the family to send off one or more members to areas of greater opportunity. The larger the family, the less often it must have recourse to paid labour, even for the heaviest, most awkward, or most labour-intensive activities. The seasonality of agricultural work is also an important consideration because it produces periods of intense labour demand occurring simultaneously on all farms;[14] the extra labour demand can be accommodated easily only by the large families who neither have to leave things undone nor pay scarcity-level wages. It also appears probable that larger numbers mean that cooperative tasks are done better, and certainly more cheerfully. Even the drudgery assumes a different air when undertaken with a son or daughter: the help is of use, the company cheering, and there is a satisfaction, and probably a value, in the training imparted. The older person may also get the younger one to do the greater share of the work, or at least the more menial and annoying tasks. "A young wife works harder than anyone else in the family and she lives more thriftily . . . she must see that her children do their share towards building up the family's economy" (Yang, 1948, p. 73.). Yang concluded from his study of a Chinese village:

> "When a son is born, even to a poor family, he is not looked upon as someone who will further divide the family's land, but as one who will add to it. When a second son is born, the parents do not worry that their small piece of land will be divided into two parts. Instead, they begin to hope that when their sons are grown up, one will be a hired labourer, another a mason, and they will earn not only their own living but add fifty dollars or so to the family every year. In two or three years, they can buy one more *mou* of land with their savings. Thus, when the parents are old, they will be better off than they are now" (1948, p. 84).

Chayanov concluded that, where there is land available, the crop, and eventually per capita consumption, rise as the family increases (1966b, pp. 67–68); and Sahlins transformed this (without pointing out that Chayanov's data and discussion were focused on the life cycle of the family) into Chayanov's Rule: "the greater the relative working capacity of the household the less its members work" (1972, p. 87).

[14] Khuda (1978) has measured seasonal labour demand in Bangladesh, showing the tendency during the peak season to exceed available labour in the average-sized household.

Whether, as most people in the region believe, highly fertile families also prosper more over time than less fertile ones is a question for which adequate longitudinal or retrospective measurement is lacking. No existing data seem to show, however, that high-fertility families are at present poorer on a per capita basis.

A key question in times of social change is how stability is maintained in productive relations (and in reproductive relations). Certainly, old men claim traditional knowledge and the traditional hallowing of their power over family members, and they claim to be either the owners or the stewards of ancestral family property.[15] Old men and women also claim to have greater knowledge of day-to-day affairs because of their long experience. They claim ultimate responsibility, and gratitude, for having arranged marriages and for having granted the precious gift of life itself. They claim, correctly, the support of religion in urging veneration for the aged and obeisance to them, and they sometimes claim to be closer to the ancestors. Similarly, with regard to male domination over females, claims to ownership of land and residence and to control over the means of production are important. The greater physical strength of males and the relative vulnerability of females because of parturition also play a role. So—and this is demographically important—does the fact that wives in the region are usually much younger than husbands and have traditionally married very young. This has been reinforced both by arranged marriage, whereby the wife's duty not to rebel is a duty she owes to her own relatives as well as to her husband's, and by patrilocality, whereby the wife is cut off from any support her own relatives might have offered.

Nevertheless, these observations are insufficient to explain why the young and strong do not revolt or why women fail to band together to protect themselves from exploitation (including reproductive exploitation). Socialization from infancy to conform to the traditional roles, and reinforcement of these roles by Moslem and Hindu family teachings, are of course part of the explanation.[16] So is the fact that a break with relatives can mean social ostracism and economic impotence, the latter determined also by civil laws governing inheritance and land tenure. Yet there are other factors of great importance. One is the life cycle element in all familial modes of production: if one bears one's present situation a little longer, then the system that has been oppressive can yield rewards instead. Sons become fathers and daughters-in-law mothers-in-law. Perhaps the most effective stabilizer is peer rivalry. Just how badly the outside observer can misinterpret the stabilizing influence of rivalry is shown by Wolf's treatment of tensions

[15] Veneration for the aged will be investigated by the author in a study, "The reversal of the veneration flow: The true context of the reversal of the intergenerational wealth flow".

[16] The same teachings are deeply embedded in traditional Chinese culture and can be found in gentler versions in Buddhism and Christianity.

within the extended family (1966, p. 68). He regards as signs of family weakness quarrels between women, which in fact strengthen male authority, and those between siblings, which powerfully buttress parental control. The unequal and difficult relationship between mother-in-law and daughter-in-law is probably the single most significant element in the subjection of women, as is the rivalry between brothers in preventing them from competing with fathers. This rivalry and indeed most forms of rivalry are powerfully supported by high fertility. More generally, age and sex dominance are fostered by assigning great importance to age gradations and to the specialization of occupational, consumption, and ceremonial patterns by age and sex; hence the stress that traditional societies lay not merely on such relationships as being "brothers" but on being "senior brothers" or "junior brothers." The larger the family, the more apparent and effective are these distinctions and gradations.

The Demographic Aspects of the Peasant Family

For the purposes of this chapter, this essentially economic analysis of the extended family is of interest only in the sense that it determines the demographic nature of the family. Indeed, this nature cannot be understood without the economic analysis. Several demographic aspects should be separately considered.

The most basic matter is that of demographic priorities, an area that existing literature shows to be almost universally misunderstood. The peasant family does not aim at reproducing as quickly as possible, with generations following close upon each other and the number of relatives within the household being maximized. If such were the case, then sons would marry at puberty or the family would be matrilocal. The truth is very different. Priority is given to preserving the structure of discipline and work within the family. Daughters in the North Africa–South Asia–China region are married out,[17] so that the generational structure of the family depends upon the marriage age of sons. In the Middle East, men usually marry for the first time after 25 years of age (United Nations, 1978), and male marriage elsewhere in South and East Asia has not traditionally been early. The major aim has been to retain a five-to-ten-year age gap between spouses, which, together with patrilocality, has ensured male dominance. The price, in terms of reproduction within the household, has been considerable. If the wife begins childbearing when the husband is around 25 years of age, the average length of generation *within* the household is about 36 years—an extraordinary period in countries where life expectancy at

[17] All these societies are patrilocal, so traditionally the bride moved into the house of the bridegroom's family. In Islamic areas, however, and especially in the Arab Middle East, the practice of endogamy means that the bride is not likely to leave her particular locality; indeed parallel-cousin and other kin marriages may mean that she does not leave the household.

birth is still often no more than 50 years (and was much less a few decades ago).

As soon as the young bride enters the household, there is much interest in her reproduction. Her husband may be 25 years old, and his father will probably be between 50 and 75, depending on whether the husband was the first or last child. The old couple will urge the young couple to have many children as soon as possible: if young children mean work, that work will no longer fall upon the old people's shoulders; if somewhat older children run messages and do services, that is precisely the help the old prize. In the traditional family, the young have little option but to be fertile. Even for them there are advantages. Only by bearing children can the young wife establish her position, work a little less hard, enjoy a somewhat larger share of food and other consumption items, and, ultimately, achieve a major breakthrough with regard to all these matters by becoming a mother-in-law. The young husband can have helpers in the field within 10 or 12 years and can shift some of the harder work off his shoulders by the time he is 40 years of age.

Several aspects of the continuous supply of children are important. A frequent pattern—perhaps the anticipated pattern—is that when a husband and wife become the major decision-makers of the family (through the death of the husband's father), the supply of adolescents will be a major factor in easing their lives. Thereafter, those who live most comfortably will be the parents who have a continuing supply of children of both sexes growing up; to meet the need of having persons of different ages to do the age-specific tasks, to engender sibling competition in providing labour during their parents' maturity and comprehensive aid during their decline, and to supply successive new daughters-in-law, who probably work harder than anyone else. Descendants are the most valued protection that a couple can have against destitution in old age. Throughout the region this consideration is paramount; the fear of land fragmentation appears everywhere to be minimal (perhaps, in part, because there is a growing nonagricultural labour market). Where land is not divided until the old die, they seem, in most societies, to be more interested in advantages during their lifetimes than in any disadvantages to their descendants. Fear of land subdivision seems to be an obsession only of western observers.[18]

From the point of view of the decision-makers, probably the most important aspect of high fertility is that it stabilizes the family. It keeps it in the expected mould. Daughters-in-law with many children will be forced to undertake the work women have always done and will need to fit themselves

[18] The actual position is more complex in many developing societies. Those without sufficient sons fear losing land to others through physical duress (see Cain, 1978). This conclusion is also borne out by work undertaken in another rural area of Bangladesh by A. K. M. Jalaluddin (in preparation).

and their progeny into the framework of the larger family. Sons with many siblings can hardly revolt if there are rivals for the inheritance. Numerous grandchildren may provide an extra source of security to whom direct appeal can be made if children are found wanting.

Decision-Making and Fertility Control

While the economic structure of the peasant family holds, fertility everywhere in the region remains high and contraception is rarely practised. There has been a tendency in some population studies to overstress traditional contraception and to imply that practices that were occasionally employed to prevent socially unacceptable conceptions or to avoid pregnancy during a subsistence crisis were also used to limit ultimate family size. The evidence for the latter contention is poor everywhere in Asia and Africa and almost nonexistent in the regions concentrated upon here.

This lack of fertility control within marriage has often been taken to be a sign of ignorance of contraception or of easy acceptance of the inevitable. There is little to support this view: high fertility is valued, especially among the decision-makers, often as a central aim of societies throughout the peasant cultures of the region. Not only are fertility decisions made, but they are stronger and occasion fewer misgivings than in most low-fertility societies. They merely happen to be for high fertility and against contraception and are undetectable in terms of trends and differentials because they maintain past patterns. It is this maintenance that gives the traditional decision-makers such strength; they could not as easily lead a fertility or contraceptive innovational trend among the younger generation.

Who are the reproductive decision-makers? Usually, they are the old, especially males. Reproductive decisions are not really separable from economic decisions, because the reproductive pattern is needed to support the economic one and to maintain the existing gradations of material advantage within the family. The patriarch, because of his ownership or stewardship of the means of production, is almost unchallenged in economic decision-making. His control of reproductive decision-making is less direct and potentially less certain, but, traditionally, the economic power has provided him with sufficient reproductive control.

This patriarchal control is more one of situation than of personality. Peasant society abounds with scandals about families in which the wife has too much say or the elder son really makes decisions; but these family members are usually powerful only if they support the traditional situation, indeed if they exhort a weak or backsliding patriarch to fulfill his duties. An attempt at economic or reproductive decision-making innovation by the patriarch's wife would probably be countered by the eldest son, or all the sons, chiding their father. A like attempt by an eldest son would probably confront a coalition of his brothers and mother. Few adequate studies of the situation have been made; such studies as exist suggest that encroachments on patriarchal power are highly exceptional.[19] This is not to deny that, even in many patriarchal societies, exhortations to reproductive conformity are made more often by the patriarch's wife to their sons and daughters-in-law, but nearly always within the moral framework approved by her husband.

Perhaps the most important question is why these decisions are obeyed. Certainly the economic power of the patriarch, the family's ability to ostracize and disinherit a son, and the possibility of forcing a divorce against a daughter-in-law are all important. Nevertheless, the strongest control against deviance in peasant society is talk—scandal-mongering, ridicule, and stronger expressions of derision and even anger and disgust—and, less often, violence. In the area of economic decision-making the villagers watch for the weak father, the overmighty son, and the disrespectful or lazy daughter-in-law; they all feel threatened by continuing behaviour of this type. In the area of fertility decision-making such vigilance is even stronger because deviation and indiscretion trespass on sensitive areas where instincts or emotions have long been suppressed. Contraception is highly suspect both because of its likely impact on fertility and because of its implications about the wife's attitude toward sexual relations; over much of the region, even involuntary infecundity or subfecundity is taken to be a personal failing justifying contempt and divorce or polygyny.

Just as the peasant family structure has long formed the pattern for many nonpeasant segments of the society—the landless labourers and wage earners, the artisans, the urban commercial classes, even traditional rulers and other nonmodern elites—so the peasant pattern of decision-making, and society's backing for these decisions, have operated in a similar fashion among these other groups.

Economic and Demographic Transition

Modes of production do not just replace each other; they usually coexist for long periods, and individuals, families, and tribes may participate in more than one system at a time.

Precapitalist modes of production other than the peasant mode include shifting cultivation, hunting and gathering, and nomadism. Although the basic units in these modes are generally networks of relatives, they usually

[19] Kubanin (1931), pp. 108–109 reported that, in early twentieth-century Russia, neither long-term nor day-to-day economic decisions were ever made against the wishes of the family head, and that the head heeded advice in only 8% and 42% of households, respectively, in these two types of decisions. Indeed, he had punitive powers over all members of the household in two-thirds of families and over all children in five-sixths.

involve economic and decision-making groupings larger than the family. In many of these groups, children are considered to belong to the group rather than to the individual parents. Further, net intergenerational wealth flows are less specifically directed from children to parents than from younger to older generation in general. Little research has been conducted comparing economic–fertility relationships in these societies with those in peasant societies, but one may speculate that the pressures for high fertility would be significantly lower in them than in the smaller units of the peasant family.

From the point of view of a demographer interested in fertility decline, the transition of most importance is that from familial to capitalist production. This transition is the most complex both economically and demographically—so complex that it has been largely misunderstood—in that it is the only transition from familial to nonfamilial production.

The term capitalist production has been used throughout this chapter instead of industrialization or modern economy or highly developed economy, because it is contended that the real reproductive divide lies between modes of production based largely on networks of relatives and those in which the individuals may sell their labour to complete strangers.[20] It is not factories and steel mills that count in the reduction of fertility; it is the replacement of a system in which material advantage accruing from production and reproduction flows to people who can control or influence reproduction by a system in which those with economic power either gain no advantage from reproduction or cannot control it. This usually occurs only with the collapse of familial production, although it can follow fundamental changes in the balance of material advantage and decision-making within the family.

The transformation from familial to capitalist production is a process rather than a sudden change. What is formed first and is sustained for long periods of time is a two-tiered system in which the two forms of economies coexist. To learn something of the nature of the transition and its implications for fertility, one can look to the historical experience of Western Europe.

Economic and Demographic Transition in the West

Capitalist production as the dominant form of production outside the home first developed in Europe, where there is some evidence that the residential joint family, and even the extended family of mutual obligations, was already collapsing, perhaps because of direct productive relations between

---

[20] Familial production may be found in the area of money and large-scale production: for instance, where a whole family act as a firm or as the employers in a firm, or where some members of a peasant family offer their labour for wages without really leaving the traditional family (in that they funnel some or all of their money to it and receive guarantees and other benefits in return).

the feudal lords and the male heads of conjugal families. Certainly, under capitalism, the ability of the husband to secure employment with adequate remuneration outside the family was decisive in the erosion of the extended family. At the early stages, however, only the husband participated in the capitalist mode of production; services within the house were provided on a subsistence basis by a familial mode of production not very different from that found in the peasant household.

To understand the nature of the supports for high fertility and of fertility decline where it has occurred, it is necessary to analyse this two-tiered system correctly. The failure to do so is, once again, primarily an unwillingness to disturb the mystique of the family. The familial system in the West depended on a sharp division of labour: the husband worked outside the home for wages or profits and almost all his input of labour was into these activities, while a wide range of activities (clothing, feeding, providing a clean and comfortable environment, child rearing) was undertaken by the wife with the help of the children (especially the daughters). In effect, then, the husband ran his own highly efficient family-based subsistence system for producing services. Fundamentally, this was a second (and at least equally important) mode of production in the society; the relations of production in the first mode were between employer and employee, but in this second mode they were between a husband and his wife and children.[21]

Originally this familial mode of production worked cheaply and well (at least from the husband's viewpoint). The cheapness was achieved by the women and children consuming less than the husband. Very real differentials in material advantage were maintained by emphasizing the importance of the husband's work compared with the familial production, by distinguishing between productive and domestic work and between paid and unpaid work, and by stressing that husbands had to have a certain standard of dress and of living to hold their jobs and that they deserved to spend some of their earnings on themselves outside the home. This discrimination between men's and women's work had another effect. Many women (and, especially early in the Industrial Revolution, children) had always worked outside the home. However, the prevailing attitudes allowed women to be paid much less than adult males, and allowed society, their employers, and

[21] Some women's-movement and Marxist writers have failed to identify these relations of production because of their desire to indict the capitalist system for exploiting the family as a whole or for maintaining a reserve army of female labour. This is less true in the case of Benston (1969) and Morton (1970) but is generally true of Mitchell (1971) and Zaretsky (1976), although the last focuses more on historical understanding. Some writers lay stress on the eternal male achievement of material advantage rather than on the domestic mode of production under capitalism—for example, Firestone (1971) and Figes (1970). The women's-movement classics also place emphasis on the achievement and maintenance of male advantage, not always even material advantage—for example, de Beauvoir (1972) and Millett (1971).

the women themselves to regard their work as marginal and "temporary", even when the work continued for years.[22]

Demographically, this two-tiered mode of production can sustain high or moderately high fertility.[23] As long as children consume relatively little and boys start earning early (and even contribute to the family budget), then high fertility is no disadvantage. This is especially the case under two conditions: first, where the wife and children can offer a great range of household productive services without effective competition from the market; second, where the wife is uneducated or little educated, where she is not affected by ideologies urging her to demand a greater place in the sun, and where she accepts her place in the household with its implications for low consumption, hard work, and responsibility for keeping child-care problems away from her husband. This is the explanation for high fertility among the urban middle class in much of the developing world,[24] as it was in mid-nineteenth-century Europe.

When this two-tiered mode of production is at its height, large family size remains desirable. Yet, the two-tiered mode of production was inherently unstable in Western Europe for a number of reasons. It depended on competing successfully with capitalist production in the provision of household services, on wives and children remaining hardworking producers and low-level consumers, on economic and fertility decision-making remaining largely with the male household head, and on household production being augmented more by women's activities in the home than by services purchased with their outside earnings. All these conditions were to be challenged by the spectacular growth in capitalist production and by ideological change, rooted in the society but fuelled by economic growth.[25]

[22] This was the exact counterpart to the outside work done by the younger members of the peasant family, even down to the handing over of most of the earnings without thereby achieving a major role in economic (or, usually, reproductive) decision-making.

[23] It cannot as easily sustain early age at marriage. As I have argued elsewhere, the increasingly accepted requirement that a man have a secure job and savings before embarking on marriage led to widespread postponement of marriage in nineteenth-century Europe. Rising age at marriage moderated fertility levels in Europe prior to the major period of demographic transition, but there is little evidence that—as others have claimed—this was its intent. Contemporary evidence suggests it was the rising cost of marriage not the rising cost of children that led to marriage postponement. By postponing marriage, a man built up the necessary savings to capitalize the domestic system of production he would create by marriage (See Chapter 6).

[24] *Note:* Caldwell and Caldwell (1978), in which the stability of high fertility in the Ibadan middle class is documented, together with the nature of the very small number of families in which fertility had been restricted.

[25] Fertility in Western Europe has been shown to have remained high in those areas where the censuses reported the most use of family labour. See Lesthaeghe and Wilson (1978). Lesthaeghe has subsequently pointed out in a private communication that evidence of this kind remains least satisfactory for France and that perhaps the most severe test for the approach presented in this paper will be provided by the analysis of changes in family authority and decision-making patterns and in the nature of the family economy and family production in that country.

Probably the decisive change in Western Europe was a fairly sudden rise in the cost of children and a decline in their labour inputs into household production. The major cause was the spread of education, together with a rise in its duration and cost. This was a product partly of the needs of the industrial system and partly of public awareness that the economy would now bear the cost. School children needed and demanded more expenditure, had less time for household chores, and were more resistant to working—the phenomenon is currently visible throughout the developing world (Caldwell, 1968a, pp. 96–114, esp. pp. 104–110). Growing parental wealth and the waning influence of religious creeds proclaiming virtue in child austerity and child labour reinforced the tendency to spend more on children and demand less from them. Consequently the net intergenerational flow of wealth changed direction from upward to downward.

At much the same time, the industrial system began a massive onslaught on home production, by offering commodities in the market that had been made at home, by offering gadgets that reduced domestic labour inputs, and by tempting the family to raise its capital input into the home. As consumption aspirations rose, the kinds of services that could be performed by dependent members of the family were devalued compared with purchased commodities. Subsistence production declined and the monetized sector of the economy expanded.

There was another source of basic instability in the system: the egalitarian strain in the modern European ideology, powerfully augmented by the spread of education. Girls were educated too (although usually not as much as boys), partly because of the demands of the egalitarian ethic, but partly because educated husbands want to talk to educated wives (an important destabilizing influence in the contemporary Middle East and South Asia) and educated fathers want to talk to educated daughters. Both consumption and decision-making became more democratic. The sex differential in wages narrowed, and married women gained greater acceptance in the workforce (as the more highly capitalized economy increasingly demanded their labour). In the family, the impact of pregnancy or motherhood on the wife began to be taken into account in reproductive decisions. As the wife's income became more important, the reproductive decision became a significant immediate economic decision as well as a long-term one. The fall in fertility was also partly the product of the continuing contraceptive revolution—one of familiarization with a different conjugal relationship as much as changing technology, and one that itself both was a product of changes in family relations and accelerated those changes.

The fall in fertility was protracted as the familial subsistence mode of production, although ever more eroded, showed remarkable resistance to extinction or even to becoming insignificant.[26]

The Conditions of Fertility Change: The Developing World

Fertility in the developing world will decline as the decision-makers no longer secure decisive material advantage from high fertility—which means changes both in the identity and authority of those gaining material advantage and making decisions and in the way in which fertility affects material advantage. These changes will be a product of economic change—of capitalist production outpacing even industrialization—and of largely imported social change (broadly speaking, westernization).[27]

In the modern world the peasant familial system of production is not stable. Wage employment is increasing and the young family member who takes up employment is ever more likely to receive sufficient income to support a separate conjugal family. Urban populations are growing disproportionately. The economic underpinning of the patriarchal joint family in urban areas has never been secure, and has been increasingly susceptible to disintegration with economic and social change. In rural areas, both pressure on the land and government land-redistribution schemes tend to disperse the patriarchal family and so to remove young couples from patriarchal authority, leading to more diffusion of economic and fertility decision-making. Ultimately the changeover to capitalist or socialist production will terminate the economic system that benefits from high fertility.

Nevertheless, it is social and ideological change that is likely to have the greatest immediate impact. In most of the developing world the familial production of household services and the authority of the family head are even more stably based than was the case in nineteenth-century Europe. However, existing differentials in advantage by age and sex are under attack from the same forces that brought change in nineteenth-century Europe: education of children, relative rise in the position of females,[28] and the lure

[26] These issues are touched upon in Hartmann (1976). Hartmann does not discuss the domestic mode of production in modern industrial society as the most efficient method of producing such goods and services from the standpoint of the chief decision-maker, the male household head. She focuses on the period before the market begins an increasingly successful attempt to compete in producing these goods and services.

[27] It can be argued that labour is of paramount value and its control of surpassing importance in economies with very low levels of technology and hence of capital inputs into farming, and that the necessary condition for both economic and demographic change, as well as increased market orientation, is technological advance in farming. In terms of the timing of demographic change, it is doubtful whether this is the case. In India, technological change has been greater in Punjab and social change in Kerala; the demographic breakthrough occurred in the latter. Even the move from subsistence to capitalistic farming is often more related to the appearance of a market for the product than to a change in technology; this was certainly the case in the Central Plain of Thailand from the 1870s, when the Southeast Asian rice market developed, and the extra production was achieved at first by greater family labour inputs under patriarchal direction. See Caldwell (1967b), p. 28.

[28] In both western and Middle Eastern Mediterranean families, the different interests of women have been identified as having the greatest potential of any factor for destroying the patriarchal family and its political, economic, and demographic structure. See Peristiany, (1976), p. 2.

of household consumption goods. The original position was more stable than in Europe, but the attack is stronger too, largely because of the European example and because of the development of a global economy and global ideologies. The messages from the media and educational systems are largely western and tend to teach age and sex equality. So do the new ideologies both of the left and of those stressing modern capitalism. Furthermore, the discussion of sexual relations and contraception is increasingly legitimized by essentially western influence. This, and the availability of contraceptives, may well make the initial fertility decline more rapid than in the West. The very discussion of contraception and reproductive decisions almost certainly does something to lessen sex differentials and hence male material advantage. This is probably also true in terms of the publicizing of the pleasures of sexual relations. As the conjugal bond becomes closer, or more sentimental, and as the mother's maternal feelings play a greater role in family decision-making, the sex and age differentials in material advantage are likely to be increasingly eroded.

Summary

The essence of all precapitalist modes of production was kin-based production, and the relations of production were those between relatives. These relations were unequal and gave material advantage to the elders. Thus high fertility yielded economic advantage. But high fertility was not the sole demographic aim of the family decision-makers; the stability of the relations of production was more important, because continuing material advantage was most important.

A complete capitalist mode of production makes high fertility economically disadvantageous. But long after capitalist production is general in a society, household services continue to be produced by a precapitalist, familial mode of production, which may involve the majority of all labour inputs in the society. It was the persistence of this mode of production, and the unequal relations of production within it, that buttressed moderately high fertility in Europe until a century ago.

Fertility ultimately fell in the West when the pattern of material advantage, and hence the net intergenerational wealth flow, decisively changed within the household mode of production—a result of social change made possible by economic change. Fertility has continued to fall as that pattern has continued to shift.

In high-fertility societies, further economic change will inevitably produce this two-tiered mode of production. Economic and social change will ultimately make high fertility uneconomic in the working of both tiers, a process that will occur faster than in the West because of the import of ideas, ideologies, and educational systems (and child labour laws) that reduce age and sex differentials in material advantage and ultimately make high fertility uneconomic.

Social scientists feel compelled to prove what members of different societies know to be the indisputable truth: high fertility in an advanced capitalist society (especially one in which the domestic mode of production has been curtailed because a large proportion of household needs are provided by the market) reduces a family's potential standard of living, while in a peasant society it does not.

This chapter was reprinted with the permission of The Population Council from John C. Caldwell, "A theory of fertility: From high plateau to destabilization," *Population and Development Review* **4**, no. 4 (December 1978): 553–577.

D

Testing the Theory in Historical Context

Co-authored with L. T. Ruzicka

6

The Australian fertility transition: an analysis

The rationale for a consideration of Australian fertility trends lies not in their uniqueness but, rather, in the extraordinary similarity between the course of birth rates in Australia and the United States (Coale and Zelnik, 1963, pp. 27–31; Jones, 1971), and the similarity between the fertility of these two societies over time and those of Britain, New Zealand, and English-speaking Canada. The diffusion of fertility control practices within single-language groups has been noted elsewhere (Coale, 1973, pp. 62–63), but perhaps its most intriguing manifestation has been that within English-language populations around the world.

As a preliminary to consideration of Australian trends, it is important, then, to observe differences between Australia, Britain, and the United States. The most striking is that of population size. Australia still has only about 14 million inhabitants, who constitute around 5% of the English-speaking world, or much the same proportion as do the people of Texas or Illinois in the United States. The white population numbered no more than a quarter of a million before the gold rushes of the 1850s, rising from 1·25 million in the early 1860s to 2·25 million in the early 1880s, and reaching 3·75 million by the turn of the century. In the critical years of the 1860s and 1870s when fertility first began to fall, this was essentially an immigrant population; less than half of all adults were native-born as late as 1891, compared with five-sixths in America at the time and nearly the whole population in Britain. If attention is concentrated on the mid-years of the second half of the nineteenth century, then the contrasts become even clearer. Australia's low rainfall and its settlement after the beginning of the industrial revolution had produced a commercial agricultural system, dominated by livestock raising, with hardly any subsistence production or traditional village life. By 1881, only 28% of the workforce was employed in agriculture, a level attained by England and Wales in 1821 and reached by America only during World War I. By world and even European, standards, the population was highly urbanized; in 1881 one-fifth lived in centres with more than 100 000 inhabitants, the level found in England and Wales in 1840 and the United States in 1910. Nor, by the standards of the time, were these poor immigrant peoples. Gold and wool underpinned an economy that continued to boom for four decades from 1850 to 1890 and was expected, as is clear from contemporary testimony, to continue unfalteringly. At the end of this period, per capita incomes were probably the world's highest, perhaps an eighth above those in the United States and double the level in Britain (Clark (1951), pp. 140–141; Kuznets (1956). See also Butlin, (1964) and (1970), pp. 266–327). A complex of factors, including the living standard, dispersion of population that reduced the transmission of infectious disease, and perhaps the mild climate, yielded an expectation of life at birth that was consistently about five years greater than that of England and Wales.

Australia provides a suitable laboratory for examining the stages of demographic transition from high to low fertility and for testing various central assumptions in transition theory. From the time of the earliest European settlements in the eighteenth century, demographic statistics for Australia are good, at least for the population of European descent, who now make up over 98% of the total.[1] The available data throw new light on a range of fertility-change theories. They allow us to examine the population of the third quarter of the nineteenth century to see if it was in a condition of fertility equilibrium intermediate between the "first European demographic transition" (the transition to later age at marriage) and the "second transition" (to lower marital fertility).[2] We can test the proposition that net wealth flows from parents to children in pretransition societies are too small to affect demographic behaviour.[3] It is also possible to present evidence bearing on theories based on threshold hypotheses[4] and diffusion mechanisms,[5] as well as a range of explanations put forward by economists and depending heavily on fertility differentials and changes over time.[6] Finally,

[1] Repeated and comprehensive population counts were initiated partly because of the origin of this population, from 1788 a penal settlement, becoming a more broadly based group of colonies but continuing to be under the scrutiny of paternal official eyes; and subsequently they were maintained because of the interest in growth and development that was sustained from 1851 onward with self-government in most of these colonies. In addition to recent analyses of these data, there exists a considerable body of information on fertility control practices and an increasing volume of material drawn from historical records and literature on social change paralleling demographic movements.

[2] The notion of two demographic transitions is elaborated in Coale (1973), p. 57.

[3] This proposition was set forth in Chapter 4. The author argued there that in primitive and traditional societies the "net intergenerational flow of wealth" (i.e., the flow of wealth in money, goods, and services between parents and children) is from children to parents. In transitional societies, the direction of this flow reverses, and fertility limitation is a rational response to the change in the impact of children.

[4] The threshold hypothesis argues that only above some minimum educational level (or income level, or level of other socioeconomic indications) will women reduce their family size; and above this threshold, any improvement in the particular indicator will elicit a fertility response.

[5] On the hypothesis that fertility limitation is largely a matter of cultural diffusion within cultural areas, see Coale, 1973.

[6] Representative works in the microeconomics of fertility include: Becker (1960) and Easterlin (1969).

the explanation of fertility decline in terms of increasingly improved contraceptive performance, in contrast to fluctuating family size ideals, can be tested with some precision.[7]

Five propositions emerge from this examination and are put forward as contributing to an explanation of fertility transition in Australia and, by extension, in the West as a whole.

1. Until the late nineteenth century, marriage postponement was due primarily to a determination to establish the family on a sound economic footing, as was popularly claimed, and not, as social science analysts are often inclined to infer, to limit fertility.

2. In the second half of the nineteenth century, a radical change occurred in parent–child economic relationships, associated primarily with the erection of mass education systems but also with secularization and an accompanying democratization of emotional and economic relationships within the family.

3. Contraception has been increasingly effective and has not been subject to major fluctuations in either purpose or application.

4. The explanation of fertility transition is essentially a historical one with one stage necessarily preceding and helping to cause the next.

5. Fertility differentials, once they are viewed in terms of (a) differential incidence of marriage, arising from causes other than the desire to control completed family size, and (b) differential incidence at any specific time of ability to practice contraception, are of little significance in explaining fertility transition although they do illuminate the historical process of fertility change. The differentials do not demand economic explanations for their existence.

These propositions provide the conceptual framework for this paper, although a detailed examination will require some zigzagging from attention to the nature of the society in various periods to fertility trends between these periods.

The First Demographic Transition: Marriage Postponement

The first proposition above, relating to marriage postponement, arises from an examination of Australian society during the third quarter of the nineteenth century. At the start of the period, the society was characterized by nearly universal female marriage and high fertility within marriage; female age at marriage rose persistently over the period. The traditional explanation for this pattern, stemming from Malthus and more recently Goode (1963b)[8] is that in the frontier conditions that characterized the start

[7] For two opposing views on this issue, see Ryder (1973) and Blake and Das Gupta (1975).

[8] Malthus so intertwined his case for reducing population growth with his advocacy of a proper moral restraint that it has been only too easy to assume that deferred European marriage was primarily intended as a check on family size. An examination of the Australian experience suggests this assumption should be reconsidered.

of the period, children were not much of a burden and may even have been productive; thus there was no need to defer marriage to limit childbearing as was the case in "more developed" European countries. As Australia became increasingly modernized, this argument goes on, children became increasingly costly, and marriage was deferred to limit family size. A closer look at fertility and marital trends and at contemporary commentary does not support this argument.

Marital and Fertility Trends in the 1850s–70s

The fertility of Australian women in this period was high, probably above that of their British forebears in the preceding two centuries (Hajnal, 1965). In 1860, although females made up only three-sevenths of the population, the birth rate was 43 per thousand population per year Australia. Commonwealth Bureau of Census and Statistics 1928 and 1947. Retrospective evidence suggests that those women who bore most of their children during the 1850s, 1860s, and 1870s averaged at least seven live births; those who married under 16 years of age and survived to 1911 averaged ten births.

The very high level of fertility in mid-nineteenth century Australia was the consequence of nearly universal and relatively early female marriage.[9] Whereas in Britain, during the second half of the nineteenth century, at least 70% of women 20–24 years of age remained unmarried, in Australia the proportion was little over 33% in the 1850s, 50% in the late 1860s, and 66% by the late 1880s. This pattern reflected the great shortage of marriageable women resulting from the preponderance of single males in the population: the proportion of single males was far above that found in Britain until the end of the century, averaging in the third quarter of the century about 60% at 25–29 years of age.

Female age at marriage rose persistently through the 1850s, 1860s, and 1870s. Yet postponement of marriage in Australia in the third quarter of the century does not seem to have been instigated to check family size. Not only did marital fertility rise by 7% between 1861 and 1881,[10] but contemporaries did not express any belief until near the end of that period that parents had any difficulties in Australian conditions in supporting a large family. Contemporary references, in literature, in the press, and in reminiscences, make it quite clear that marriage was deferred because of the costs inherent in marriage itself. In conditions where women were in very limited supply and where also the demand for personal services far exceeded what was

[9] Marriage data throughout the paper are largely drawn from McDonald (1975).

[10] This rise may have been no more than an automatic reaction to steep falls in the proportions married in the main reproductive ages in a society where the first period after marriage exhibited unusually high age-specific birth rates, partly because the number of pregnant brides was considerable and partly because very few women gave birth shortly before marriage.

available, wives were needed not only for sexual relations but also to maintain any kind of domestic unit; and on the farms they were nearly indispensable in a wide range of activities.

For men, society rewarded establishment in an occupation, attained through long hours of work when young and attention to matters such as dress. Marriage meant extra expenditure, especially extra initial expenditure. Because the population contained so many young adult immigrants, marriage required the immediate establishment of a new household in a much higher proportion of cases than at that time in Britain, where young couples commonly lived for a time with parents. There was a "proper time to marry," and it meant precisely what the expression says and was not a euphemism for the proper time to reproduce. Deferred marriage meant smaller families, but that does not seem to have been the purpose of the deferment, and, at least until the end of the third quarter of the century, lower fertility apparently was not planned or even probably economically beneficial.[11]

Economic Impact of Fertility

Because marriage postponement in the first stage of the European demographic transition has so persistently been interpreted as a response to the rising costs of children, it is important in the case of Australia in the comparable stage of transition to examine why high fertility was not economically disadvantageous. Up to and throughout the third quarter of the century, it is clear, with the exception perhaps of farmers, that the general opinion was not that fortunes increased with family size, but rather that there was little relationship between the two. The reason was neither that individuals had not yet fully developed a modern sense of economic rationality nor that they did not apply it to the family. Australia was a land of immigrants who had come to make their fortunes and who had a strong sense of economic advantage about all their concerns. The modern reader of the preserved letters of a century or more ago often flinches at the careful cost-accounting attitude and the sense of getting ahead. Nor was it that the society was largely agrarian. There were no peasant farms, and, throughout the period, employment in farming and livestock raising remained constant at only 30% of the workforce.[12] The solution to the problem lies in a consideration of the cost of raising children, children's work, the services they provided, and the alternative possibilities for parental expenditure.

[11] Evidence of contemporary comment here and elsewhere in the paper is drawn from an unpublished file compiled by Pat Caldwell, of population references in the *Sydney Herald* and *Sydney Morning Herald* during the nineteenth century and from references in contemporary literature. The evidence on this point is necessarily mostly negative; the complaints about the burden of large families that appear from the 1880s were not expressed earlier. Prior to the 1880s, distressed families seem commonly to have been families in which the male head was deceased or incapacitated.

[12] It fell slowly to 26% at the end of the century. See Butlin (1964) p. 194; Ford (1970), p. 91.

An examination of the records of life of a century or more ago suggests repeatedly that the important element in the economic valuation of children was the cheapness of their keep. Clothes were handmade by mothers, aunts, and elder sisters. Most children had a pair of shoes, but they were often "Sunday best" and, until the end of the century, bare feet were more common than shod ones. Food was essentially free on farms. Elsewhere it tended to be simple and of the type that was made in quantity so that an extra plate made little difference in the quantities thrown into the pot. Apart from meat, which (especially mutton) was cheap until the end of the century, and eggs, which were usually home produced, meals were dominated by porridge, potatoes, bread and jam (or the cheaper golden syrup, which was a by-product of cane sugar refining). Cakes and bread were baked at home. A description of the home of a carpenter around 1880 makes the point that he was well housed compared with his fellow tradesmen who did not migrate from Britain, but goes on to describe the house as containing, in addition to the kitchen, a room shared by the two youngest children with the carpenter and his wife, and an adjacent small room for the four older children (Twopeny, 1973, p. 46). Children rarely saw doctors or dentists.

Contemporary reports do not regard these conditions as implying great poverty. Nor do they regard it as invidious that the children of even moderately well-off parents lived a frugal life. It was looked upon as "good for them" and as an essential part of their upbringing; anything more would have amounted to "spoiling them." Neither children nor their parents believed that the former should have parity with the latter in consumption or pleasures or even that such a comparison should be made.

Assessing the value of children's work is a more complex matter, and, until near the end of the century, statistics are rare. Clearly children and wives worked endlessly on the farms, and investigations of rural fertility must try to determine why fertility came down as soon as it did. In the towns the balance between breadwinners and nonearning dependents was less clear. Until the early 1890s any boy could earn money for skilled or semi-skilled work, and the abundance of such work was often quoted to explain the native-borns' disdain for apprenticeship (Fry, 1956, vol. 1, pp. 388–389). Those who did earn contributed fairly generously to the household. With sons tending to stay home until marriage, in a society in which only a minority of males were married at 25–29 years of age, families often had several wage earners. The household provided most of its own services, and, except among the very well-off, both daughters and mothers did the chores.

Many school children, apparently the great majority of working-class boys, earned some money outside school hours. Furthermore, even in the mid–1880s, daily school attendance averaged only about 60% of enrollments and absences soared, particularly in rural areas, during peak periods of labour demand. From around 1880, with the spread of factories, many women, listed as dependents, took in outwork, especially from the textile and leather industries, and distributed work to their children whether they went to school or not (Fry, 1956, pp. 121–150; Cannon, 1975).

This system in which children were raised frugally and expected to contribute to the financial support of the household remained stable throughout the third quarter of the century. The culture was saturated with strong views on the morality of a strict and frugal upbringing for children, a morality that had strong religious sanctions. A major component of the explanation of subsequent fertility transition may well lie in the decline of an ethic that expected children to work hard, contribute to the household, and demand little. In modern Australia children are expensive: a greater share of income is spent on them, and they contribute less in money and services to the household. Historical demographers have thought of declining religion and growing secularism as making parents more aware of the possibility of controlling their own familial economic destinies. It may well be that a much more important effect was the undermining of a morality that kept children in their place, and a relatively cheap place at that.

Early Stages of the Second Demographic Transition

Our second proposition is that in the second half of the nineteenth century a radical change occurred in parent–child relationships and that this change was a primary factor in the onset of fertility decline.

Timing and Nature of Fertility Decline

Overall fertility declined continuously in Australia during the second half of the nineteenth century. A reduction in the proportion of the reproductive span that females spent in marriage between 1861 and 1901 was responsible for three-fifths of the total fall in fertility during that period; however, the portentous change was the beginning of a sustained decline in the fertility of married women from the 1880s.[13] Taking the 1881

---

[13] Two major sources of statistical data can be used for timing the fertility change: the censuses held in the first year of each decade until 1921, and the annual numbers of births registered. These exist in the form of colonial censuses until 1891 in the six colonies; state censuses in 1901 in the six states; Commonwealth of Australia censuses from 1911 including cross-tabulations of the parity of married women by age in 1911, 1921, and 1947 (all issue in 1911, issue of current marriage in 1921 and 1947); Colonial and State birth registrations; and summaries in the Commonwealth of Australia, *Yearbook* and *Demography Bulletins*. The statistical analysis is detailed in Ruzicka and Caldwell (1977).

level as a baseline, marital fertility fell by 8% by 1891 and a further 18% between 1891 and 1901, and this decline showed surprisingly little variation by wife's age.[14]

In an effort to identify leading groups in the fertility decline, it seems logical to begin by examining fertility in this period by country of birth of mother, since over 50% of the adult population were immigrants. The picture looks simple at first sight: the fertility of immigrant British women began to decline as early as the late 1870s, while that of the Australian born did not do so until the 1880s,[15] suggesting that British immigrants imported the fertility control practices then underway in Britain and these spread through diffusion to the Australian population. It is not in fact quite as simple as this. Data on residence by age (Ruzicka and Caldwell, 1977) suggest that the large majority of the British-born had been in Australia for all their childbearing years, and most since childhood; in fact the distinction between those born in Australia and Britain was frequently that between the younger and elder siblings in the same immigrant family. Furthermore, the native-born were more likely to be living in rural areas, where fertility was higher, and were—in keeping with the shortage of women in Australia—likely to have married earlier than British women who married before migrating. (It might also be noted that the lower fertility of the British-born has persisted until the present day, averaging about 10% less than that of the Australian-born in each cohort in recent decades.)

Socioeconomic status is another possible factor in differential fertility decline. Information is available for this period in Australia on the number of live births of wives by age and occupation of husband; and estimates can be made of the average age of wives and the timing of their major reproductive periods.[16] Two facts stand out. First, nonrural workers recorded surpris-

[14] Thus, in New South Wales between 1881 and 1891 marital fertility rates fell by 13–14% among women aged 25–29 years, with falls of 8–9% being recorded by women under 25 and over 39; between 1891 and 1901 the rates fell by 22–27% for women aged 30–44, with falls of 16 and 5% among those aged 25–29 and 20–24, respectively. Based on age-specific marital fertility rates for New South Wales computed for each census year, Royal Commission on the Decline of the Birth Rate and on the Mortality of Infants in New South Wales, *Report* (1904), vol. 1, Appendix, p. 90.

[15] Comparing the 1831–36, 1836–41, and 1841–46 birth cohorts (aged 35–39, 30–34, and 25–29 in 1871, 45–49, 40–44, and 35–39 in 1881, and 75–79, 70–74, and 65–69 in 1911), we find that the average number of live births of the Australian-born women rose between the first and second cohorts but fell by 2% between the second and third, while that of women born in the United Kingdom fell by 1% between the first and second cohorts and 3% between the second and third. See Banks (1954), Royal Commission on Population (1950), pp. 202–206. Crude birth rates for England and Wales adjusted for under-registration of births by Teitelbaum (1974) suggest a possibility of a slight decline in the crude birth rate in the decade 1871–80 in comparison with the decade 1861–70, followed by a more rapid fall of the birth rates during the subsequent decades e.g. 1861–70 (34·98), 1871–80 (34·40), 1881–90 (32·33), 1891–1900 (29·08), 1901–10 (26·25).

[16] Wives are assumed to be three to four years younger than their husbands (see McDonald, 1975, p. 82) with a mean age of childbearing of 29 years. In terms of proportional fertility decline by five-year periods after the early 1880s (i.e. using approximately 1883 as a baseline and estimating fertility declines by 1888, 1893, 1898, and 1903), two groups stand out: that where the husband's occupation was professional, domestic or commercial, which had declines of approximately 10, 20, 30, and 40% respectively up to each of these dates; and that where the husband's occupation was in transport and communications, industry and primary production, which recorded falls of around 6, 12, 23, and 33% respectively.

ingly similar fertility at the beginning of fertility transition. (Their fertility was markedly lower than that of rural workers, approximately half the difference being attributable to a differential in the wives' age at marriage and the other half to one in marital fertility.) Second, fertility transition affected all parts of society at much the same time; the poorer and less educated classes lagged somewhat behind the richer and more educated, but the lag was small (about five years) and of progressively less importance. We will return to these findings later in the paper in our examination of the fifth proposition, that the fertility differentials do not demand economic explanations for their existence.

Causes of Fertility Decline

If fertility limitation is largely a matter of cultural diffusion within cultural areas, and if those areas are likely to be linguistic ones, then the English-language area deserves special attention for at least three reasons: its size may allow innovations to arise somewhat more readily and may encourage chain reactions; diffusion to noncontiguous areas is involved; and, in the period under review, parts of the area were subject to unusually rapid change either because of industrialization or because of commercial relationships with industrial areas. Australia's small population meant, and still means, that most books read were written elsewhere and that newspaper and magazine articles presenting new ideas about behaviour usually discussed imported ideas. In the nineteenth century, much of the adult population regarded itself as overseas British: indeed, a court action in 1888 on the freedom to publish contraceptive information essentially upheld the right of overseas British to live as those at "home" did (Haire, 1943, p. 19). The important question, then, is whether Australia's fertility transition was wholly the result of the diffusion of birth control ideas and practices, or whether conditions in the late nineteenth century were conducive to family limitation.

It is difficult to postulate an explanation for Australian fertility transition in terms of either income or mortality levels. Employment for children and for the unskilled was probably even more readily available in the 1880s than in the 1870s. Infant and child mortality had already fallen in the pretransitional 1860s and 1870s to levels that were not attained in Britain for another 30 years, well after British fertility decline had begun.[17] Nor can either characteristic of the society explain why large families were regarded as being no problem in the third quarter of the nineteenth century, but an increasing problem in the last quarter.

[17] Australian data from 1911 Census, Statistician's Report, Pell (1867 and 1879), Burridge (1882 and 1884) and Young (1969). Data on England and Wales from Keyfitz and Flieger (1968), pp. 520–528.

One visitor to Australia in the early twentieth century talked widely to Australian women about the decline in the birth rate and concluded that the primary cause was the education of children and the greater effort being put into the training of each child (Ackermann, 1913, pp. 94–96). Certainly the letters to the press during the last three decades of the nineteenth century support this assertion. It is also the one change that radically altered life in the second half of the nineteenth century and had a similar impact in Australia and Britain, as well as other English-speaking areas.

Mass schooling used to be suggested as the major cause of fertility decline in Britain (Leybourne and White, 1940), but enthusiasm for this explanation has waned in recent decades, partly because the timing seemed wrong and partly because the extra necessary expenditure did not seem great enough and the proof that schooling prevented children from working did not seem sufficiently strong. Australian evidence tends to support the original hypothesis.

The problem of timing is largely that incipient fertility decline can be detected in sections of British society as early as the 1860s, Report of the Royal Commission on Population (1950), pp. 202–206, while compulsory education was not legislated until 1876 (in Scotland in 1872). In fact such legislation in Britain, as in the United States and Australia, did not inaugurate a new era, but rather completed the achievement of decades during which governments became increasingly involved in financing education and an ever-growing proportion of children entered schools. In Britain the timing problem has largely disappeared as a result of the debate of the last decade on the history of education (West, 1965 and 1975; Lawson and Silver, 1973), which has shown that most children had some schooling by the 1860s and probably even by the 1850s. This situation can be shown to have obtained in Australia as well (Ruzicka and Caldwell, 1977).[18]

The real cost of schooling to parents is far greater than the earlier examinations suggested and may well be the primary factor in the fertility decline. It is probable that schooling upset the whole parent–child relationship and balance of expenditure so that the position described above as still largely persisting in the third quarter of the century was never regained. This interpretation is in keeping with the discussions in Australian newspaper letter columns and elsewhere in the last quarter of the century; and it has been described with reference to the contemporary developing world (Caldwell, 1968a, pp. 96–114). Schooling costs something in terms of books and perhaps fees, but often more in standards of clothing required or encouraged. Parents make both financial and emotional investments in education that encourage them to make more. The education of children

---

[18] Important sources were Rankin (1939), Griffiths (1957) and Colonial parliamentary papers including annual reports on the education systems.

provides a direction for effort, much as the occupational advancement of the male household head does. Parents are far more likely to take pleasure in introducing the educated child to some of the experiences or consumption delights of the adult world than is the case with the uneducated one. The concept of the spare and rigorous upbringing waned rapidly toward the end of the century, especially when the upbringing was in the hands of parents who had themselves been to school. Schooling did not make other employment impossible. The great majority of children were in day schools and attendance was lax: only 50% of enrollments per day in the mid–1870s and 60% by the end of the century; but schoolchildren were likely to resent working considerable hours in unpleasant occupations, and parents were increasingly reluctant to force them to do so. Schooling emphasized the concept of dependency.

Education also became a self-sustaining process. The Australian population had not been illiterate even before mass schooling; in 1851 the census revealed three-quarters of the males and two-thirds of the females were literate. Furthermore the community's level of skills in both letters and numeracy was probably adequate for the great majority of jobs until the end of the century. However, employers demanded educational qualifications as these became available, and competition for higher qualifications became inevitable. Another factor also played a role: analysis of recent survey data shows the strong disinclination for parents to give children only as much education as they received themselves, let alone less,[19] and it seems probable that a similar attitude has been maintained over the last century.

While fundamental changes were occurring in family relationships—ones that would make children a net cost and one alternative in consumption choices—the family began to be subject to temptations that were previously rare. Newspaper advertisements and catalogues offered few luxury goods before the 1880s; however, the 1880s witnessed an expansion in the availability of furniture made by craftsmen, pianos, buggies, sewing machines, ice chests, and, as the century drew to a close, bicycles and even cameras. Thus, a change in the net intergenerational flow of wealth, brought about largely by the costs of schooling and the changes in aspirations of parents for their children, combined with aspirations for new consumer goods, produced for the first time in Australia a widespread demand for fertility limitation.

---

[19] Although only 19% of respondents and 25% of their husbands in the Melbourne Survey had completed secondary school, 64% expected their sons and 55% their daughters to attain at least this level. Although only 3% of respondents and 7% of their husbands had been to university, 38% wanted their sons and 29% their daughters to have such education.

The Means of Fertility Control

Our third proposition is that contraceptive use has been increasingly effective and has not been subject to major fluctuations in either purpose or application. Support for this proposition can be drawn from Australian experience over the last 100 years. Evidence as to the means by which fertility was controlled is available from the 1880s onward in newspaper advertisements, parliamentary debates, references in medical and other literature, evidence presented to the 1904 Royal Commission on the Birth Rate in New South Wales, and, more recently, from retrospective data from the 1971 Melbourne Survey and further surveys in depth in the mid–1970s.[20]

Methods regarded by the turn of the century as having been long in use include abstinence, prolonged lactation, withdrawal, and rhythm. Indeed, it was believed that by that time, prolonged lactation was being employed to a lesser extent than previously. There were also chemical pessaries, spray douches, syringes, condoms, spring pessaries, sponges, chemical abortifacients, and physically induced abortions. Abortion was known and used to a limited extent both within marriage and outside it. Terminal abstinence or near abstinence played a considerable role in Australian contraception until World War II, particularly in the Irish Catholic working classes among whom it was common for the husband to retire to a back room or verandah to sleep once his wife was entering middle age (frequently late thirties) or had borne a large family (Ruzicka and Caldwell, 1977).

It is our contention that the introduction of contraceptive ideas and practices would not have found such receptivity but for a major change in the closing decades of the nineteenth century in the cost of children. Nevertheless, there can be little doubt that the rapidity of the spread of birth control during that period owed much to diffusion—to imported British advertisements and devices, increasingly common in the late 1880s, and to the influence of people with first- or second-hand experience of Britain. Advertisements for contraceptives and abortifacients became more common in Australia in the second half of the 1880s, and contraceptives imported from Britain were increasingly supplemented by local manufacture. The evidence seems to be that when contraception was wanted in Australia it was available. There is little evidence of prolonged and massive use of withdrawal, abstinence, or rhythm prior to the 1880s.

[20] The 1971 Melbourne and Queanbeyan Surveys and more recent surveys were carried out by the Department of Demography, Australian National University, and reported in Caldwell and Ware (1973) and Caldwell et al. (1976). Additional fertility data are from Hicks (1971) and from Pat Caldwell's file of references from the Sydney Herald and the Sydney Morning Herald.

For the three-quarters of a century after the initial fertility decline, the contraceptive methods available were not very efficient. In fact, the methods available in the 1880s and 1890s remained virtually unchanged, except for improvements in commercial packaging and tablet manufacture, for decades. They represented 85% of the methods of fertility control in the late 1930s, 80% in the late 1940s, and 71% in the late 1950s; they did not fall below 50% until 1970 (Caldwell and Ware, 1973, p. 17). Indeed, withdrawal, rhythm, and abstinence made up 40–50% of all birth control until the late 1960s. The Dutch cap and the diaphragm were not used by more than 12% of contraceptors even at the end of the Depression of the 1930s and usage did not rise above 20% until the late 1950s. The Gräfenberg ring attained a level of 3% during World War II and 6% in the 1950s in Melbourne (but probably no more than half these levels in the whole country). The real change came only in the 1960s. Pill users increased from 19% of all contraceptors in the early 1960s, to 39% in the mid–1960s, and 48% in the early 1970s. By the latter date over two-thirds of the youngest contracepting wives were using the pill, and half of all contraceptors and three-quarters of the youngest were employing pills or IUDs.

The fact that much the same methods of contraception were used for half, or even three-quarters, of a century after the 1880s does not mean that the efficiency of contraception did not improve. All the methods, except perhaps the condom, needed considerable cooperation between sexual partners and were most suited to use within marriage. Even within marriage, contraception in the community as a whole became more efficient as it became more accepted and respectable: as contraception could be discussed more easily between partners, between friends and occasionally between mothers and daughters or fathers and sons, and between clients and doctors or pharmacists. This was a continuous process, but the fertility and contraceptive record bears witness to the efficacy of the great crises in Australian society in speeding up practice of contraception. The burden of children became greater in the intense economic depressions of the 1890s and 1930s, as did the fear of further childbirth.[21] Contraceptive practice appears to have risen substantially too during World War I and demonstrably did so during and after World War II.[22] and parallel to the population and women's debates from the late 1950s onward. Not only was contraception more efficiently employed, but the proportion of married couples

[21] So did a man's difficulty in setting himself up in marriage, although the decline in proportions married was only one-third as great as the proportionate decline in marital fertility in the 1890s and only one-fiftieth as great in the 1930s, comparing indices of 1901 with 1891 and 1933 with 1921.

[22] The Melbourne Survey retrospective data showed that among wives in their mid-twenties the proportions practising birth control in 1935–39, 1940–44, and 1945–49 respectively were 45, 58, and 70% (a decade later it was only 72%), while the proportions for wives around 30 years of age were 53, 71, and 78% (a decade later it was only 81%).

contracepting at all continued to increase, as did the proportion of couples doing so early in marriage. In the 1930s only about half the couples in which the wife was under age 30 and not knowingly infecund had ever used contraception; by the late 1950s, 75% were doing so; by the late 1960s, 85%; and by the early 1970s, 95% of such couples were contracepting.

According to the 1971 Melbourne Survey of Family Formation, most methods of contraception exhibit strong educational (and associated socioeconomic) differentials in acceptance. Thus, use of the condom as the principal method of contraception in the late 1940s and early 1950s ranged from 18% among wives with 0–9 years of education to 31% among those with 13 or more years; use of the diaphragm during the 1950s ranged from 19% among the lowest educational group to 30% among the highest; and use of the pill in the first half of the 1960s ranged from 25% among the lowest group to 35% among the highest. Since the 1940s the use of withdrawal has exhibited an inverse relationship with education, but it is likely that it exhibited a direct relationship during the late nineteenth century. These differentials reflect both personal acceptance of innovation and the ability of couples to communicate ideas and experiment with new practices. They may also reflect differences in the pressures exerted by large families. Nevertheless, these kinds of differentials in the ability to employ innovations, doubtless accompanied also by a differential in the ability to employ them efficiently, are easily sufficient to explain fertility differentials in early transition, without having to posit differences in the impact of the large family on the various socioeconomic classes.

The Successive Stages of Fertility Transition: Cause and Effect

We can now examine the proposition that the explanation of fertility transition is in terms of historical stages, one necessarily preceding and contributing to the next.

In the third quarter of the nineteenth century, Australia was a British immigrant society. It was religious, predominantly Protestant, and very earnest. Children were raised fairly strictly and austerely, being admonished with religious precept, proverb, and adage. It was not a society in which most gained by high fertility. The population was drawn from a culture in which most gained by high fertility. The population was drawn from a culture in which the family had long largely nucleated economically and emotionally and in which the breadwinner usually could not look to the extended family for help in times of need. This nucleation had been intensified by migration.

The society, like its parent culture in Britain, strongly favoured the establishment of the young adult male securely in an occupation before he married and fathered a family. To achieve this, male marriage had been deferred in Europe over the course of the previous centuries. In the Australian colonies, with their perennial shortage of women, deferment was longer still. From mid-century until the beginning of the 1890s the median age at first marriage for men was about 27 years in Australia, compared with around 25 in England and Wales. That for Australian women had probably been under 23 in the 1850s compared with about 24 in England and Wales. The similarity of marriage ages in Australia and Britain testifies to the extraordinary extent to which the migrants remained bound by their culture, for, although the British "marriage market" throughout the period evinced a deficit of males of around 20%, Australia had a surplus of around 200% at the beginning of the 1860s, of about 50% a decade later, and of 30% as late as 1891.[23] The real impact of this imbalance was on the proportions of women married at each age, and hence on fertility. In the 1850s, almost two-thirds of 20–24-year-old women in Australia were married compared with less than one-third in England and Wales, and 97% of 45–49-year-olds compared with 87%. Considerable margins persisted until the end of the century.

The establishment of males in their occupations was an undertaking that changed over time. Increasingly, as the economy industrialized, a higher proportion of males found themselves working in employment that was characterized not only by more stringent requirements in education and skills for initial qualification but by successive targets of advancement or promotion throughout a working lifetime. This was especially the case in white-collar occupations, which comprised about 9% of the workforce in 1861, 11% in 1881, 20% in 1901, and 31% in 1971.[24] A large family might well hinder such advancement as early marriage had once hindered initial establishment.

During the third quarter of the nineteenth century, a significant social change took place: the introduction of schooling for nearly all. It was not a single change but a continuing process: half the children probably had some schooling in the 1850s, three-quarters in the late 1860s, and nearly all by 1880. In the century that has since passed, there has been an almost uninterrupted increase in the average period of full-time education provided children and in the proportion of the enrolled school-children in attendance each day.[25] It is argued here that the trend toward universal education had a

[23] McDonald (1975), p. 70 and 95, employing a formula that takes into account both the proportions unmarried and the age gap between spouses. The data for Australia are from New South Wales, Victoria, and South Australia.

[24] Figures for 1861 and 1881 from Victorian Censuses, and for 1901 and 1971 from census data for all Australia. There are problems of definition in each census and major ones between censuses.

[25] Caldwell et al. (1976), and also responses to educational questions in the Melbourne Survey.

profound impact on fertility. It was not the direct impact that counted so much as the changes in the relationship between parents and children, especially in the economic relationship (i.e., in the net intergenerational wealth flow). These changes took time to develop and probably accelerated when the parents themselves had enjoyed some schooling, as was probably the case in the majority of families by the last two decades of the century.[26]

From the 1880s began a long period of familiarization with the new methods of birth control: an increasing proportion of couples being able to suggest or agree on use, more being able to use them efficiently, and more retail outlets being available for contraceptives. The Depression of the 1890s accelerated this early spread, just as that of the 1930s came close to maximizing the efficiency with which nearly the whole society could use these methods.

The nature of the fertility change in the 1890s may provide an important key to the reasons for early fertility decline. The most significant evidence is that fertility fell at all female ages. It seems likely that in the early to mid-1890s this limiting of fertility was not based on a desire to achieve a lower completed family size, but rather was a response to an immediate burden, both in terms of the lower level of earnings of the household head and of the fear (where he had not already lost his job) of unemployment and immediate destitution. In a society experiencing very harsh times, but still for only a limited period after four decades of high prosperity and ready availability of employment, postponement of childbearing was a rational response. It was as if it were suddenly no longer the proper time to bear children.

As the decade wore on and was succeeded by the economic relapse of the first years of the present century, a different reason for the fertility decline may have come to the fore. Confidence in the long-term future had been profoundly shaken (as most Australian historians aver), and the large family was now seen as a danger to living standards. Couples were so aware of the imperfect nature of their contraception that they realized that only sustained efforts to avoid pregnancy at every stage could lead to a moderately sized family.[27]

By the beginning of the present century there was a growing confidence that early marriage did not necessarily entail having a large number of children. The proportion of women ever marrying has been rising over this century: the

[26] In 1861, more than half the children aged 7–12 years in Victoria were enrolled at schools. Victoria, Papers Presented to Parliament by Command, Session 1862–3, vol. 3, paper 15, p. 5 and vol. 4, paper 44, p. 6; Census of Victoria, 1861.

[27] The role of economic depression, particularly of the threat and reality of unemployment in bringing about fertility limitation in the late nineteenth century as it had not in the hard times of the 1840s, is clear. South Australia alone witnessed considerable unemployment in the late 1870s and marital fertility declined between 1876 and 1881 by 4%, compared with a rise in Queensland (the only other State with 1871 population data); Western Australia alone enjoyed prosperity in the early 1890s because of huge new finds of gold) and recorded a level of marital fertility in 1891 above that of 1881 in contrast to a decline in all other Colonies.

1921 census recorded 17% of women aged 45–49 as never married in contrast to 4% in 1971. Female age at marriage has been falling since the 1930s.[28] These changes probably owed much to a growing secularism and belief in participating in the pleasures of this world and more still to the changing attitudes toward sexual relations, themselves at least partially related to diffusion of contraception. It is also tempting to conclude that the greater contraceptive skill induced by the Depression of the 1890s made the movement toward universal female marriage possible, and that induced by the Depression of the 1930s initiated the move toward younger female (and male) marriage. Both changes were to mean, in turn, a greater demand for more efficient contraception.

The chain of cause and effect can be seen extending the analysis to the present day. The fertility decline inevitably has had important secondary effects, and has probably been a major cause of the collapse of the domestic society in the modern era. Women born during 1906–10, after weathering the Depression of the 1930s, averaged in their mid-thirties (during World War II) only 1·9 children, and in their mid-forties (in the early 1950s) only 2·3 (Spencer, 1971). This was not the only respect in which their families were smaller: women born in the first decade of the present century, after the fertility decline of the 1890s, averaged about three siblings compared with at least double that number for women born a generation earlier. The domestic society underwent further transformations in the 1950s and 1960s: more transport by car meant less neighbourliness; regional shopping centres and huge impersonal stores replaced local centres and smaller shops where the customer was known; church attendance and community life built around it declined; and families moved to new neighbourhoods more often (Ruzicka and Caldwell, 1977).

In these circumstances, a growing proportion of women prepared not only to work throughout much of their lives, but to expect and plan advancement in their work.[29] The withdrawal of an increasing proportion of women from the homes was a self-sustaining process in that it reinforced the isolation of wives who were not working and the down-grading of the domestic virtues.

Thus, close to universal contraception encouraged early marriage, which led to increasingly high rates of labour force participation of wives and mothers. This participation stepped up rapidly in all age groups starting in the early 1960s,[30] partly, it seems likely, because of better contraception.

[28] McDonald (1975), pp. 186–187.

[29] The collapse of domestic society was not the only reason that married women joined the labour force in larger numbers. The nature of employment available had changed dramatically over the century: office and shop-assistant jobs had multiplied, as had lighter and cleaner jobs in manufacturing. Girls' education, with all its implications of preparation for a career, was extending. The manpower crisis of World War II had brought great numbers of married women into the workforce in response to government pleas to their and their husbands' patriotism. See Australia Department of Labour and National Service, (1970), p. 13.

[30] Data are analysed in Alberto (1976). See also Cooper (1969).

The change began almost a decade before the arguments of the women's movement impinged strongly on the society. Indeed, it is easier to argue that the move toward females having lifetime working careers produced the women's movement than to present the argument in reverse order.

The continuing chain of cause and effect produced two more changes in the 1970s. The first was the postponement of the first birth within marriage. Survey evidence (Caldwell et al., 1976) indicates that this has arisen partly from the desire to establish the home, especially to pay off the second mortgage[31] and to buy furniture: residential nucleation of families right from the time of marriage has increased dramatically in the last three decades.[32] However, surveys also report a great number of young women explaining the need to establish a career and to demonstrate before their first pregnancy that they have mastered the career and are suited to either re-employment or continued employment. Without question, they are describing "the proper time to reproduce".

The second change in the 1970s has been the perfection of birth control by contraception and abortion to the point that sexual relations can be safely divorced from marriage and that such improved control no longer reduces the age at marriage but may increase it in a community where most still regard marriage as the preliminary to childbirth but not to sexual relations. Attitudes to marriage are certainly changing, but whether age at marriage (or, perhaps more appropriately, legal marriage) has begun to increase is still a matter of debate.[33]

Fertility transition in Australia over the course of the last century can almost certainly be seen as a phenomenon induced by birth control and propelled by better birth control. However, it can be fully understood, especially in its time dimension, only in terms of the series of interacting changes described above.

The crucial period of change was that from the 1850s to the 1880s. Australian evidence suggests that period witnessed a significant movement in parental–child relationships, which rendered children relatively more expensive. Growing secularism, the beginnings of the consumer society, but, above all, the impact of education on both children and parents, were

[31] I.e., the short-term, high-interest rate, second loan for purchasing a house. By the early 1970s, some finance companies were sufficiently certain of the efficacy of birth control and of women's commitment to the workforce to grant second mortgages on the condition of wives' continued employment.

[32] Only 40% of Melbourne Survey respondents who had married prior to 1950 had begun married life in an unshared house or flat; but the proportion for 1950–54 marriages was 49%, 1955–59 marriages 53%, 1960–64 marriages 55%, 1965–69 marriages 65%, and 1970–71 marriages 79%. Interviews of the unmarried in 1975/76 (Caldwell et al., 1976) showed a strong belief that such separate accommodation should have top priority.

[33] McDonald interprets data to the present time as showing no more than that the trends toward earlier marriages and more universal marriage have finally come to a halt. However, for an interpretation suggesting that the trends may already have been reversed, see Hall (1976).

the cause of this change. That parent–child emotional and economic relationships alter subtly, but profoundly and irreversibly, with the arrival of mass schooling can be shown to be true in much of the contemporary Third World (Hull and Hull, 1977; Caldwell, 1968a), but needs more historical research in the West.

Reassessing the Significance of Fertility Differentials

The Australian experience suggests that too much can be made, and has been made, of the existence of statistically significant socioeconomic fertility differentials during fertility transition. The real significance of that experience was that the fertility of all groups began to decline at roughly the same time, and that, with the exception of a differential between Catholics and non-Catholics, each lower level of fertility attained by the leading groups was matched within a surprisingly short time by the other groups. Changes within the family and society that made children an economic liability—and yielded an unequivocal wealth flow from the older to the younger generation—reached a critical point in the last decades of the nineteenth century. Even the religious differential may be explained at least as much by differences in attitudes toward family relationships and child rearing as by opposing views on the permissibility of contraception.

Once these fundamental changes had occurred, children—any children—were unquestionably an economic liability to parents. Fertility did not fall immediately to replacement or below because the initial fertility declines, and the means used to achieve them, interacting with economic and occupational change, sparked off a chain reaction that has taken about a century to reach zero population growth and may take longer still before fertility and family structure reach a new position of equilibrium. In terms of major social change, this has been a very short period indeed.

Inevitably, changes in the proper time to marry, in familiarization with contraceptives, in the collapse of the domestic society, in women penetrating the occupational structure (especially as far as careers allowing for a ladder of advancement), and in parent–child emotional and economic relationships proceeded at somewhat different rates according to socioeconomic status. But to employ socioeconomic fertility differentials at any particular time during this period of transition to argue the differential value—economic or otherwise—of children to parents of different social classes (let alone to try to measure the magnitudes involved) would appear to be an enterprize that underscores the fact that much contemporary social science is fatally flawed by its ahistorical approach. Such differentials are, however—and this is the fifth proposition—a valuable source of evidence for the social historian in determining the way social changes move through a society and occur over time.

The history of the fertility transition during the last half-century has also had its fascinating aspects and provides important support for the theses argued above. It can be shown that fertility, when measured by the fertility of married women by the period of exposure to conception, very largely declined in a unilinear fashion during the whole period, and that the apparent swings of reproductive fashion with the Depression of the 1930s and the so-called post-war "baby boom" were artefacts of the fertility indices employed rather than evidence that fertility would, in a society that had achieved complete reproductive control, rise and fall with fashion. That too is an ahistorical interpretation and has been analysed fully elsewhere (Caldwell and Ruzicka, 1977, Chapter 6; Ruzicka and Caldwell, 1977).

The Australian experience is unlikely to differ significantly from those of other English-speaking countries of European origin, or indeed from those of other populations in Western and Northern Europe. But this needs to be established by the detailed investigation of family and social change over the last century and a half. We believe that it will be shown that the period witnessed a profound change in the nature of parent–child emotional and economic relationships and that the spread of mass education was an important aspect of this (see Chapter 4). The demonstration of the validity of this hypothesis is important because it has implications for all fertility transition and not merely that which has occurred in the West.

This chapter was reprinted with the permission of The Population Council from John C. Caldwell and Lado T. Ruzicka, "The Australian fertility transition: An Analysis," *Population and Development Review* **4**, no. 1 (March 1978): 81–103.

7

The mechanisms of demographic change in historical perspective

In several earlier papers I have attempted to analyse fertility transition.[1] My aim was both to present a general theory of change and also to explain why, though fertility remains high in many contemporary Third World countries, it may well begin sustained decline without having to await further fundamental economic change.

The major tenet of the argument was that, within upper and lower limits, fertility in all societies is rational, given the identity of the decision-makers and the nature of the socially determined goals. An effort was made to show why high fertility was advantageous in pre-capitalist economies and why it is eventually not so as a capitalist labour market develops.

Several lines of attack on the theory have been developed,[2] but significantly not the one most anticipated. Nearly all the controversialists appear to assume that where fertility is high the reason is that such levels bring advantage at least to those in a position to influence fertility. The most trenchant critic, Thadani, writes, "A reversal in wealth flows from parents to children is, thus, not contingent upon (family) economic nucleation, but is an aspect of it, and both are a function of the social-structural conditions" (1978, p. 490). This is most intriguing in view of the apparent strength only a few years ago of the view that all people in all high-fertility societies would benefit from a decline in family size and only outworn lore prevented them from perceiving the fact.[3]

[1] See Chapters 4 and 5 in this volume. These papers footnote other papers investigating change in Ghana and Nigeria. The findings of research into the fertility transition in Australia are summarized in Caldwell and Ruzicka (1978).

[2] See especially Thandani (1978) and Hawthorn (1978), pp. 9–10. The latter criticism is somewhat confused and the author appears to believe that the changes outlined are "mere fashion", while at the same time putting forth a rather extraordinary theory that family transformation in Ghana and Nigeria "is caused by men wishing to assert some control over their wives".

[3] C.f. Mueller (1976) who may also remain an exception to the above generalization.

The main attacks have stressed the following points: my most recent formulations of my position appear to stress relative advantage within the family at the expense of the advantage of high fertility to the whole family (or clan); I have too distinctly separated the social and the economic and have ignored the primacy of the latter; I have acccounted for neither the absence of extremely high fertility in pre-transition Europe nor the presence of moderate, rather than minimum, fertility in the West for generations after the transition; I have downplayed the fact that young—or very young—children probably do have some net cost everywhere; and my own research provides only a slender empirical base for the wealth flows theory.

All but the last two areas of apparent conflict seem to arise in three ways. The first is a misunderstanding about my increasing concentration on the conditions immediately prior to the onset of sustained fertility decline. The second is a more general problem of time-scale. The third is a tendency by some critics to treat each society as autonomous and to ignore the movement towards a global society and economy.

All these problems will be dealt with below, but will be treated in such a way as to generate a more general theory with a more satisfactory time dimension.

The Advantage of Numbers

Among warring clans, and even families, prior to the establishment of larger organizational units, numbers were presumably once almost the only guarantee of security from attack and of the ability to take resources from others (the position of hunters and gatherers is complex because significant natural increase can also threaten their resource base). This condition, where numbers meant safety and hence a degree of prosperity, was not suddenly succeeded by another where such factors played no role; there was a long period of overlap which in many societies has lasted until the present day.

In most of the Third World a secure residence is one which is never empty and is always guarded by the presence of a few family members bustling about, with others within summoning distance if necessary. An even temporarily deserted house is taken to be an invitation to disaster. Every house is a castle which, in many societies, is rarely or never entered by anyone except relatives (Fernea, 1976, p. 109). Bangladesh is a typical example of a culture where relatives cluster their houses together within villages in case disputes leading to conflict spring up (Jalaluddin, in preparation). In the same country Cain has demonstrated the role of family members in protecting family property during such critical periods as that surrounding land inheritance following the death of the patriarch (1978, pp. 427–428). The ability of an old man to put forward his view and to influence policy in an African village meeting may well depend on his having strong sons in the audience (Kabwegyere and Mbula, 1980). In rural Mexico, "the Zapotecs do not enjoy solitude and never live alone by preference; the more household members, the more secure is the household from physical acts of aggression" (Chiñas, 1973, p. 88). In Indian villages, where all members of a family usually belong to the same *jati* faction, it is the numbers in the faction which often help to achieve both governmental preference and personal safety for members (Cohn, 1965; Mandelbaum, 1970a, pp. 240–252; Epstein, 1962, p. 130). Physical force is still much more pervasive in the world than is usually assumed in social science models; the reason is a personal and national sensitivity about reporting such matters to outsiders.

Even when overt physical force is less needed, the family can act like a small State and can secure advantages from numbers. Most Yorubas take it for granted that large families prosper because they have the contacts, because they are more likely to to able to pressure others into favourable commercial agreements, and because they have disproportionate say in the allocation of communal resources (see Chapter 3, pp. 104). In India, "domestic rites and celebrations can be staged more elegantly by a large family, and the resulting prestige enhances all within the family" (Mandelbaum, 1970a, p. 37); indeed, even with regard to modern Bombay, the *potlatch* aspect of ceremonial occasions, and the consequent advantage of numbers, has been stressed (Lannoy, 1971, p. 300). From Chad (Reyna, 1975b) to Bangladesh (Cain, 1978, pp. 426–427), the large family has been shown to benefit from its ability to diversify its labour force and even to use this ability to exploit the possibility of windfall gains from unusual circumstances in the neighbourhood or beyond it.

In each situation the family gives a guarantee of protection and safety—of individuals not going to the wall alone—because of its continuity. There is a parallel with the protection offered by the viable State. In Mexico,

"Families are strong and cohesive, held together by traditional bonds of loyalty, common economic strivings, mutual dependence, the prospect of inheritance, and, finally, the absence of any other social group to which the individual can turn . . . without a family the individual stands unprotected and isolated, a prey to every form of aggression, exploitation and humiliation" (Lewis, 1960, p. 54).

A major reason why wealth flow analysis cannot concentrate solely on intrafamilial flows and relative situational advantage is the parallel existence of this older complex of demographic advantage. Indeed, it is a complex that is not extinct in some post-transitional societies where children are clearly a net loss in terms of intrafamilial economic transactions.

Successor systems: Modes of production where there is some guarantee of external security

If the only advantage of high fertility had been its ability to sustain physical force, either overtly or in its more sophisticated and hidden forms, birth rates would have been more affected by the rise of powerful States—often enforcing moralities with a theological basis and being supported in post-classical Europe by a powerful church—than has in fact been the case. The other advantage (at least to the decision-makers) has lain in the nature of the familial production mode. This has been argued at length in a previous paper,[4] and an empirical analysis (Caldwell *et al.*, 1981). In any case the conclusions about the effect on fertility of familial production do not seem to be in dispute; the attack has been on the postulated conditions of fertility change.

At its least perceptive, the attack has taken this form: "From his own account, in which he admits that the flow of goods from children to parents is actually greatest among the more prosperous and secure, it is difficult to see how a mere change in fashion could induce prosperous, prospective parents to renounce the possibility of future benefits" (Hawthorn, 1978, p. 9). At its more sophisticated, the thrust has been: "Family nucleation and intergenerational net flows of wealth toward children can be seen to be different aspects of the same phenomenon, the phenomenon of the emergence of the modern form of the family, nuclear in structure and autonomous in its economy and external relationships" (Thadani, 1978, p. 489). "To isolate the 'social' and the 'economic', as in Caldwell's analysis, and to identify the 'social' as the sole causal agent of the changes in the economic sphere, is to equate an aspect of the subsystem with the subsystem" (Ibid., p. 481).

The basic assertion is that the economic nature of a society determines its institutions and that "fashion" or "sentiment"[5] cannot take the lead in inducing change. This probably approximates the view of most contemporary economic historians and sociologists of the functionalist school, and dates back to Marx:

"The totality of the relations of production constitutes the economic structure of society, the real foundations, on which arises a legal and political superstructure

[4] See Chapter 5 in this volume, where there is also a definition of modes of production.
[5] Thadani's term, derived from Stone (1977).

and to which correspond definite forms of social consciousness . . . At a certain stage in development, the material forces of a society come into conflict with the existing relations of production . . . The changes in the economic foundation lead sooner or later to the transformation of the whole immense superstructure" (Marx, 1975).

This is a position which I only partially dispute. It is indisputable that a settled, largely subsistence economy based predominantly on familial production will have high fertility (except where there are pathological problems, e.g. in the low fertility belt of Middle Africa), and that it was inevitable that a capitalist society with a fully developed labour market producing nearly all goods and services would have low fertility. It is not this tautology that is important for our times. Rather is it whether there can be lags or accelerations in the chain from the material forces of production to the modes of production to such parts of the superstructure as family structure and fertility behaviour, and whether, as in the Third World (and parts of the West), imported social concepts can change the local superstructure at a different rate than would have been dictated solely by the movement of the economic base in a culturally autonomous society (and also, though it is not necessary for the argument, whether such changes in the superstructure can actually modify the base). The critical change is one which extends so far that high fertility is no longer economic. These quibbles might mean a difference of decades in pin-pointing the onset of fertility decline and billions in the estimates of the size of the eventual quasi-stationary global population, as well as significant differences in the interpretation of demographic change in the nineteenth century West and the contemporary Third World.

A Recapitulation and Restatement of the Wealth Flows Theory

In terms of its ultimate impact on fertility, the significant aspect of the economy is whether production is based on the familial organization of labour or whether there is a free and monetized labour market (i.e. capitalist production). The long history of familial production is not homogeneous—hunting and gathering bands may have been typified by wealth flows from the younger to the older generation without a specific child–parent flow, and fertility may have been valuable more in terms of numbers and security than in terms of production before the external imposition of greater security—but such production never favoured highly controlled fertility. Familial production is not confined to subsistence agriculture but has long typified pre-capitalist artisan and commercial families, as well as the families of landless labourers—and, in a sense, even the nobility and administrators in such societies can organize their families in this way.

The familial organization of production was maintained even in urban areas because of the strength of the cultural superstructure—based on the needs of subsistence agriculture but working effectively outside it. The central point that must be emphasized is that for most of human history the cultural superstructure has been overwhelmingly concerned with matters that maintain the modes of production—with how people adhere to or stray from the behaviour patterns expected in terms of their age, sex, relationship to each other and so forth.[6] The praise, excitement and scandal of the village is very largely about such things. Music and art may to some extent have a life of their own, but they usually reinforce these themes, and religion very largely does so. The parallels with our own society are not at first sight so clear, but they are there, and will be spelt out below.

The superstructure is then very powerful. In a society which is isolated or little affected by outside cultural influences—which has been the situation of the leading segments of the West for a millennium—that power is likely to be a conservative one. Where there are strong external cultural influences then the course of change is much more open.

Some of these points will be clearer after we examine the familial and capitalist cultural superstructures. The need to do so arises because the economic value of children to parents is determined by behavioural patterns monitored by these superstructures. It is also pertinent to consider whether the superstructures are all of a piece, or whether segments can be modified (with implications for fertility) without immediately endangering the mode of production.

Familial Production—The Cultural Superstructure

The fundamental aspect of familial culture is the emphasis on the family itself—on its primacy, on its home as its castle, on its continuity, and on the maintenance of its internal relationships. Continuity is expressed and reinforced by rises of birth, puberty or initiation, marriage and, above all, death, for it is the funerary observations which link the living with the ancestors, reinforcing continuity and emphasizing the importance of the old (c.f., in Europe, Davis (1977) p. 93). This is true even where there is no ancestor worship as such (although it should be noted that, over great

---

[6] The role of conversation in maintaining the modes of production has been investigated during 1979–80 by the author and Pat Caldwell, first in Bangladesh in collaboration with A. K. M. Jalaluddin, and secondly in South India in collaboration with P. H. Reddy and others in a joint project of the Department of Demography, The Australian National University, and the Bangalore Population Centre.

stretches of Asia normally described as adhering to one or another of the major religions, aspects of ancestor worship exist in the village household religious observations while in sub-Saharan Africa such practices are usually maintained even in societies apparently converted to major religions). Stories, pictures, songs, myths and proverbs tell of good sons and daughters, faithful wives and the wise and venerable old.

The stabilizing element in familial production, and that which ensures larger returns to its productive and reproductive decision-makers, is the segmentation of the family and society by age, sex, marital status and relationship. The fact that the family is a producer as well as a consumer-unit means that it is widely typified by patriarchy (Shanin, 1972, pp. 28–29). Such rule may not be absolute; Lewis reported of the Mexican village that, "The most even-tempered marriages are those which follow a middle course: the wife does little to challenge the authority of the husband and the husband is not too overbearing toward his wife (Lewis, 1960, p. 55). Indeed, the more powerful may be constrained by the need to behave in accordance with that power; Mandelbaum stresses the necessity in India for the old to retain their dignity before the young (1970a, pp. 59–60). Indeed, "with family authority goes responsibility", and with its lack goes a right to protection and care (ibid., p. 40). So pervasive is the system that those within it are usually unable to perceive the real differentials in production and consumption;[7] in Morocco a neighbour describes the nearly incapable wife of the patriarch thus: "She may be old and nearly blind. But it's she who takes care of them. She runs the house. She manages the money. Her sons give her their wages, they are good sons, and she takes care of everything" (Fernea, 1976, p. 102). "That's [her granddaughter who] wants to get married, but [the grandmother] won't agree because there is too much work around the house" (ibid., p. 101). The segmentation also takes the form of stressing blood relationships over affinal ones, and of duties to parents and siblings before wives, thus maintaining the strength of the family of origin.

They are also often unable to distinguish the real foci of power and decision-making. Much authority, which in the last resort could be reassumed by the patriarch, is delegated to his wife, and is exercised most strongly over daughters-in-law. Not only command but also complaints appear to originate most frequently with women; sons who wish to split up joint-family households are content to blame it on the friction (which undoubtedly exists) between their wives and mothers, thus admittedly freeing the essential lines of male cooperation from bitterness (Mandelbaum, 1970a. pp. 90–94). Authority can be direct; in Mexico control of

[7] Although we are at present attempting to remedy this in the Bangladesh Control of Activity Study.

children may be violent, but, significantly, usually only for two crimes, "flouting the authority of his parents or for unwillingness to work" (Lewis, 1960, p. 60). Indeed, straying wives, in Latin America and elsewhere, may be killed.[8] Usually social pressure is sufficient to ensure that women and children remain in their place. The concept of "reputation" is found everywhere. In India, a wife should walk behind her husband, avoid using his personal name and greet him ritually with gestures of respect and deference, while children should show their parents deference, respect their authority and avoid contradicting their will (Mandelbaum, 1970a, p. 39). In many societies of this kind, women are expected to reveal little excitement in sexual relations. Often the male reputation is judged by the morality of their female relatives. Not only are those who would flout convention kept in line, but so are those who would relax the rules; local ridicule keeps a gentle husband or soft parent from the failure to exercise his rights. Indeed, so strong are the conventions that the weak can frequently exercise strong negative authority by adopting a "holier than thou" posture.[9] Such conventions have become embedded in manners, morals and religion, for religion can rarely avoid supporting—and reinforcing—what is recognized as a virtue. In fact, the rules are not only restrictive, but they also provide reassurance and can be used as a weapon.

Most matters of moment occur, and most emotions are felt, within the ambit of the family. The extreme form of the familial system is experienced within the residential extended family, but no aspect listed above of the cultural superstructure of the familial production system is impossible where nuclear family residence is practised—as it often is either among part of the population for life-cycle reasons or more widely as a way of life. Nevertheless, joint residence can reinforce such views and practices, partly by reducing the amount of overt emotion that can be expressed between spouses or parents and children. Women indeed are often expected to stay inside the house, or to leave it rarely, sometimes only if the mother-in-law accompanies them,[10] or, at the most, to have a much more restricted pattern of mobility than their husbands.

Ultimately, authority rests on the control of the means of production—in rural areas on land, and, sometimes, animals. Hence the importance of the rules of inheritance, and of the conditions for disinheritance. Safety is ensured not only by such possessions but also by relations with other families, and therefore the importance of marriage, especially the arranged marriage. Within the family, authority is reinforced by segregation and division, by differentials in duties and rights; "divide and rule" operates and

[8] C.f., on Columbia, Richardson (1970), p. 88.
[9] In India, wives frequently refuse to cook meat for their husbands.
[10] Cf., in Turkey, Fallers and Fallers (1976), p. 250.

sibling jealousies and hatred between the women are frequently part of the system.

Capitalist Production—The Cultural Superstructure

Direct parallels can be drawn often in the form of contrasts. Clearly, in this case, the superstructure is not nearly as hallowed by time, and hence by religion and lore. Furthermore, in most societies and in all Third World societies, it is still in the formative state and contains many elements— sometimes modified and sometimes transformed for its own purposes—of the familial production superstructure. Both in the West and in the mortality that the West is exporting, it contains some elements that were fashioned as much, or more, by Western history (such as aversion to polygyny or to arranged marriages) as by the demands of the capitalist mode of production. It also shows development over time—as was doubtless also the case when the morality suited to hunting and gathering was giving way to one suited to settled agriculture—with successive stages fitted first to a capitalism creaming off some labour in a society where familial production was still important and schooling was not, then to one where adult males sold their labour in the market while their wives sustained a domestic subsistence system for household services, and children devoted most of their time to schooling, and finally to one where the labour market attempts to engage all members of the household who are not still being educated.

Even early capitalism is forced to challenge some aspects of the hitherto monolithic family. The employer usually has to emphasize that the contractual relationship is between himself and an individual member of the family and that, for the purposes of work, family authority does not compete with his own, and also that his obligations end with the employee and do not extend to the whole family (there have, of course, always been some situations where the employment of the household head implied work from and some obligations to entire households). Whereas the family usually demanded scrupulous honesty in internal transactions—at least in dealings with those higher in the family pecking order—the employer had to emphasize that this applied even more in his case and that honesty in this relationship was bound by the laws of the State.[11] Similarly he had to turn the work ethic from the family to himself, but, if his enterprise was larger than a family and its activities located so that he could not always keep an eye on all at once, he had also to emphasize initiative, individualism and self-reliance

[11] See Banfield (1958), who discusses the conflict between familial and extra-familial morality without apparently recognizing its economic base, but instead viewing the familial morality solely as an economically retarding factor. Cf. also Weber (1930) where there is a greater appreciation of the importance of the extent of capitalist development.

to an extent that would have been abhorrent to the traditional family and against the interests of its more powerful members. He has to develop a respect for work rather than the dominant attitude found in familial production which gives primacy to respecting and observing the hierarchies of intrafamilial relationships with regard to work.

The conflict between familial morality, suited to familial production, and extra-familial morality, suited to the capitalist labour market, can be extreme during periods of transition. Both tourists and development experts who have wandered into a society of family production are likely to decide that the lack of "development" arises from an inadequate morality. At the same time, parents with children tending to obey the new extra-familial morality are likely to regard them as a testimony to an inadequate upbringing.[12] Until the morality transition takes place, the direction of the wealth flow is not likely to reverse.

Early capitalism eagerly accepted the family's willingness to impose a firm upbringing in order to induce the ability to work hard and without complaint. It also appreciated the family teaching its less powerful members that it was good for them to live austerely and that there should be no resentment of differential treatment and privilege. Indeed, if the family taught honesty and diligence better than the State it was a good thing. There was no problem in maintaining the sanctity of the family; in fact the decreasing need for organizing productive relations between its members reduced the internal tensions. However, the fact that the family bread-winner in the labour market had to be of working age meant that the recognition of the head of a family was likely to be extended to the head of the nuclear component even of an extended family. Sometimes the employer placed more emphasis on virtues like thrift and sobriety than had been the case in the traditional family.

This position, whereby the traditional family retained its ancient morality and produced obedient employees for a system not based on family production and not fundamentally needing much of its morality, proved surprisingly stable. There were, of course, reasons also at the family level for maintaining the system. If the young were employed outside the family but handed over most of their earnings, then the patriarchal system could survive almost intact—but the young had to be exhorted more, for no longer were the sanctions such simple ones as denial of access to land and food. If the womenfolk would continue to live modestly and work hard to produce household domestic services, then the household could obtain these products more cheaply than they could be acquired from the outside

---

[12] Cf. Wiser and Wiser (1971), pp. 263–267, for an excellent description of a man in rural India who became an exemplary village headman to the disgrace and heartbreak of his parents when it became obvious that he was not placing his family's interests first.

market—but the family had to reach new heights in emphasizing the difference between the things that men were suited for and those that lay in the female sphere. High fertility helped: it emphasized the female role, it kept the mother tied to the home, and it supplied her with extra helpers. Capitalism could hardly but approve; it was able to obtain a man's labour for lower wages than would have been needed by his family to obtain all their needs directly from the market. The parallel is striking with the situation described by Meillassoux whereby foreign firms in Africa paid low wages knowing that subsistence support would be supplied by the workers' extended families (1972, p. 102).

Ultimately, as the labour market expanded in the industrializing West, this stability was to be undermined. The need for higher levels of skills, and the temptations of relative affluence, meant that children were put into school on a mass scale, with complex and ramifying effects (see Chapter 10). The school presented children with new authority figures; it undermined the ability of the old to claim greater wisdom; it substituted virtue in being diligent in schoolwork for diligence in household activities; it raised consumption expectations; and ultimately it encouraged parents and children, as well as husbands and wives, to see each other in new lights with an inevitable tendency towards egalitarianism.

At the same time the position of the wife lost its earlier stability, first in the middle classes. In England (here we seem to be picking up a specific Western thread which probably accelerated global demographic transition) parents had not lived with their married children and intervened between them for a very long time and mothers-in-law had not kept daughters-in-law in their place (Macfarlane, 1978). Over centuries "affective individualism" and sentiment developed (Stone, 1977), spurred by growing wealth and probably by the decline in familial production. The culmination of this process with nineteenth century affluence has been described well by Ann Douglas in "The Feminization of American Culture" (1978) (even if one disagrees with her distinguishing of the central mechanism). The decades up to about 1880 witnessed in the English-speaking world an almost frantic attempt by the media to convince middle class women that their place was in the home—no longer because of dire need or even so much moral imperative but because they were essentially gay, frivolous, decorative creatures who took dresses more seriously than industry or ideas.[13] By the second half of the twentieth century the market was competing strongly for the labour even of married women with young children and was increasingly offering to produce most household needs.

Inevitably moralities had changed towards those more suited to a fully developed capitalism. The stress of the rights of the old had almost disappeared and that on male prerogatives was declining. Morality had passed successively from being chiefly the concern of the family to that of the Church and

---

[13] Unpublished file compiled by Pat Caldwell on nineteenth century Australia from the *Sydney Herald*, the *Sydney Morning Herald* and *The Australasian*.

ultimately the State. More importantly, in terms of the likely impact on fertility, it was concerned ever less with intrafamilial relations. This meant a declining chance of an economic return from children in later life, which, together with the fact that their productive usefulness when young had crumbled, turned the wealth flow downward and made low fertility inevitable.

Contradictions and Change

Clearly, except in long ages of stability, there is not likely to be a superstructure that exactly fits the needs of the current state of the modes of production. Although there has been a persistent family mystique, the family—especially that which controlled production—has always been marked by tensions, some inevitable and some equilibrating. Such tensions should be distinguished from the bitterness which marks rapid changes in parts of the Third World during which some family members feel not that their position is invidious but that they have been robbed of age-old rights (Kiray, 1976). Much of the interest and excitement of village life—the essence which keeps life from being so miserably poor and dreary as outsiders often assume—lies in observing the skill with which some villagers observe the traditional mores and niceties in contrast to the daring with which others bend the rules or the crassness with which some break them. This carries through into life with capitalist production; much of English manners, literature and humour centres on the degree of skill in noting and observing social class differences.

Nevertheless, there are stress points in the traditional family which are of crucial importance with either evolutionary or imported social change.

One is the incompatibility between the high value placed upon the family built up by reproduction and so sustained by full blood ties and the need to maintain a production unit of efficient size in conditions of capricious mortality and accidental subfertility or a sexual imbalance in the births. Thus many of the most family-conscious societies tend to be marked by remarriage, step-parents, half-brothers and sisters,[14] fictive kin and adoption.

Another is the incongruous position of the partriarch. In order to maintain his position of awesome respect from a distance, and because of the related delegation of authority, he tends to become increasingly isolated. He avoids intimacy, he cannot talk to his sons as he would to other men, and he has to allow his wife to run the household almost as if he were not present. Where segregation is substantial he may have to spend much of

[14] Cf., on pre-modern France, Davis (1977), p. 87.

his time out (in Turkey he frequents coffee shops) because the house has become a woman's place.[15] There are difficulties in the father–son relationship; as parents grow older they usually tend to assume more managerial roles (hence the upwardly flowing wealth flow) especially if the family is wealthy,[16] but the real intergenerational strain can come later if an increasingly senile old man tries to maintain his control over a son at the height of his powers. The power delegated to the older women often becomes real in practice, and the alliance formed between her and her son may undermine the ideal family structure and serve as an instrument for change.[17] The problem of senile old men—and the problem of unduly delayed inheritance—is increasingly aggravated by a demographic factor, declining mortality.

The greatest potential for conflict and change arises from the peculiar position of women. Women are a major—and underestimated—part of the workforce. In fact—and this point is rarely taken into account in demographic literature—patriarchs do not distinguish very much between the labour inputs of wives and children (and they can substitute for one another, a potentially important point in the timing of demographic transition). Precisely in those societies, where all respondents tell the researcher that women are of so little value that the birth of a daughter brings no joy, are girls so socialized to obey and to work that they become, when married out, the backbone of the family labour inputs. This is often obscured by emphasis being placed on the managerial role of the mother-in-law or on an artificial analytical division between "productive work" and "household activities" (as in Connell and Lipton, 1977). In India, "though the young wife is taken to be a person of little consequence in the family, her role is one of great importance. Few family roles are subject to such close scrutiny and so liable to such quick redressive action" (Mandelbaum, 1970a, p. 93). Indeed, her own family is supposed to participate in that process by upbringing, instruction at the time of marriage, and even subsequent intervention if necessary (ibid., with a reference to Ranade, 1938). It might be noted that daughters, even though married out, retain a certain value by this very fact in that such marriages help create family alliances.

With regard to women, there is one curious parallel between the superstructure of traditional familial production and of two-tiered capitalistic production where women work in the household. In each the male position is most secure, and stability is most easily maintained, if women are kept divided. There is strong male pressure (and supporting jokes and folk wisdom) against too much "sisterhood" developing.

[15] Cf., on India, Mandelbaum (1970a), pp. 58–61; on Turkey, Fallers and Fallers (1976), p. 247; on Mexico, Lewis (1969), pp. 56–61.

[16] Cf., on Bangladesh, Khuda (1978).

[17] Cf., on Turkey, Kiray (1976), pp. 266–267.

The peculiarities of women's position stem partly from the delegation of male power to the mother-in-law with a consequent frequent bitterness, and even hatred, between the older and younger woman that remains a standing threat to the whole family structure. This is reinforced by the fact that the younger woman usually adopts a position which is closer to the real long-term interests of her husband than is the position adopted by his mother. The situation is stable only if the bond between the younger husband and wife is kept weak, partly by emphasizing the husband's prior obligations to his parents and siblings, but necessarily also by downgrading the pleasures of marital sex, reinforced in many societies by an insistence that the wife display little emotion during sexual relations with her husband. The maintenance of this situation depends to a considerable degree on arranged marriage.[18] The maintenance of power by the older generation has important implications for reproduction, because it separates reproductive decision-making from those biologically involved.

A related issue is the purity of wives. In Mexico this may mean a diminution of all external family contacts (ibid., p. 57), the husband's as well as the wife's, and may have direct demographic consequences: "Men feel most secure when their wives are pregnant or have an infant to care for; thus to have one child follow upon another is a desirable state of affairs from the men's viewpoint" (ibid., p. 58).

A highly portentous weakness of the superstructure generated by familial production is the almost inevitable strain between its morality and that of the major religions which are likely to have strongest hold over its urban or elite populations (one of the distinctions between the Little and Great Traditions in India (Redfield, 1955; Redfield and Singer, 1954; Marriott, 1955)). A religion which is not wholly family-based is likely to make some appeal directly to individuals rather than always through the patriarch, and it is likely to put some stress on individual moralities applying to one and all rather than in gradations by family position. The same is true of all legal systems, and of most other actions which a State might take.

With economic change, a crucial weakness is the attitude towards instilling, or allowing, competitiveness and individual initiative in children during their upbringing. Traditional child-rearing opposes such concepts which can weaken the traditional family. As capitalism develops, employers are increasingly forced to demand such attributes. Eventually, tempted by the chance of external income, many families allow their children to develop such characteristics so as to compete successfully for jobs in the market place. In these circumstances the direction of the wealth flow changes quickly. The willingness of families to make this change in

---

[18] Cf., on Mexico, Lewis (1960), p. 58.

upbringing depends not only on the economic temptations but also on the stress the culture has traditionally put on children knowing their place.

Most of the discussion has assumed patriarchy and has implied patrilineality and patrilocality—rightly in terms of the great majority of Third World societies. But there are areas, especially in Southeast Asia and parts of tropical Africa, where matrilinearity or matrilocality or neolocality are quite common. Such societies may resist change less readily when faced with Westernization (furthermore, Western inheritance and land law codes and attitudes tend to produce confusion and consequent change in matrilineal societies).

Problems in Interpreting the Course of Western Fertility

The major problems in applying wealth flows theory to the West are: (1) the relatively low fertility in Western Europe prior to the final sustained decline, and (2) certain populations with an earlier fertility decline, (3) the surprisingly late start for general fertility decline, (4) the sudden beginning of sustained fertility decline in a range of countries in the short period from the 1860s to the 1880s, and (5) the long, slow and interrupted decline in fertility over the last hundred years.

One point should be made at the outset. The West was the one culture that received no models from other cultures (except—and this may be important—certain models transmitted by Christianity, which, though transmuted and reinterpreted in many ways, originated in the classical world or even in Hebrew society). Hence there were lags that are unlikely to be seen again, first in creating a superstructure where high fertility disadvantaged reproductive decision-makers, and secondly in substituting easier for more difficult forms of contraception. We are unlikely to witness again a society with as little familial production as characterized England of the 1870s without low fertility, and we are unlikely to find in future Third World transitions the level of use of withdrawal as a contraceptive method as was found in a substantial part of the West earlier this century. Neither the Western capitalist development, nor the superstructure, nor the pressures on it to change, were the same throughout the West. Much remains to be discovered about cultural interchange, and the West still has cultural leaders and followers. But in much of the society there was a homogeneity compared with contemporary global society.

The West had for long not maximized upward wealth flows (a fact of fundamental importance in the world demographic transition). Families and households had not generally been multigenerational for centuries. According to Macfarlane's analysis (1978) which is taken back to the beginning of the thirteenth century, part of the explanation, at least in England, may have been a much earlier reduction in familial production than was once assumed. Part may have been because the complex family is rendered easier to form by arranged marriage, an institution forbidden by canon law (Davis, 1977, p. 106). Macfarlane appears to hint at reasons reaching back through Saxon culture to German tribal patterns which had never fully adjusted to the conditions of a peasantry. Some of the cause must lie in the nature of the strong post-Conquest State and of the feudal system, but some may well lie in the existence of a strong Church with behavioural (superstructural) concepts formed in the urban areas of the Roman Empire at its height, when much production was not familial (the external nature of the Church would not have rendered that a crucial point in any case). Certainly, an examination of nineteenth century Australian society suggests that fertility remained high, at least at that time, not so much because large families added greatly to economic well-being but because they did little to detract from it (see Chapter 6; Ruzicka and Caldwell, 1977). (Frequent references will be made to the Australian transition, not because it was atypical of the Western tradition but because it seems to have been very typical, and we happen to have done some work on it of a kind that we hope will soon be duplicated in other Western societies). Yet marital fertility in the pre-transition West was high even in terms of the contemporary Third World.[19] Moderate fertility was achieved largely through the postponement of marriage, and the writer believes that this will eventually be shown to have had little to do with any effort to restrict the ultimate size of the family (prior, at least, to the second half of the nineteenth century) but to be concerned almost entirely with the achievement of economic security and a sufficiency to capitalize marriage and its domestic economy.[20]

However, there is evidence of a measurable degree of marital fertility control for the nobility of Geneva and the aristocracy of France, from about 1700 (Henry, 1965, pp. 451–452), and of more general practice accompanied by declining marital fertility in France from the last quarter of the eighteenth century (Bourgeois-Pichat, 1965, p. 482). In contrast, marital

---

[19] In Australia an I_g of around 0·7 until the 1880s (Caldwell and Ruzicka, 1977, Appendix A); in Belgium an I_g of over 0·8 until the 1890s (Lesthaeghe, 1977, p. 102); in Germany one of over 0·75 until the 1870s (Knodel, 1974, p. 39); and, for comparison, an I_g of 0·76 in Mexico in 1960 and 0·66 in Taiwan in 1930 (Coale, 1967, p. 209), 0·56 in Korea in 1925 (Coale et al., 1981), and 0·55 in Ibadan, Nigeria, in 1973 (Caldwell and Caldwell, 1980, p. 19).

[20] Chapter 6, p. 186 and findings from an ongoing project by John and Pat Caldwell. There is a myth that Ireland was different and early postponed marriage severely in order to restrict fertility. Actually its I_m index in 1870 (immediately before the onset of the Western fertility transition) was 0·42, the same as Sweden and lower than Norway, and its I_g index was 0·67, just below England and Wales and well below Norway and Sweden (Coale, 1967). The postponement of marriage in rural Ireland was a problem of land shortage and land inheritance, and hence of the proper time to marry. By 1900 Ireland's I_m was the lowest in Europe, but by 1900 Western Europe had changed and the wealth flow was everywhere downward.

fertility did not fall anywhere else in the West (or the world) before the 1860s,[21] and there is no evidence of marital fertility restriction even among the British aristocracy before this date (Hollingsworth, 1965, p. 373).

Now, it is possible that there were downward wealth flows among the French aristocracy by this time (although children were valuable for the delegation of power) but it is unlikely that financially it mattered. Familial production was declining in France, but was not as low as in England, and in any case some of the early falls in fertility appear to have occurred in predominantly family-farming areas of Normandy and the Gironde.

This means that one other factor must be reconsidered: the locus of fertility decision-making. In the multigenerational family, whether co-residential or not, that locus was likely to be found in the generation older than the one actually involved in reproduction, and, if the flow of wealth was upward (or even close to zero), the result was high marital fertility. The position was much the same in the two-generational family if it inclined toward male dominance. The remaining case for consideration is that where there was a significant degree of female participation in the two-generational family. One reason for this qualification is that nearly every fertility study of pre-transitional populations has shown that wives are less likely to favour high fertility than their husbands.[22] Women may well have a material interest in avoiding very high fertility even before the wealth flow changes decisively downward, in that frequent births inconvenience and even immobilize them, as well as tending—especially in pre-modern societies—to erode their health.[23]

A greater role in female fertility decision-making would itself imply an important transition in the superstructure—toward a greater belief in female co-participation or companionship in work or social activities, and perhaps evidencing and accelerating a decline (perhaps with increasing secularization) in strong moral or religious views on the separate roles of the sexes and the sanctity of maternity. Changes of this kind may well have occurred among the French nobility (described by Sauvy as "that brilliant and corrupt aristocracy which introduced forbidden practices . . . from the

[21] Between 1860 and 1890 marital fertility began to decline in most Western and Central European countries and in English-speaking countries of overseas European settlement.

[22] Females had lower ideal family size, or a desire for longer birth intervals, or a lesser desire for the last birth or the next one in India (United Nations, 1961, pp. 137–158; Sovani and Dandekar, 1955, pp. 105–106), in Kenya (Dow, 1967, pp. 784–791), in East Java (Gille and Pardoko, 1966, pp. 514–517), in Turkey (Kirk, 1966, p. 577), in Tunisia (Morsa, 1966, pp. 583–584), in Sri Lanka (Kinch, 1962, pp. 90–91) and in Ghana (Caldwell, 1968a, pp. 85–91). The exceptions, where the men desired fewer, were Taiwan (Freedman *et al.*, 1963, pp. 226–228), and Malaysia (Coombs and Fernandez, 1978), close to or after the beginning of fertility transition, as well as a range of contemporary Western countries.

[23] The joint project of the Department of Demography, the Australian National University, and the Bangalore Population Centre, cited in footnote 25, which combined demographic and anthropological approaches, has produced a great deal of evidence for this assertion.

world of prostitution into that of irregular unions and adultery, and from there to the marriage chamber" (1969, p. 362), but were they so likely among the mass of the people? Something very significant had certainly happened in France among the latter who, by the mid-nineteenth century, probably had marital fertility levels of around two-thirds of those in other Western European countries (Lesthaeghe, 1977; Knodel, 1974; van de Walle, 1974).[24] Nevertheless, what had happened was probably distinct from what was to occur towards the end of the century, when France fully participated (in spite of the demographic myth that France's long slow fall in fertility was a substitute for the later sharper falls in other parts of the West) in the general fertility transition—in the thirty years from 1850 to 1880 French marital fertility fell 9% in contrast to a fall of 32% in the next thirty years from 1880 to 1910 (which was, for this latter period, a slightly smaller decline than that experienced by Belgium but a greater one than those in Germany, Netherlands and Australia).

My interpretation of late eighteenth and nineteenth century French social history is that there is as yet no convincing demonstration of greater male–female partnership during that period. Evidence may well be forthcoming, for one of the persistent strains in the struggle for greater female rights in England and Australia in the second half of the nineteenth century was the claim that the French woman worked beside her husband instead of being relegated to the nursery.[25]

The real proof that the superstructure can move at a significantly different rate than the modes of production is provided by the fact that marital fertility did not fall decisively until the 1870s or 1880s in any Western country except France. By this date only one-fifth of the British male workforce was in agriculture (Mitchell, with Deane, 1962, p. 60) (it had been only one-third half a century earlier), and a much smaller proportion in agricultural familial production or any other type of familial production. The argument being put forward here is that the lag in the superstructure— in the way of life controlled by the mores and attitudes of the society—was so great that children were not an appreciable economic disadvantage (that is that the wealth flow had not turned decisively downward) until this time. Two other explanations can be put forward. The first is that the wealth flow had changed but that the only mechanism for adjustment that the society at first knew or was prepared to countenance was delayed marriage. This appears not to have been the case. The proportions married had not been falling in Western Europe (indeed, they appear to have been rising over the preceding half-century),[26] and may well have been at a level that had typified

[24] All comparisons are in terms of I_g (Lesthaeghe, 1977; Knodel, 1974; van de Walle, 1974; Ruzicka and Caldwell, 1977); the 1880–1919 decline was 41% in Belgium, 26% in Germany, 24% in Australia, and 22% in the Netherlands.

[25] See footnote [13], p. 213.

[26] Cf. R. J. Lesthaeghe (1977) p. 102. The I_m index for Belgium rose from 0·375 in 1845 to 0·435 in 1880, that for France from 0·516 in 1840 to 0·538 in 1880, that for Germany from 0·454 in 1865 to 0·501 in 1880, and that for the Netherlands from 0·389 in 1850 to 0·469 in 1880 (in each case the first estimate is the earliest available).

Europe for centuries[27] well back to a period when the wealth flow had certainly been upward. There is no evidence in Australia that prior to the 1880s delayed female marriage was regarded as a method for containing family size.[28] The second is that there was a specific lag in either facing the fact that children had become uneconomic or that contraception could be used or was acceptable. Here again the Australian evidence for the period 1850–1880 is that large families were not felt to be economically oppressive and that family size was not thought to be a factor determining success in life (see Chapter 6). This was in marked contrast to premature male marriage which was widely believed to be an economic indiscretion that was subsequently exceedingly difficult to remedy. When high fertility joined early male marriage as an economic indiscretion—from the 1880s—then contraceptive practice became increasingly acceptable and marital fertility began to decline rapidly. Something had happened in the 1870s or 1880s—not earlier in the century.

What did happen in the 1870s and 1880s? The contemporary Australian material reveals three significant trends: the enforcement of universal, compulsory schooling; an intensification of the movement for women's suffrage and for more equal rights for women; and an increase in the availability of the wares of the consumption society and their advertisement. In contrast it did not exhibit a steep decline in infant or child mortality or any marked change in occupational structure (there had never been subsistence agriculture, and familial production made up a very small part of the whole economy). The populace were becoming more worldly but there seems to be little indication that they were becoming less religious until close to the end of the century. Contemporary observers felt that it was schooling that changed the impact of children on the family, and they were almost certainly right. The reason why even fee-free schooling made children costly has been argued elsewhere (ibid., pp. 88–90)[29] and will not be repeated here. What has not been said, but does seem possible, is that there was a complex interaction between husbands, wives and children. Prior to schooling, the domestic workforce had been the wife and the children. Once the latter went to school, more of the household work was thrown on to the wife's shoulders, and the specific female case against repeated childbirth probably became more intensified. Furthermore, children could hardly live less austerely without their mothers also doing so; this was especially the case once an increasing proportion of mothers had themselves been to school. Fertility fell at much the same time in a score of countries because universal schooling was implemented at much the same time in all. This was largely a

[27] From the seventeenth century, according to Hajnal (1965); from at least the thirteenth century in England, according to Macfarlane (1978).

[28] Ongoing project by John Caldwell and Pat Caldwell.

[29] On the Third World, see Caldwell (1968a), especially pp. 96–114.

social decision, based on increasing affluence—the economy at the time was not expanding at such a rate as to need this sudden rise in educated persons. Fertility within countries also often fell from about the same year across a broad spectrum of society irrespective of the role in the economy played by the parents.[30]

Fertility continued to fall for another hundred years partly because the traditional family with its segregated roles and its justification of such segregation took this period (and more) to dismantle. As the wealth flow toward children increased, large families were described by all as unbearably expensive. Looking after children became far more emotionally draining, partly because of the extra thought given to their welfare, and partly because of the increasing clash between less restrained children and far more expensive and fragile housing and household possessions. Efficient use of contraception did not occur at once, and its effect was partly negated by the fact that it allowed more universal and earlier marriage. Not all the movement was in the superstructure. Elsewhere the two-tiered structure of production has been described (see Chapter 5). At least as much labour input went into the subsistence production of household goods and services as into production outside the home during most of these hundred years. Slowly the market overcame the complex problems of competing efficiently in producing many of these services. Slowly, too, but faster by the 1950s, the expanding labour market began to tempt women to go outside the home to work. Increasingly the superstructure changed to justify this transformation, inevitably with friction and some bitterness.

Problems in Interpreting the Course of Third World Fertility

The process in the peripheral areas of the West and in the Third World has not been, and could not be, like that just described. The central fact of our times has been the ability of the dominant Western economy to establish a global economy and society. This transformation has been based on the strength of the Western economy. The export of its society has not been based on similar social strength but rather on two other features: first, the ability of the paramount exporting economy to sell its society as well, and second, the fact that the Western society was ahead in accommodating itself to the more capitalist economy and hence offered a model for change

---

[30] W. Brass reports (personal communication based on a chapter in press) that fertility began to decline in every county of England about 1876. Ruzicka and Caldwell (1977) pp. 171–176, reported fertility declines commencing in all Australian occupational groups during the 1880s.

when traditional social relations fitted increasingly ill with new modes of production.

There is a tendency among more economically determinist social scientists of a functionalist persuasion to interpret the parallel between economic change towards a more Westernized model and social change towards the same model as demonstrating the governance of that social change by the economic change. This, I suggest, is a major error leading to a fundamental misinterpretation of what is happening, and what is likely to happen, in the contemporary world. It overestimates the impact of the economic change alone, and accordingly tempts researchers to measure demographic and social change with economic indices alone or predominately. It explains highly significant transformations in family relationships in occupational terms, when even the participants are keenly aware that imported social models have played a major role and even made the acceptance of new occupations possible. It neglects the fact that some Western economies had so changed in the early nineteenth or even eighteenth centuries that the availability of seductive external models of family relations could have changed family relationships to the point of rendering high fertility economically disadvantageous without any faster movement in the economic base (although such family changes may have speeded up the movement). If greater egalitarianism had developed between parents and children and between husbands and wives in emotional relationships and in consumption (and possibly production) decisions, fertility may well have fallen much earlier.

The Western society, and above all the Western family pattern, is not for the Third World merely an external pattern. It is largely imposed. Western richness has been identified with the Western way of life. Missionaries, colonial administrators, imported legal systems, the media and schools have all taught it. International programmes, especially the family planning ones, both assume and, almost unconsciously, advocate the Western family. In United Nations statements about the 1975 International Women's Year and the 1979 International Year of the Child no concessions were made to family relationships that were not contemporary—even avant-garde western ones. The West has also exported a view of life and a secular scepticism of religion and traditional ways and ethics that has powerfully catalysed its direct teachings on family change.

Mass schooling has probably had a greater impact on the family than it had even in the West. There are several reasons for this. First, mass schooling has come in many countries at an earlier stage in terms of the economic and occupational structure than it did in the West. Secondly, the message that schooling means an access to Western riches and the Western way of life has been almost universally received. Thirdly, Western schooling assumes and teaches the Western way of life—especially the Western family—almost exclusively. Even teachers who do not live a very Western family life believe that they should not deny the validity of the Western family message when teaching their students. Fourthly, traditional families treat educated members quite differently than they treat uneducated members (Caldwell, 1979)—invariably educated children cost more and give less. Most demographic and social surveys of the Third World yield measures testifying to the extraordinary impact of formal schooling—even patently poor schooling—but little has been done to investigate the nature of that impact.

The literature on the nature of family change in Third World countries is still limited—there is actually more concentration on the traditional situation—but what exists is instructive, especially in the clarity with which it, usually inadvertently, reveals for many societies that children's economic value ultimately declines with such change. Examples will be taken here from studies of three societies subjected to a substantial amount of external influence: Eregli, a small town in Turkey on the coast of the Black Sea, as studied by Mübeccel Kiray (1976) in the 1960s; Tepoztlán, a highland village in central Mexico, as studied by Oscar Lewis (1960) in the 1940s and 1950s;[31] and K'un Shen, a village on the south-west coast of Taiwan, as studied by Norma Diamond (1969) in the 1960s.

The parallels are striking in spite of the three populations being found equi-distant around the world, and the differences few and not very significant.

First, the young people, especially the sons, are restless. They have learnt of a different way of life. Their style of clothing is changing somewhat faster than their parents approve, largely one gathers because of the implied threat to authority. The children are noisier than they were and a stage known as adolescence can be discerned—a fact not unrelated either to schooling or the media.

There is not only implied challenge, but actual challenge. Sons are restless working for their fathers on the family farm or in the family business, partly for the social reason that they resent the imperious paternal authority, and partly for the economic reason that they could earn more money elsewhere than the pocket money they are allowed from the family production. Because of the isolation and pride of the patriarch, the mother often mediates, strengthening her alliance with her son and subtly changing all family relationships.

Daughters are constrained to take their examples from their mothers, but those examples are changing. Indeed, among women, it is the authority that has been given to older women that is allowing change. "As they grow older

[31] The village was also studied by Redfield (1930) in the 1920s.

they become more self-assertive and oppose their husbands' attempts to limit their freedom and their business ventures. . . . The present trend in the village is for the younger women and even the unmarried girls to take on the more independent attitudes of the older women" (Lewis, 1960, p. 56).

Amongst the young, spousal bonds are tightening. In Taiwan the "love marriage" is appearing; in Mexico the proportion of arranged marriages is declining; while in Turkey, the arrangement of marriages without the consent of the future spouses is now rarely attempted. A potent factor is female education. In Taiwan, "The increasing amount of education as one moves down the age scale . . . gives a woman an advantage over her mother-in-law compared to earlier times" (Diamond, 1969, p. 62). In Turkey, "Many husbands even stress that they prefer their wives' advice to that of older members of their families who have been unable to keep up with today's fast-changing relationships, institutions and values" (Kiray, 1976, p. 270). There are clearly parallels here with the situation which has been described for sections of Ghanaian and Nigerian society (Caldwell, 1968a; Caldwell and Caldwell, 1976 and 1978). In all societies these new balances within the family are increasingly militating against the establishment or maintenance of the multi-generational household—a fact with implications for both emotional relations and for productive ones.

Relationships are changing—sometimes leading to bitterness, as distinct from the stresses and even hatreds of the traditional family. In Taiwan, "K'un Shen recognizes that sons have an obligation to support their parents. . . . Yet allegiance to parents is not sufficient to hold the household together. . . . There is considerable bitterness among some of the older people, who feel that they have no authority over any of their sons' households, and their presence is resented. It is not often that a man over 50 or a widow with a married son can maintain a position as household head. The leadership passes to the next generation and the elders become subordinates" (Diamond, 1969, p. 64). Another account of Taiwan reports "a new uncertainty about relationships within the family, a recognition (though not necessarily an acceptance) of a new emphasis on the husband–wife relationship and its threat to the traditionally more important relationship between parents and sons" (Wolf, 1972, p. 129). In Turkey, "Generally a son takes his mother's side in any conflict between her and his wife" (Kiray, 1976, p. 267). Nevertheless, "Sons who change their behaviour towards their fathers (and this is becoming common) also begin to change in their actions towards their wives and their mothers. Consequently, often a mother can no longer count on supreme power over her daughters-in-law if her son starts to take his wife's side against his mother" (ibid.). Often, the extent of change is not faced; in Turkey, "Fathers usually do not admit that such conflict exists, and are very reluctant to concede that their rights and duties have changed with the times [read *Westernization* for *times*] . . . both parties can usually be led to believe that neither's role has changed and so authority can formally be retained" (ibid., pp. 265–266).

The unity of the traditional family was also based partly on force, and this too is being undermined. In Mexico, "Severe punishment is traditional. On the whole, Tepoztecans agree that punishment has become less severe and that there is a greater toleration toward children's faults. This is particularly true among the more permissive and better-educated younger generation" (Lewis, 1960, p. 60).

These changes have important economic implications, not least for the value of children (and hence, also, children-in-law). In Mexico, "The custom of having daughters working in the home is a deeply ingrained one. . . . Many mothers exploit their daughters, particularly the oldest" (ibid., pp. 62–63). In Turkey, a mother, fearing weakening further her emotional bond with her son, nowadays not only is likely to consent to separate households, but often takes the necessary action to see that it can be arranged, "although she has no desire to see her son leave or be deprived of the help of his bride" (Kiray, 1976, p. 265).

A Problem in Calculating the Economic Value of Children

There is an important and curious problem that often besets the researcher when trying to draw up a balance sheet of the economic gains and losses from children. Its solution has implications for the timing of the reversal of the wealth flow.

Rural, or even poor urban populations, often deny that children cost anything, even when they are fairly explicit about long-term benefits gained from them. One explanation, that I have stressed in Chapter 2, is the wide-spread concept of "more mouths, more hands"—they join their mothers from a young age in helping to grow food. Another is the fact that children's costs are shared—in Africa they wander from relative's cooking pot to relative's cooking pot. A third is that the whole process is seen as dynamic and not static; infants grow so quickly into children whose value offsets or exceeds their cost, and their births are so frequently regarded as investments from which gains will shortly flow, that parents without a young child can easily feel economically deprived.

Yet a reworking of survey results suggests that this explanation is not enough, and that it is not what many respondents are implying. What some do seem to be saying is that there are no costs within a family—that that is what a family means. The argument appears to be that there is no parallel between deliberately putting some income aside—putting money in a bank which could be used to buy food or clothing or more frivolous things or subtracting a greater proportion of food produced for sale in the market—and tightening one's belt a little more as children multiply in order to make the same amount of food or clothing go a greater distance. The latter is regarded as enforced saving, and hence easy to achieve compared with the more difficult voluntary saving represented by the first examples. It is, of course, common that it is the children, or they and their mother, who do the most belt tightening, and hence there is no real cost to the decision-maker.[32] (It is, also, possible that such tightening increases child mortality,[33] but, once this is noted as a major problem, the chances are that both the emotional and wealth flows have turned decisively downward.) Thus the ensuing benefits from children are received without any appreciated initial outlay. There has been forced saving and investment at no felt cost.

If this calculus is common, then the point where the wealth flow is felt to swing toward the children is clearly displaced to a later date. The calculus probably is common, but the displacement is probably much rarer, because the family and its economy have so changed from the traditional pattern by the time the reversal is near that forced savings are really felt. But the calculus may be important in explaining the great stability of high fertility well before that divide is reached.

The Lessons

The fundamental point is that the fertility declines of the last century have been one of our most significant indicators of a massive change in the human condition. They are not the product of anything more deep-seated than change in ideal family size or of acquaintance with contraception or of a sudden and belated recognition that children were contrary to the family's economic interests.

This brings us to perhaps the central mystery of population studies. The statistical techniques are ever more impressive and are both needed and valuable in that they measure the true demographic position and the direction and speed of change. But in themselves they do not tell us anything about the nature of that change. Attempts to apply survey techniques with questions about reproductive attitudes and behaviour have told us something about short-term Western fertility change but the findings have often been fairly trivial and the resulting published volumes curiously

[32] Merrylin Wasson reports that this was the usual case in the poor quarter of Old Delhi where she worked for a number of years (personal communication).
[33] Evidence for this is the higher child mortality often found in larger families (Wray, 1971).

unexciting even to professionals in the field. The application of the same techniques to non-Western societies has probably been misleading while producing results which are equally unexciting. This is unusual in the social sciences where most fields tend to produce from time to time spates of work which do seem to cast new light on human behaviour and the nature of human societies. The lack of excitement is also surprising in view of the historical significance, and the importance to individuals, of the phenomena being investigated.

A correct theory of stable high fertility and of fertility decline will be essentially a theory of social and familial change. The attempt in this paper may often miss the exact mark. Nevertheless, the truth lies somewhere in the general area it has attempted to traverse. High fertility was not uneconomical in the traditional family engaged in familial production, while it is uneconomic in contemporary societies with a dominant non-familial labour market. The cost of children, or the balance between gains accruing to parents and losses experienced by them because of having children, depends very greatly on the conventional emotional and economic relations within the family—that is on the superstructure. This superstructure may lag behind changes in the method of production—nothing else will explain the lateness of the Western fertility decline—or it may move forward surprisingly rapidly, when the relations of production are changing, as a result of imported values and behavioural patterns as is at present occurring in much of the Third World as a global, Westernized society is being created.[34] Certainly there may be lags, but they are lags in family relations which prevent fertility from becoming uneconomic as early as might otherwise be the case. They are not lags in the recognition that children are uneconomic—the "props" of Notesteinian demographic transition theory whereby religion and social creed hid reality from parents. This means that, if demographers wish to explain the phenomena they study, they must either become real social scientists or alternatively confine themselves to measuring what other disciplines might be asked to explain. They must also approach fertility causation with a more sophisticated apparatus than the largely tautological one of "intermediate variables" (Davis and Blake, 1956)—originally an intriguing concept and one which still serves graduate students well as a check-list, but one which also convinces many of the same students that they have done all the explaining that needs to be done.

Such an apparatus will have to give priority to studying families with fundamentally different relations of production. The failure to do this has produced not only Westernized, and basically false, pictures of Third World

---

[34] The Soviet Union and China have not been overlooked. It will be argued elsewhere that, in terms of the relations of production, they have been Westernized at least as fast as any other society.

fertility behaviour, but also similarly Westernized and unhelpful pictures of the sociology of the family—pictures which suggest that the family structures of the world could be adequately described in terms of continuums of such characteristics as inheritance, marriage payments, combinations of relatives living together, and so on, without a proper picture of the relations of these characteristics to the whole, and the varying natures of that whole.[35]

In terms of fertility change in the Third World, the rates of economic growth and of occupational change are relatively easily measured, and predicted with somewhat greater difficulty and inaccuracy. What will determine the timing and speed of fertility decline is the rate at which family relations are Westernized. This is not merely a function of the level of cultural flow from the West. It is also very much affected by the receptivity or opposition of the receiving cultures. The areas of the world where high fertility persists longest will not necessarily be the poorest. It is likely that they will be the Islamic world where Koranic injunction serves to insulate the existing family structure,[36] and sub-Saharan Africa where the lineages retain a surprising amount of their strength even while welcoming Western imports which do not impinge on family relations. It is clear that family planning programmes hasten fertility falls in some countries (Mauldin and Berelson, 1977) but it is not equally clear that they can initiate falls. It would be unwise to assume that this represents a simple case of contraception meeting a recognized need. The fact of such programmes and governmental backing of them suggests new spousal relations and tends to legitimize such trends. The use of contraceptives, even with a degree of duress, can also change family relations.

It is also unwise to talk of societies with high child mortality and consequent high and compensating fertility. A central reason for high child mortality is that the direction of the emotional flow has not changed (Caldwell, 1979). Stress is still on the importance and needs of the older generation. It follows both that child mortality will be relatively higher than it might otherwise be and that high fertility is not economically disadvantageous and is likely to characterize the society.

The current debate as to whether the West ever had family structures or relations like the contemporary Third World is almost irrelevant. What is relevant is the impact of contemporary Western patterns on contemporary Third World patterns. Nor is the lack of homogeneity in either the West or Third World of much importance. Clearly parts of the West have greatly affected other parts.[37] Clearly also Westernization is a relative concept.

[35] See, for instance, Nimkoff (1965).
[36] This refers mostly to the Islamic heartland, and not to Indonesia or Malaysia.
[37] In evidence given to the Royal Commission on *The Decline of the Birth Rate and on the Mortality of Infants in New South Wales* (1940) vol. 1, it was testified on more than one occasion that the leading influence was that of the French.

Even the West's leading edges are changing rapidly, partly because the labour market is tempting members of the family never before attracted and is increasingly proving to individuals within the family that they need ever less protection from its structure. Nevertheless, the nature and pace of change is not solely directed by the market—the European cultural heritage plays an important role. For instance, the egalitarian ideological element in that heritage has allowed the market demands on individuals to be interpreted in very specific ways. The arguments of women's movements, and those of the younger generations, are often conceded partly because opposition to them would betray much older principles.

These changes can be researched. Even in terms of the empirical base for my own suggestions, Thadani has probably underestimated its size,[38] modest though it may still be. There are already very substantial findings on the nature of differing societies and their families, and also on change, little used by either demographers or others as yet to interpret fertility levels or fertility trends.

Certain central conclusions should be stressed.

The first one is that a society based on familial production cannot but emphasize high fertility to take uncontrolled fertility for granted. Such high fertility provides labour, and keeps the women in a position where they are family-centred, work hard, and do not demand to compete with their menfolk in consumption. When the emotional and wealth flows are both from young to old (and they must both flow in the same direction except during brief periods of traumatic change), children also work hard and consume relatively little. Any relaxation in the veneration for the old and the male would fundamentally change the production and consumption system, and, in a society of predominantly familial production, would be automatically reversed as the system became less efficient from the viewpoint of the older male decision-makers. Such societies exhibit high infant and child mortality, not merely because they do not have adequate modern health services, but also because greater care lavished on children would upset the priorities assigned to different individuals within the family structure, alter the time allocation of labour, change the balance of consumption, and render the young less likely to accept the direction of their labour or to work as hard. A society based on the labour market does not need an upward flow in either veneration or wealth. Ultimately the need of the employer to appeal directly to all individuals, and of the producer to attempt to maximize consumption among all by direct temptation, and of the strong state necessary to impose the community-based morality means that such a society not only does not require the same family priorities but inevitably causes their erosion. In the end, children become an economic

[38] One analysis omitted was Caldwell and Caldwell (1976).

burden, and, with the emotional flow directed towards them, a large number often become an emotional burden too.

This change is accelerated by the imposition of mass education systems. This was so in the West. It is much more the case in the contemporary Third World, where the arrival of mass education has occurred at a time when the move towards a global economy, together with a more rarely noted but equally important move towards a global society, has meant a major attack on the old family system. That system could not change if the system of production were not altering at the same time, but the external intrusion speeds up the rate of change in the superstructure (which, in turn, as children are more likely to seek work elsewhere or to keep a larger share of their earnings, inevitably accelerates the transformation of the system of production). We will not have an industrialized world by the end of the century, but it is unlikely that there will be any substantial parts of it where fertility is still high and has shown no decline.

This paper has attempted to demonstrate just how intricate and compelling are the mechanisms that sustain high fertility in pre-transitional societies. Those mechanisms are the fundamental sinews of the society, and uncontrolled fertility is not merely an aspect of the society, but the central aspect of the cultural superstructure that maintains the relations of production. Accordingly, the study of fertility transition is the study of the transformation of familial production into production through the labour market, of traditional society into modern society. There can be no discipline of "population studies" in the area of demographic transition which is not the discipline devoted to studying social and economic change in all aspects. Conversely the failure of social and economic change theorists to recognize the central role of demographic transition, both in terms of its occurrence and timing, in explaining the transformation of traditional society, is not merely an unfortunate omission in their explanations, but evidence of the basic inadequacy of those explanations. This is treated more fully in Chapter 9.

8

An explanation of the continued fertility decline in the West: stages, succession and crisis

Over the last one hundred years fertility levels in most countries of Northern Europe and of Northern European settlement overseas have more than halved. Total fertility rates have fallen from five or more to under two. The fall has not been continuous: the crude birth rate typically declined from the mid-30s around 1880 to near 15 in the 1930s, rose by 1960 to near 20 in Northern Europe and 25 overseas, and subsequently declined, moderately in the 1960s and steeply in the 1970s, ultimately falling below the levels of the 1930s. By 1978 most of these countries recorded net reproduction rates below unity.

Three aspects of this fertility transition particularly trouble its theorists. First, why did birth rates rise during the 20 years after the Depression of the 1930s by up to one-quarter in Europe and up to one-half overseas—the "baby boom"—if a real transition were underway? Second, why did fertility begin to decline again in the prosperous years of the 1960s and plummet during the 1970s in conditions of economic adversity which could not compare with the 1930s? Third, did the rebound in the 1930s from a net reproduction rate of just below unity (together with the current appearance of a similar phenomenon in parts of Eastern Europe) provide evidence to support the Blacker–Notestein view of a transition that was destined to bottom out at replacement levels again?

In recent years post-transition fertility theory has seemed to be in greater difficulties than pre-transition theory. In April, 1980, the *Committee on Comparative Analysis of Fertility* of the *International Union for the Scientific Study of Population* held a seminar in search of "major theories and new directions for research". The final hours of discussion of that meeting appeared to be in danger of leading to the view that we have coincidentally lived through two unrelated fertility declines, each needing its own theory to explain its mechanics, that of the half-century from the 1880s to the 1930s, and that of the last two decades. In between was a significant but inexplicable phenomenon, the "baby boom". Just how different the two transitions might be was underscored by Philippe Ariès' view that the first transition was the end-point of a European tradition of half a millennium, the move towards making the child the king, whilst the last two decades have been the product of the child's sudden and unpredicted dethronement. Clearly the meeting did not consider the theories at present being offered—Notestein's theory of demographic transition (1945 and 1953), the Chicago Household Economists' explanation of fertility change in terms of both differential investment in children and the value of women's time (see Schultz, 1973), or Easterlin's theory of alternating generations raised in either depression or boom (Easterlin, 1968 and 1976)—as being capable of dealing with a canvas of this size and intricacy. These theories will be discussed toward the end of this chapter when they can be put into the perspective of the argument presented here.

The standpoint of this discussion is that no theory of fertility decline will ultimately be found to be satisfactory that does not offer a comprehensive explanation not only for both periods of fertility decline and the intervening "baby boom" but also for the contrast between the preceding condition of high fertility and the transition that followed. The same basic forces should persist and there should not be reliance on adventitious occurrences to explain segments of the transition. There should be a recognition that a century is a comparatively short period for a major social transition. However, there should also be a realization that a transformation of this type must be viewed in terms of social changes that must necessarily precede other social changes, rather than in segments determined wholly by the relative levels of fertility and mortality as in classical demographic transition theory. Finally, the theory should allow (and attempt to explain the mechanisms) for the influence of one society on another and not imply autonomous changes in a range of societies characterized by an extraordinary coincidence in their timings.

The purpose of this discussion is to argue that the "wealth flows theory"[1] of fertility decline can provide a satisfactory explanation of the course of fertility decline, and can be used for prediction, even though it was developed to explain stable high fertility and the onset of transition—indeed, one of the above postulates states that, if it is satisfactory for one purpose, it must be for the other. The exposition will rely mainly on the Australian experience about which we have an unusually rich fund of

[1] See Chapters 4, 5, 7 and 11 in this volume.

information.[2] The details of that experience, previously described (in Chapter 6), will not be repeated here, but instead they will be employed to build the model. The Australian demographic experience was similar to that of Northern Europe, and extraordinarily similar to that of the United States. In addition there is a certain advantage in the fact that, because of its population size, Australia could hardly have been the leader in fundamental innovational change, but must have in some way participated in social movements that yielded such demographic behaviour.

The fundamental concept in wealth flow theory is that of a cultural superstructure determined by the mode of production but capable of lagging behind it in the course of change so that at any given time it specifically determines the advantages and disadvantages of children. It is not claimed here that children were a net advantage at any time after say 1875, but it is claimed that the degree of disadvantage changed. Nevertheless, the rate of change in disadvantage was not the chief determinant of fertility decline— the chief determinant was the time needed to dismantle the society found immediately prior to that date. The first concern of this paper must be the nature of that society.

The Nature of Society at the Onset of Fertility Decline

Historically, nearly all production, certainly since neolithic times, had been family production. This had been characterized by marked differences in type of work and consumption according to sex and age, with the advantage tending to go to the old and the male. Such discrimination was justified by popular morality, and religion was interpreted as enshrining it. This cultural superstructure was not ephemeral and is still being dismantled.

By the late nineteenth century the West was characterized by a massive labour market outside the family. The transition from wholly family production had been marked by two developments.

The first was an increasing tendency for some members of the family, usually males but sometimes females, to work full-time or part-time outside the family for wages. One result of this was an emphasis on the family budget, with all the wife's earnings, and much of the children's earnings, being put into a common pool largely under the control of the male household head. This, of course, had been implicit in subsistence production, because the patriarch had owned or controlled the land and his

---

[2] Much of which has been gathered by the continuing Australian Family Formation Project of the Department of Demography, The Australian National University, Canberra. Major sources employed here are the 1971 and 1977 Melbourne Surveys and the following Project Monographs and Papers: Macdonald (1975); Caldwell et al. (1976); Ruzicka and Caldwell (1977); Caldwell and Ruzicka (1977).

wife, and had given the children the gift of life. But, as the outside labour market developed, it had to be more explicitly stated in terms of obligations (and affection) within the family, usually so successfully that the net positive economic value of children persisted longer than would otherwise have been the case and was often even enhanced.

A more important result—with vast ramifications even to the present time—was the development of a two-tiered production system whereby the male head of the household worked outside the home for wages while the wife, with considerable assistance from her daughters and some assistance from her sons, produced a range of household goods and services which, during the nineteenth century, increased rather than decreased as society became wealthier and houses larger. The moral basis for this system was a subtle selection from and transformation of the pre-existing morality of family production. Its central pillar was the distinction between "the bread-winner" and the rest of the family. Adult males were bread-winners and accordingly the outside market felt the obligation not only to employ them before wives and children but also to pay them more. Bread-winning was so honoured that both its effort and the importance of the task were usually thought to be much greater than that which went on in the home, and even of a different order and incommensurate with it. So important was bread-winning that the male household head was expected to do very little work when at home and he received a disproportionate share of both household services and of the outside goods and services bought with his wages. The Australian research showed that, through much of the nineteenth century, even middle class children lived so frugally—on the moral justification of "not spoiling them"—that the wealth flow was not indisputably downward. In point of fact, household production in the nineteenth century (and well into the twentieth century) probably absorbed more hours of work than did the outside labour market, and produced a range of goods and services that capitalist production could either not provide at all or could not match.

However, the system was unstable. The virtual disappearance of family production outside the home meant that the universality of a system of morality which was an integral part of it could easily be attacked. Worse still, large-scale production (in contrast to employment in small-scale enterprises which could be run as quasi-families with strong emphasis on familial morality) required a different and, in some ways, competing morality, with emphasis on individual obligations to outside authorities. If children's chief advantage was the relatively small amount that had to be spent on them, this could be just as easily achieved by reducing their number. There were advantages to the bread-winner of high fertility as well, but they were the kind of advantages that characterize the end of an era. If the domestic virtues were to be stressed, then wives who were kept in a traditional state—and were tied to the home—by repeated pregnancies and a lifetime of child rearing were less likely to challenge the system. Similarly children in a large family, where their peers for comparison were each other rather than their father, were less likely to demand (or receive) more equal intergenerational treatment within the family than were children in a small family. The situation was complex because the dichotomy between the bread-winner and the rest meant that there was a relationship between the situation of the wife and that of the children both in terms of production and consumption—when one became disaffected or the situation changed then the other could hardly remain unaffected.

The Persistent Forces

There were fundamental forces in the society that would force it toward a dismantling of familial morality and toward lower fertility. An unsettling element in the cultural tradition had always been the concept of equality, usually applying to areas outside the family but always with a potential for providing an ideology for challenging the existing morality of interspousal or intergenerational relations. The concept of as much equality as could reasonably be expected in given circumstances underlay the Australian (and other) concepts of *fairness*, used to assess most situations. Another was the concept of individualism. Christianity's main appeal had always been to the individual rather than to the family. Capitalism's appeal had to be this way, both because it usually offered jobs to individuals (and was apprehensive of a morality which claimed that a person had obligations to his family which might override those to his employer) and because it sold its products by tempting all, often by appealing to individuals to buy and not to be held back by the constraints imposed by the whole family. A third force was the growth of the industrial system. Ultimately it would be tempted to compete in all aspects of household production and would do so ever more successfully, not necessarily at first offering finished products but part-way products (especially in food preparation). Ultimately, too, it would have enough employment capacity—partly because of the expanding invasion of the household sector—to be forced to offer employment to wives as well as husbands.

The apparently stable system of the mid-nineteenth century would in the end prove its own undoing. Women were kept in their place by the argument that their household work was inferior to their husband's work in the market place; during the twentieth century, they would first, when confined to the household, challenge the argument, although somewhat half-heartedly, while later they would increasingly accept the argument and attempt to enter the market place. The same system built an ever more complex educational structure, largely to train bread-winners for ever more complex jobs, saturated with a philosophy that implied that education fitted one more for market than household work. Yet, for a range of reasons (equality, the need of men for educated companions, the need of the state for an educated electorate) daughters, too, were taken into a system that soon became universal and compulsory.

It was probably the advent of mass schooling that determined the timing of the onset of fertility decline (see Chapter 10), although it had that effect at first more because of its impact on child costs than because it changed females' perceptions of their work roles. Yet, even in the first generation, the changed attitudes toward dependency, especially that of daughters, altered work loads, perhaps critically increasing those on mothers, and implied a certain relationship between education and household work which may have increased the feeling of the relative lack of honour for such work. The advent of mass schooling would, over the coming century, have at least three separate impacts. First, it increased the cost of children while reducing their immediate productivity, thus leading to declining fertility. Second, it provided an unrivalled extra-familial system of child care, which would eventually assist mothers to enter the extra-household labour force. Third, it would eventually go far toward bridging the gap between childhood and adulthood so that female choices between occupation and reproduction could occur at about the same age.

Many of the changes that led to the onset of fertility decline were further accelerated by the decline itself. Small families are necessarily more intimate, and hence egalitarianism by age and sex is more difficult to keep at bay. The attainment of low fertility also needs a degree of cooperation between husband and wife to achieve, which also reduces the distance between the sexes.

The reason that fertility fell is clear enough: children became a decisive economic burden. The critical question (and one intimately bound up with an understanding of present trends) is why it did not fall to replacement level almost immediately—why it has taken a century with fluctuations of fertility on the way. The obvious answer is almost certainly the wrong answer; that is that the change had to move through the society from the most innovational groups to the least. Some of the work on fertility differentials and also the assertions about quality parents wanting quality children (Becker, 1960) seem to imply this. Yet, when measured by the time taken during periods of change for one group to reach the fertility levels of the next higher group, both occupational and educational fertility differentials in Australia—and, I think, elsewhere—were of little significance. Indeed, it is the small difference that is meaningful.

The real answer is almost certainly that change of this order takes time because it consists of a series of institutional changes which must follow each other in a certain order. Distinguishing that necessary order should be a prime activity of demographers and an attempt will be made here.

Key Institutions

One can start by identifying some of the institutions that are involved in the change. The first is the industrial system itself. It has taken a century of development to be able to compete with the household in terms of what can be produced and the price at which it can be sold. The second is the educational system. It has taken all the present century for the proportion of children 5–19 years of age in full-time education to rise from 59% to 81%, thus increasing their dependency costs, removing much of the need for mothering during the daytime, and increasing the implication for females that they would be wasting that education if it were not subsequently used in a job. The reason that the education system expanded only at the rate it did was the dependence of that transformation on changing social values, changing occupational demands, changing external models, and an increasing ability of the economy to afford it.

Another simple solution—in a sense partly correct—is that contraception improved. Technically it did not really do so until the 1960s; the low birth rates of the 1930s were achieved with basically the methods available in the 1880s—indeed, the so-called natural methods formed almost half of all Australian contraceptive practice until the late 1950s (Caldwell and Ware, 1973; Caldwell, in preparation). What did change was the readiness to practice contraception and the efficiency with which it was practiced. This arose partly because of the increasing economic disadvantages of large families, and partly from a decline in the view that contraception was immoral. The latter is not, of course, a fundamental change; it owes its existence largely to an accommodation to the fact that large families had to be avoided, an accommodation helped by the spreading knowledge that others were doing it and by an increasingly secular view of life.

Nevertheless, the account just given is very superficial. These changes rested largely on fundamental alterations in family relationships, in the undoing of the system described earlier as having obtained immediately before the fertility decline. In the traditional agrarian subsistence family, the emotional link between husband and wife was relatively weak, and it was kept this way so that it did not challenge the husband's obligations to his parents or the wife's to her children. One mechanism was the downgrading of the importance of sexual relations between spouses. To this end females were reared, and conditioned within marriage, to regard sex as more of a duty than a pleasure. Indeed, their moderate sexuality was regarded as a sign of purity—an advantage in keeping the spousal bond from becoming paramount in relationships (and an advantage in preserving male rights by keeping wives from straying).

We often tend to assume that relationships a century ago were much more similar to those of today than was really the case. The 1971 Melbourne Survey (Caldwell *et al.*, 1973; Australian Family Formulation Project, 1972) showed, for women reaching adulthood between the mid-1920s and the beginning of the 1970s, a sustained rise with declining age in the proportion claiming to have a stronger emotional relationship with their husbands than their children (a trend probably even stronger in reality than in retrospective reporting because of older women having changed their attitudes over the years). There is no doubt that this trend can be projected backwards in time. An important aspect of intergenerational relations is that people who feel their relations with their children to be a major link usually also take this attitude with regard to their relations with their own parents. The Melbourne Survey also revealed a major increase with age (and certainly not just changing with age) in assent to the proposition that enjoying motherhood is more important than enjoying sex—from less than one-quarter of those who reached adulthood after 1960 to a majority of those doing so between the Wars.

The past century has, then, witnessed a strengthening of relations between husbands and wives at the expense of relations between the spouses and their own parents. This has allowed husbands and wives to feel greater freedom in discussing contraception and sexual relations with each other, and to make decisions about using contraceptives, having fewer children, and postponing the birth of the first child, without first glancing over their shoulders in a guilty fashion to ascertain the feelings of their parents. Traditional parental influences on contraceptive decision-making (and even on spousal sexual relations) have lingered longer, and have retained greater strength, than we are usually prepared to admit. Indeed, our reluctance to admit its full strength is a sign of how long the revolution against age domination has taken—for the reluctance is basically a reluctance of spouses to admit to each other that the other influences still exist. Ultimately, as we shall see, the weakening of intergenerational relations, with a complementary strengthening of age–peer relations, was to have another impact of great significance.

First, however, a transformation took place that was of major importance, and which might seem anomalous in view of the discussion above, but which is in fact very much related to it. One might assume either from the change in the direction of the wealth flows or from the rise of Notesteinian individualism, that obligations to parents were followed by obligations to self. The change was not as simple as this—certainly not in the case of women—and it began long before the nineteenth century. In the society of family production, women spend little time looking after their children—it is a responsibility of all relatives and is often carried out mostly by the children's sisters. With social change, through the development of a middle class or urbanization, one of the first gains sought by women is the right to spend more of their time on their own children (Caldwell *et al.*, 1981; Galal el Din, 1977). This is partly an assertion of their individuality, but it is also an assertion of their rights as against their parents and parents-in-law. Later, and this was certainly the case in the late nineteenth and early twentieth century West, wives went further; they would forge a powerful weapon for weakening their husbands' bonds with their parents by arguing that the children must come first, that they are *their* children. This weapon was particularly potent as mass schooling came into existence. Men already had a ladder of targets in the world—their job or jobs; married women would not have this for several more generations, not until they, too, flocked into the non-household labour market. Now children had a ladder of targets provided by the schooling system, and mothers could identify with their children's success, and could ensure that their husbands felt the primacy of these goals. Thus mothers identified with their children in order to forge a genuine emotional nuclear family, and because they themselves had nowhere else to go. In the process children became an ever greater economic liability; they cost more and probably did even less in the home.

This is now the place to discuss the remaining two continuing forces of change in the society. From the time of the first fertility declines the intergenerational wealth flow was downward, but, nevertheless, its flow was not constant but increased with time. This arose from the egalitarian ethic (increasingly freed from the countervailing needs of an ethic required to enforce familial production), from the demands exerted by the educational system, and from the situation with the nuclear family where mothers could play an even greater maternal role and see that their husbands played a greater paternal one. The 1971 Melbourne Survey found that 90% of Australian women believe that the total fraction of family income now being spent on children has risen since their own childhood, and, among those who were children between the Wars, that proportion was 95%. Another factor also played a role, and this was the burgeoning of the consumption society. This was largely a product of the growth of industry. Nevertheless, the growing consumption rights of wives and children almost certainly played a role in its rapid spread. The position is even more complex than this for three reasons. First, parents, especially male heads, had an increasing option of forgoing some service provided by the household production system for some preferred pleasure bought from the market for money—money which could often be obtained only by reducing the outlays that were capitalizing the system of household production. Second, as children became more dependent, parents often obtained great pleasure from their children's consumption of toys and other goods, which could be maintained at an adequate level only if there were fewer children. Third, as household possessions accumulated and individually became more valuable, and, as houses and their contents became more expensive and fragile and were often acquired earlier in the marital life cycle, the necessary level of care per child rose steeply, increasing the cost of children in terms of mothers' time, and separating the identity of mother and child by highlighting the differences between mother's needs and child's needs.

The Stages of Fertility Decline

We are now in a position to examine how one stage necessarily followed another in what is often regarded as a long-drawn out fertility decline, but which has so far taken only four generations, a comparatively short time when alterations in intergenerational relations form a prime mechanism in the process.

We start with the fundamental factors, a society where children were already a net economic disadvantage to parents, and one which would increase over time but about which something already had to be done. The household production of goods and services was efficient and was controlled by a morality which was suited to the purpose but which could change without endangering the conventional living standards of even male household heads in a way that would have been impossible for the morality that controlled subsistence peasant agriculture.

This was a society with a morality which ensured that the older generation still played a marked role, where younger wives could erode that role by emphasizing their and their husbands' primary obligation to their children, where spousal emotional links were still confused by an emphasis on female purity and limited interest in sexual relations even within marriage, where wives and children lived relatively austerely, and where household work was held to be inferior to bread-winning.

Outside the family things were changing. The industrial system would be able to offer an increasing number of jobs, an ever higher proportion neither dirty nor gruelling, categories thought particularly unsuitable for women; more consumption goods were becoming available; more goods and services were able to compete successfully with household production; the education system was providing a new way of life for children and new implications about what they would do as adults.

Many of these changes allowed underlying—but only slowly more effective—forces in the culture to operate: movements toward egalitarianism and individualism, and toward goals of happiness and pleasure if the case against could not be spelt out in realistic terms. The latter must be seen in the context of a diminished role for religion, a change which both assisted the dismantling of the old family morality and was probably itself accelerated by that dismantling.

The central theme of this paper is that, once children were a net economic disadvantage, the major influence on the rate of fertility decline was the time taken, and the ordering of successive stages, in the transformation of the family morality. Three important points should be made. The first is that the family morality did not primarily change because of the increasing cost of children. Some of the change occurred because of the spreading of contraception, and some because the smaller family size necessarily affected the nature of maternal tasks. But most occurred because of movements, inspired by demands for fairness or equality, that had little or nothing to do with demographic pressures. The second is that these movements did not operate evenly, but change usually occurred as a result of a period of crisis, often centring on women's rights, as during the suffragette or women's liberation movements, or on intergenerational friction, as during the protest movement against involvement in Vietnam. The third is that these protests of rights are very easily exportable, partly because the family economic systems that brought into being the institutions being opposed have largely deteriorated by the time the protest is made.

The last point leads to a central truth. Immediate export, in undiluted form, is possible only to a range of countries with very similar family cultures and with very similar histories of past change. The group that seem to move together are found in Europe north of the Alps and the Pyrenees and west of the Slavonic area (apart from Ireland); in North America, they consist of the United States and Canada; and in Oceania, of Australia and New Zealand. The turning points in their fertility movements often occur in the same year; their fertility levels are often very close. This implies the fast export of demographic behavioural models; the implication is almost certainly wrong—what are exported are models of relationships. Export is not quite the right word. Initial movements nowadays are most likely to come from the United States (as they came from France and Britain in the nineteenth century), but the whole area serves as a mixing bowl to achieve the final blend. The movements that were most closely related to pure demographic behaviour were the various stages of the legitimation of the use of contraceptives (in the 1880s and 1890s, in the Depression of the 1930s, during the introduction of the pill and IUD in the 1960s and greater acceptance of abortion and sterilization in the 1970s) and the discussion of population explosion (1950s and 1960s) and of environmental protection (1960s and 1970s). Nevertheless, even these movements were minor aspects of much more profound movements in family relations which they supplemented. The reason that Mediterranean Europe did not exhibit fertility change at the same time as this primary fertility-decline bloc was not lesser industrialization or more Catholicism but a different family system. What the bloc has in common (Protestant influences? the Teutonic family?) lies outside this paper.

Successive Stages in Australia

(1) *1881–1901*

The period 1881–1901, which was marked by a fall in fertility of 23% as measured by the crude birth rate and 31% as measured by the Princeton I_f index, the index of total fertility,[3] provides valuable information as to what was happening. Prior to 1881 there is little evidence that children were a burden, and there is little evidence of fertility restriction within marriage (the I_g index, that of marital fertility, had been slowly rising for at least two decades). Universal elementary schooling was established in the major states by 1880 and during the rest of the decade fertility fell slowly. By 1891 there were growing sales of contraceptives (following a pattern which had been established in Britain during the previous decade) (Hicks, 1978, p. 22). Most of the fertility decline in the 1880s was caused by increased fertility restriction within marriage, doubtless by a minority of couples (I_f fell at only 1% per annum and 92% of its decline was explained by the fall in marital fertility, I_g).

This pattern probably would have persisted, slowly steepening, but for the occurrence in the 1890s of an extraordinary intense economic depression causing a sharper decline in fertility during these years than in any other country of the primary fertility-decline bloc. Fertility (as measured by I_f) fell by one-quarter, and mass birth control had clearly begun. From our point of view, the point of most interest is that two-fifths of the decline can be explained by the movement in female marriage levels. Never again, not even in the Depression of the 1930s, was marriage to be used as a major means for reducing fertility. Much of the delay in marriage was probably caused by greater difficulty in capitalizing a household. But the movement in marriage rates is probably also evidence that, though the community was

[3] The Princeton Indices of Overall Fertility, Marital Fertility and Marriage are described in Coale (1967).

beginning to accept fertility limitation, and the means for contraception were fairly widely available, many couples did not have the kind of relationship that allowed their use.

The massive fall in marital fertility in the 1890s—greater than in any other decade except the 1970s—undoubtedly owed much to the ideological basis laid in the 1880s; if a major economic depression had occurred in the 1870s it probably would not have had nearly such an impact on fertility. The important question is what began to happen in the 1880s—why did couples increasingly come to the conclusion that they could cooperate with each other in restricting their fertility without worrying a great deal about the views of their more pro-natalist (or, at least, less fertility interventionist) parents. One reason is probably a marked upswing in the position of women—or, at least, a feeling that their views should be heard in public and in private to an extent that had not previously been the case. The suffragette campaign of the 1870s to the 1890s was the strongest and socially most unsettling women's movement prior to the 1970s. Clearly it was interrelated with movements in Britain and the United States. In Australia it not only received strength from the socialist and republican ferment of the time (as the women's liberation movement did from the New Left, three-quarters of a century later) but it gave much to these other movements. It is difficult to imagine the development of Australia's greatest nationalist poet, Henry Lawson (1867–1922) without the influence of his feminist mother (who brought out the radical journal *Republican* in 1887 and founded and edited the feminist journal *Dawn* from 1888 until 1905) and wife. Women obtained the vote in South Australia in 1894 (after years of near success in Victoria—and subsequent to that achievement in New Zealand in 1893 and Wyoming in 1869) and in the new Federal Parliament in 1902. This latter success brought a decline in women's political agitation—and in its social repercussions—long before the suffragette movement reached its major goals in North America and Western Europe.

(2) *1901–1939*

The period from 1901 to the Second World War is the critical intermediate period in both demographic and family terms. It was not an era of booming prosperity and national self-confidence, as the 1880s had been and the period from the Second World War to the early 1970s was to be. Just before it began and towards its end, in the 1890s and 1930s respectively, severe economic depressions had made fertility particularly perilous and had hastened mass familarity with contraception. The social convulsion of the First World War undoubtedly weakened intergenerational links and increased those between age peers including those between spouses. The main reason was the sheer size of the Australian participation in the War from 1914 to 1918 (from a population of less than five millions, almost half a million young men enlisted, resulting in one-third of a million being sent overseas, of whom nealy one-fifth were killed and one-half injured). Clearly the young had to be treated as persons with rights to unfettered decisions of their own, and equally clearly many of the young came to regard life as more ephemeral than society had traditionally regarded it.

During the 1890s both overall and marital fertility (when these terms are used, reference is to the Princeton indices) had presumably been displaced by crisis below the long-term trend-line of the decline. Hence during the first decade of the present century (when some deferred births were probably taking place) there was no fall in either measure. However, between 1911 and 1933 (these are census dates) both measures fell by around 40% at approximately 2% per year. In retrospect it is clear that the fertility level of the mid-1930s was below the century-long line from 1880 to 1980, and it also now appears—from what happened in the prosperous years after the Second World War—that it was below the level it would have reached had there been no economic crisis. In the 1930s peak unemployment in the male adult labour force reached 25%, compared with 7% in the 1970s (a comparison cannot be made of the female labour forces because of their very different structures). Australia was relatively badly affected because of the high proportion of its work force in secondary industry (40%) and because of the vulnerability of its export-oriented primary industries to the collapse of overseas markets.

Nevertheless, the period 1901–1939 is one that demands the answers to some very important questions. It did not seem to presage the baby boom that began only a few years after its end, nor the massive movement by married women into the labour force that accelerated with the 1950s, nor the spurning by younger married women of predominantly household roles that gathered force from the late 1960s. Why not?

The demographic data certainly provide clues, most strikingly in the trends in marriage (McDonald, 1975; Caldwell et al., 1981b; McDonald, forthcoming).

Perhaps the most interesting, in a society which had through the whole period a male surplus resulting in immigration (McDonald, 1975), was the movement in the proportions of females who never married. Taking their marital status at 45–49 years of age as an index of spinsterdom, and relating this to the date at which 50% of their cohort had married once, one notes a rise in the proportion who would remain single from 7% in the early 1870s, to 10% in the early 1880s, 15% in the early 1890s, and 19% after 1900. Thereafter, a long, but slow, decline commenced to 15% before the First World War, 13% in the 1920s, 11% in the 1930s, 8% at the beginning of the 1940s, 6% in the late 1940s (and probably 4% in the 1950s for which the cohort evidence is not yet complete).

Several points are striking. The marriage revolt began before the fertility revolt, and was well underway by the early 1880s. The turning point did not come until the first decade of the present century, when fertility had already fallen by one-third and the possibility of contraception was known throughout much of the community (helped by the publicity given by the New South Wales Royal Commission on the Birth Rate of 1903–4, established to try to arrest the fertility decline) (Hicks, 1978). The decline in proportions never marrying continued through the 1930s, showing that marriage levels this century have had little to do with economic conditions, and became really low after the Second World War. It is difficult to avoid the conclusion that the contraceptive revolution eventually produced a sexual revolution but that it was a long time coming. Indeed, the women's movement of the 1880s and the beginning of the birth revolt may well have raised the proportion of women who were less than enthusiastic about marital sexual relations (or about reproduction)—earlier, girls had been raised to be pure (and doubtless the seeds of sexual apprehension lay there) but it was less obvious that they had any choice or that the community had much place for those who did not marry. Thereafter, the number of spinster daughters living with ageing parents or maiden aunts living with their sisters' families increased, while the urban boarding houses that had long housed bachelors continued to spread (until they largely disappeared after the Second World War).

The second type of nuptial lag, evidenced by the median age of female marriage (again, the age when 50% of the cohort had married once), was even more prolonged. That age rose until the end of the nineteenth century and remained remarkably stable at around 25 years until the Second World War, falling steeply during the War and afterwards to about 21 years in the early 1970s. The concept of a proper time to marry continued for two-fifths of the way through the present century, perhaps artificially prolonged by the economic rigours of the 1930s. Those marrying were waiting—"responsibly"—to save enough to establish a household, in the sense of securing housing and furniture, and banking enough money so as to be able to care for children when they arrived, as well as to ensure that the husband had a secure job. I find it difficult to accept that this pattern prevailed so long merely because of the serious attitude of the young to their future, without a significant element being the responsibility expected of them by their parents (just as I feel that the issues of *population explosion* and the *preservation of the environment* in the 1960s and 1970s must be seen as rationalizing low fertility behaviour not only to those involved but also to their parents—but with a lesser feeling of the need for justification). If this is so, we are concerned still with intergenerational morality and its decline. Similarly, it is possible that the youth revolt of the First World War consolidated the trend toward an ever greater proportion marrying (especially if proportions ever married are related, when dating the trend, not to the year when half the cohort had married but to the years of the later marriages).

These high ages at female marriage go far toward explaining the lack of movement toward a greater proportion of working wives and mothers. Indeed, during the first decade of this period, 1901–1911, the proportion of wives in employment fell, evidence that working wives had been a sign—to the community and to the women themselves—of near family destitution, a situation reduced as prosperity returned after about 1903.

(3) *1940–1959*
The period 1940–1959 forms the theoretical nub of the question. Why did mid-twentieth century women, in the middle of a long secular decline in fertility and just prior to a massive debate on women's rights, settle for almost universal domesticity and larger families? Any theory that cannot take the baby boom in its stride is insufficient. By the 1950s female marriage would be more universal in Australia than it had been since the frontier days of the mid-nineteenth century when potential wives were relatively scarce; during the whole period from 1940 to 1959 the crude birth rate rose by 26%.

The Second World War played a decisive role in the move toward younger and more universal marriage. Once again—and for six years this time—the appeal was to the young and they carried the greater burden. Intergenerational differences weakened and the older generation surrendered ever more prerogatives—not always unwillingly, for they, too, had been socially radicalized by the decline of religion, the greater emphasis on pleasure and on sexuality, the soul-searching of the 1930s, and much else that preceded the War. The young wanted to move out of the parental home and to be playmates together. There were still constraints: the great majority of couples were not expected to live together, and indeed would not do so, without formal marriage, and most women still did not have sexual relations while single.[4] The answer was early marriage. The contraceptive revolution had proceeded sufficiently far (in 1945–49 over 70% of wives 20–29 were using contraception compared with less than 50% in the 1930s (Caldwell and Ware, 1973)) for them to be less fearful than their parents of continuous childbirth, and the related sexual revolution meant that marital sex was now feared by comparatively few (indeed, there was a growing fear of appearing to be apprehensive about it).

There was another aspect of these changes. One element of the revolt of the younger generation was a sharp reaction against the careful way their parents had planned the future. This was a wartime phenomenon that outlived the

---

[4] Projecting back from the more recent reports by the group at Johns Hopkins University on changing levels of premarital sexual relations (Zelnik *et al.*, 1979).

War. It had a certain poignancy, for the revolt was carried out by those guaranteed full employment (and ultimately housing by governments, through Housing Commissions, moving to ensure that no-one was left completely homeless) against those who had often faced horrific difficulties—and the revolt may not have been sustained but for continued prosperity.

Demographically, the baby boom was not quite as spectacular as crude birth rates and the popular memory has it (they were not entirely wrong, for those rates did accurately measure the subsequent demand for schooling and housing). Marital fertility rates did not increase as much as crude birth rates, for a larger proportion of women were marrying and hence were sharing the births that did take place; cohort marital fertility rates rose more slowly still for the boom, especially its earlier stages, was partly a product of the coincidental fertility of overlapping cohorts as childbearing started ever earlier among the young, and was also completed by some of the older women after Depression or War postponements; conceptions per marital year (especially when weighted for the years when conception is most probable) rose more slowly still, for women, marrying younger, now faced many more potentially reproductive years (an important consideration if, in a period of imperfect contraception, a significant fraction of all births were unintended). Female cohort fertility, cumulated to 35 years of age, increased from 1·75 for the 1980 birth cohort (which bore its children during the Depression and ultimately reached 2·21 by 1953) to 2·79 for the 1934 birth cohort (marrying in the mid-1950s)[5] (Caldwell and Ruzicka, 1977), an increase of 59%. There remains an increase of 50% if we adjust for the proportion of women who never married (but do not adjust further for the total number of married years of reproductive age)[6] and perhaps of 30% if we regard the fertility of the 1908 birth cohort as having been depressed by economic disaster below the long-term trend line and attempt to ascribe a "normal" position on the trend line to the cohort.

There is, then, something left to explain. The explanation is probably the youth revolt, for this is how most of the survivors seem to see it. Couples had always married and had children, but now they would do it as soon as they liked, and they would set up their own households, with comparatively little intrusion from grandparents and other relatives. Female revolt was not as absent from the whole phenomenon as is sometimes now implied in retrospect, for, as the magazines and newspapers of the time reveal, the concept of a qualitative difference between bread-winning and household

---

[5] The denominator for cumulative fertility is currently married women.

[6] Some adjustment is undoubtedly necessary in a period of imperfect contraception. A full adjustment completely explains the baby boom (see Caldwell and Ruzicka, 1977), but in a partially contracepting society a full adjustment is probably not warranted (see Trussell et al., 1981).

subsistence-type activities was under attack as never before (or since). It was the period when women's magazines regularly published articles showing, perhaps more in pride than in bitterness, the relatively longer hours worked by women than men and the total value of a wife's work if imputed from the costs of those services on the open market (usually astronomical, in much the same way as the calculations of a later era were to be of the cost of raising a child).

To a large extent the intergenerational battle had been won. Even if women had different household tasks from men, the 20-year-old married woman running her own household had established herself as an adult—if only as an adult woman—to an extent that was not true of her peers of the same age and sex who were unmarried and still living at home, even if they worked outside the home for wages during the day. There were still strong prohibitions against these unmarried young women being away from their parents, particularly strong against them living alone and condemnatory against them living with young men. This explains why the young married earlier than their parents but not necessarily why they exhibited higher fertility. The answer may well be that such a lesser care about the containment of fertility was necessary, defiantly so, to proclaim the absoluteness of their control over their relations with their spouses and the children who were the products of their union. The defiance had to be upward in terms of child numbers, in contrast to the care of the "Depression" generation who preceded them. It was assisted—and even permitted—by prosperity and by the longer years of potential reproduction spent within marriage. Yet this is probably not the whole story. Paradoxically, the movement towards females justifying their work activities vis-à-vis males may, in the last period before wives could easily work in the market place, have resulted in a determination to do more child raising in order to exhibit equality, and in order to demonstrate their vocation. The 1950s certainly were not merely the mirror image of the 1970s, and the baby boom was not a capricious whim.

For a number of reasons, the whole system—like the systems before it—was unstable.

One reason was that the new generation, which had scorned the careful ways of the old in saving before marriage for houses and other comfortable appurtenances of married life, now found that, if the wife too, were to contribute money towards these ends, she would have to do so from within marriage rather than from savings from pre-marital work—indeed, it was often now more urgent because the husband had not had time, either, to accumulate pre-marital savings. Easterlin's satisfied generation was growing up. A silent revolution began—silent because it was still undertaken stealthily, the ideological justification having not yet been argued, but with vast implications for the future: between 1947 and 1961 the proportion of the Australian female workforce made up by married women rose from 19% to 38% (and by 1971 it was to be 57%). The silence of this revolution—a behavioural change which was not loudly defended—has obvious parallels with the move to contraception in the late nineteenth century; both changes would subsequently develop ideologies which would reinforce them.

This slow change not only threatened the ideological underpinnings of the age of sexually differentiated (but theoretically equally respected work) but it began to erode its material basis. The system had depended on women not being isolated in the home but being able to consult others working on the same specialized tasks of housekeeping and childbearing in the suburban neighbourhood (and Australian society was little else). Slowly, as more wives went to work, as the gardens around houses grew larger, the use of cars more frequent, and shopping was transferred from the corner store to the supermarket, suburbia began to become lonelier (in reality, as well as in perception). By the mid-1950s newly married women were members of the reduced cohort born in the Depression; they had few siblings—and most had no sisters—to provide family visiting companionship.

There were two other problems.

The *King Child* was in the ascendancy and he received ever more care, often irritating even the most earnest of mothers. As affluence grew, the family possessions multiplied and keeping the children from destroying them became more time-consuming. Furthermore, the load fell ever more on the mother because the King Child had King Siblings who were ever less likely to be ordered to assist. Nor did the husband give much help, partly because of the enshrinement of the division of labour.

The other problem—inherent in the move from the family system to individualism, and, in some ways, occurring surprisingly late—was that the King Child, himself (or, more significantly, herself) was growing up. From the early 1950s the proportion of Australian females receiving full-time tertiary education continued to increase until, by the late 1970s, it reached almost 25% of the 18 to 21 year olds. The average gap between the end of female education and marriage had fallen in a quarter of a century from a decade to from two to four years. There was an increasing feeling that the promise of their complex and studied upbringing, and their longer and better education, should be put to use in the same generation, instead of being recycled into even better training for the next generation (in one sense, a revolt against continued human investment).

The better known descriptions of these two decades (drawing on sources which are American but which nevertheless had an impact on Australia almost immediately after publication) tend to be of its troubled latter stages, when these stresses were becoming stronger: for instance, Betty Friedan's description (1963) or Marilyn French's novel (1977), concentrating at first on suburbia of the late 1950s (and strongly influenced by the views and analytical approaches of the 1970s).

The period may have produced the same birth rates as the mid-1920s but it was by no means a return to it. Girls no longer lived in their parental home for a decade after their education was completed, learning housecraft as apprentices together with their sisters. The early marriages were much more spontaneous and the remaining vestiges of the parentally approved marriage had largely disappeared. Young women (and young men) possessed their own biological family, not in any sense a segment of the lineage. This was, in fact, what the young mothers were demonstrating by turning so definitely, in some cases almost defiantly, toward their own children. Much of the battle to reduce intergenerational differentials had been won, perhaps at the expense of the reduction of inter-sex differentials.

(4) *1960–1980*

The next two decades, 1960–1980, witnessed two series of interacting events.

The first set consisted of the debate about the "population explosion" which began in the 1950s and that on the preservation of the environment which gained force from the late 1960s. These issues soon became part of the popular culture. The 1971 Melbourne Survey found that 87% of respondents had decided that population growth should be discouraged in poor, crowded countries, although only 29% held that Australians should be discouraged from having more than two children and only 10% believed that Australian couples having more than six children were behaving immorally. Almost two-thirds knew of arguments relating population growth and pollution. Such views do not seem to have led many people to having fewer children than they really wanted. But they provided valuable weapons against parents (or spouses) who held that it was moral or worthy to bear children. They provided a rationalization for low fertility, or even for remaining childless, and allowed preferences in childbearing to be acted on fairly easily. They provided valuable weapons that prevented parental pressure from being exerted at a time when the older generation was probably more pronatalist than the younger one, thus preventing a lag from occurring in the movement to lower fertility levels, rather than being the major influence in fixing the newer levels.

The population debate also had another impact. It accelerated the development of new contraceptives, especially oral contraceptives and the IUD (which have probably prevented more conceptions to date in industrialized countries than the Third World—particularly if China is excluded), and it led to the greater legitimation of contraception. By the late

1960s the use of contraception was almost of moral priority, a very different position from the private and somewhat guilty practice which was typical in the early decades of the century and persisted until after the Second World War. The 1971 and 1977 Melbourne Surveys revealed that each new marriage cohort was more likely than the previous one to be practising contraception from the beginning of married life (around 90% by 1971 and close to 95% by 1977, with the pill accounting for around three-quarters of all methods used by these young couples).

That these changes were mechanisms rather than underlying forces is suggested by the movement of the fertility indices during the 1960s. The baby boom was definitely over, but, in spite of the massive new respectability, and even encouragement, for fertility limitation, fertility (as measured by the total fertility rate) fell only 13% during the decade, and at its end was at the same level as it had been in 1962 and 1928. Indeed, the total fertility rate was constant at 2·86 from 1967 until 1971.

More fundamental change in the relations between the generations and between the sexes was emerging—indeed, was almost exploding—by the end of the 1960s. The Vietnam War, and Australia's implementation of compulsory military service for young males, led to sharper intergenerational tensions than the country had previously experienced (the change in intergenerational relations in the two World Wars had been largely by consensus). The feeling of alienation between the generations has subsequently waned, but the conviction of the young that their morality might well be superior and that they had a right to act upon it without waiting guiltily for approbation has not. The new morality includes not only judgements about wars, but also about the need for formal marriage, the need to have children and the need to have them soon after marriage, and the legitimacy of the mothers of young children working outside the home. Australian women who return to work after the birth of a child most frequently do so soon after the birth of the child or three or five years later, the intermediate period now becoming more common, perhaps a sign that the care provided by schooling is increasingly thought to cover pre-schooling.[7]

These changes in attitudes toward mothers working occurred as a result of a revolution which is misunderstood and which has already generated much of its own mythology. To a very large extent the Women's Liberation Movement was called into being by the existence of vast numbers of wives already in the workforce suffering from all kinds of disabilities and frustrations because of the unequal treatment of the sexes. The Women's Movement did not have a strong impact in Australia until almost the end of the 1960s. Yet the proportion of married women at work rose from 9% in

[7] For an analysis of women returning to work, by age of children, see Young (1978).

1947 to 18% in 1961, and doubled again to 36% in 1971 (and reached 40% in 1975)[8] (Ruzicka and Caldwell, 1977). The proportion of the female workforce who were married had risen from 9% in 1921 to 19% in 1947, 38% in 1961 and 57% in 1971. By the latter date 32% of the workforce was female and 19% consisted of married women. The 1917–21 female birth cohort (24–28 years old in 1945) showed a minimum level of work at any age (i.e. the prime baby rearing age) of 8%, while the 1947–51 birth cohort (24–28 in 1975) is unlikely to fall below 40%. These changes partly reflected the capacity of the economy to provide jobs: between 1950 and 1975 the population increased by 54% while the number of jobs grew by 69%.

The late 1960s and early 1970s displayed a remarkable ideological resemblance to the 1880s and 1890s. In each period radical political movements and radical women's movements interacted with each other and assisted each other. In the late 1960s the increased proportion of women in the non-household labour force brought the Women's Movement into existence, but the ideology of the movement owed much to the New Left. The coincidence around 1970 of a reduction in both intergenerational and inter-sex differentials and influences—or a determination that they should be reduced—was to have momentous social and demographic repercussions through the 1970s and beyond.

The Women's Movement did not put young wives and mothers into the workforce but it did much to legitimize the change. What put them there was a previously slow interaction between the temptation (or need) for two wages, and the fact that this behaviour pattern was becoming more common and more accepted in the community. The Melbourne Surveys and other research have shown that the majority of wives work for money rather than through a feeling that such activity was the only worthy life style. A retrospective analysis of the Melbourne data showed that unplanned participation in the workforce (doubtless often because of family needs) reduced the fertility of wives by 0·4 children but intended participation lowered it by one whole child (Ware, 1976, p. 422).

This double attack on the age and sex differentials in authority and rights, still remaining from the society we began by describing as existing in the mid-nineteenth century, had certain new aspects—which brought society much closer to the individualist society which was the inevitable goal. The ideological intergenerational struggle had always been between young adults and older adults. Real children's liberation movements have not proved to be possible, although the speed of fertility decline can undoubtedly be explained by ever more successful demands by children for a more equal share in family consumption and pleasure and to do less work in household production—actions based on comparison with peers and

[8] Employing data provided by Alberto (1976).

owing something (both in being put forward and being accepted) to the ethic of egalitarianism. Nevertheless, the real victories have been to the young adults, and always will be. After the Second World War, the establishment of tight companionate marriages and more emotionally nucleated families was the most immediate attainable goal for young women. Children benefited in treatment (and rose in numbers), their gain being a byproduct of the goals of their elders. Much the same can be said for the establishment of mass schooling in the latter nineteenth century. But in the 1970s the female half of this young adult generation could move closer to reducing inequalities between the sexes by reshaping their activity patterns much closer to those of males—an action made possible by more reliable contraception, more equality in education, an economy that continually provided more jobs until it began to stagger in the mid-1970s, and by supporting ideologies.

There were anomalies in the situation with immediate or potential demographic implications. The radicalism of the 1960s had assailed the work ethic, while the Women's Movement had often found it advantageous to adopt an almost Protestant respect for paid work outside the home. Admittedly, this was argued in terms of lack of dependence and guaranteed longer term security, but the line between the moral value of having work and the moral value of working was often thin. The major ethic was not against having children at all—indeed, in their ability to do this women showed superiority over men, but children could often be very inconvenient if other targets were to be met. Australian interviews show very few couples wanting no children or one child at the time of marriage (most now desire two), but it later transpires that other priorities—the wife's work, career or gaining of qualifications (the third ladder of targets)—mean that many accept the impossibility or inconvenience of having any (Caldwell *et al.*, 1976). One reason is that working wives still do the majority of housework in most families, and children add to that load. There is some evidence that, when the sharing of household work becomes more common, husbands are as reluctant as wives to increase the total by adding children to the family.

We have stayed so closely with the analysis of the main forces that we have almost ignored some important supplementary changes.

The contraceptive revolution, together with the medical and attitudinal transformation of the danger of venereal disease, have long made it inevitable that sexual relations would become ever more separated from reproduction, and also from purity and guilt and from family relations. The sexual revolution has been a mechanism, and another result, in the dismantling of the nineteenth century family, but is not an underlying cause. Similarly the ideological revolutions of a decade ago have helped win battles for easier abortion, and they (together with a fear of the possible long-term effects of the pill) have greatly increased the resort to sterilization—but these two are mechanisms. The ideological and sexual revolutions, together with the continuing erosion of the efficacy of religious sanctions, have led to some decline in the incidence of formal marriage from about 1973, but the Australian pattern of change has been much less spectacular than those of North American and Scandinavia and much closer to those of other primary low-fertility bloc countries (Caldwell *et al.*, 1981b). Nevertheless, there is no parallel with the decline in marriage of the late nineteenth century, for that meant the deferral of the onset of sexual relations for much of the female community, and the contemporary marriage changes do not. Similar forces have increased the divorce rate markedly, so that perhaps one-quarter of recent marriages are likely to be eventually dissolved by the courts (Caldwell, 1980). Both the new marriage and divorce patterns will probably have some depressant effect on fertility, but each is merely another aspect of greater emphasis on the individual and less on the family, and the impact of each is likely to be relatively small compared to the impact of the attempt to build a female educational and occupational structure as close as possible to that of males.

By the early 1970s all these forces were in operation, and, after 1971, Australian fertility fell steeply, by almost one-third (as measured by the total fertility ratio) in eight years to below replacement level. Survey interviews left little doubt that the main reason was the clash between female work (whether preferred or felt necessary), training or life style on one hand and reproduction on the other (Caldwell *et al.*, 1976). One demographic manifestation of this was fewer births in the first years of marriage (Ruzicka, 1976, p. 15) a phenomenon which could doubtless be explained partly as a transfer of the pattern of childbearing to longer marriage durations, but it was very doubtful if the displacement of reproduction was the sole explanation.

Generations earlier it had become clear in most marriages that one partner could not impose the use of contraception on the other without agreement. During the 1970s the society moved much closer to the situation where one partner could not impose the absence of contraception without the agreement of the other (Caldwell *et al.*, 1976, p. 335).

Australia had not spontaneously produced either the angry youth or the women's debate, but the social conditions existed for both issues to have a major impact with the import of some ideas and subsequently with the interaction between imported and locally generated views—a position not very different from that obtaining in much of the primary low-fertility bloc and even most parts of the United States.

A Theoretical Synthesis

The argument of this paper is that the inevitability of continued fertility decline came about as soon as children became a definite economic disadvantage to parents, but that the time taken for the transition has been a function of both the economic nature of the mid-nineteenth century family and of the cultural superstructure that defended that type of family and determined how it operated. The two key elements were, as they had been in the traditional peasant family, differentials in work and consumption patterns by age and sex.

The system had none of the stability of agrarian families carrying out subsistence agriculture where the family system was needed to make the production system work. Much of the population already worked in non-familial employment, and the household production system was being undermined by the industrial system competitively offering to produce similar goods and services and by it offering paid employment to wives and children.

Subsistence agriculture was a family system. The industrial system with an open labour market involved offering individuals employment and tempting individuals to buy its products. This system, whether capitalist or socialist, meant that the family would move toward atomization. The capitalist economy, endlessly looking for new markets, is eventually propelled into seeking separate markets for its products among young people or amongst females; the force here for continuing to weaken family ties can hardly be overestimated.

Economic forces were basic but the extent to which they affected fertility in any given period depended on how long it took to dismantle the system of age and sex differentiation and the morality that supported it. At most times the system was surprisingly stable, partly because participants in an inegalitarian system have advantages as well as disadvantages—rights as well as duties—at every level, and are usually the main influences in pulling their aberrant peers into line. Nevertheless, the structure was too unstable to be maintained against the fundamental egalitarian forces operating ever more strongly as the society grew richer and more educated, and operating between persons in close contact and with strong emotional links. Even the changing of family relations had a substantial degree of cooperation: when the young demanded change they achieved more because their parents' views were less rigid than those of their grandparents had been, while the successes of the Women's Movement in the areas of legitimizing wives' work outside the home and greater job-sharing within has partly occurred because of its direct appeal to males.

The dismantling of the system and the resulting fertility decline took a century (or more) for two reasons.

The first is that some changes took a long while to work through the system. For instance, the loneliness in suburbia in the 1950s and 1960s, which helped bring about the flight of young wives into the workforce, was partly a product of declining fertility in the 1920s and 1930s.

The second, and more important reason, is that age and sex differentials, regarded as almost natural and usually taking the form of close emotional links, are, like many other social institutions, changed more in periodic crises than by slow erosion.

Age differentials faced four decisive periods of crisis. The first, the only one primarily between dependent children and their relatively young parents, dominated the last third of the nineteenth century and has persisted ever since. It was produced by the movement to a system of universal education, and almost certainly determined the timing of the onset of fertility decline. The remaining three crises each concerned the relation between young adults and their parents, resulting on each occasion in the young adults being able to go their own way more easily with less influence from the older generation. The three crises were the First and Second World Wars and the Vietnam War. Our society is not wrong in regarding the Wars, which have only occupied one-tenth of the last hundred years, as the great turning points of our era involving irreversible social flux of great consequence.

Sex differentials faced two periods of crisis. The first was the battle for the vote, inflamed in Australia by the achievement of full manhood suffrage in the early 1850s, reaching floodtide in the 1880s and 1890s, and dying down at the end of the century. Many of the issues raised again almost a hundred years later were discussed by the feminists and suffragettes of that time. The second, equally political but without a political goal as its prime end, was the Women's Movement of the 1960s and 1970s. It is argued here that this arose primarily out of occupational conditions, but it has built up a case against sex differentials in the family and society of a completeness which has not been attempted for age differentials. It has enormous continuing implications for the activities of young wives and for fertility.

The movement toward individualism with minimum age and sex differentiation appears to be the basic social change of our time consequent upon a fundamental change—perhaps the only fundamental change—in the relations of production. It is difficult to see women turning away from outside jobs and it appears improbable that fertility will again rise. The baby boom was almost certainly not the first of a series proving voluntary control over fertility—the ability to opt for more or fewer children just as fads come and go for consumer durables—but a unique step in the destruction of the older sexual and economic morality with its postponement, and even cancellation, of the beginning of sexual union, and in the destruction of family influence extending beyond two generations.

The social conditions for change pre-exist every crisis and the ideologies produced by crisis. Those conditions are the unstable age and sex relations. It is the similarity in these relations—or in their condition of instability— that makes fertility in primary low-fertility bloc countries change in such a similar way in terms of timing and even of level. Any explanation based on their very different income or educational structures is doomed to failure. Such simultaneity depends, of course, on the communication of ideas, and necessarily the United States, with its population size (and the size of its university communities) and a social structure that throws up innovation and clash, has initiated many of the new trends in recent times. Nevertheless, the ideas and new behaviour patterns are spread around the whole bloc and beyond, are reinforced, and develop new forms. It is partly the sheer size of the whole population involved, with its insatiable mass media, that explains how rapidly new movements (new reactions to crisis) build up, as if on a great sounding board. Any theory which treats each society as a distinct phenomenon cannot provide adequate explanation.

One important matter has until now been largely ignored, and that is social class. The discussion has tended to assume a largely homogeneous society, although it could be argued that the analysis presented so far is applicable to alterations within the relationships of the middle class family resulting in such behavioural changes as increased fertility control which diffused into the working class. The evidence for Australia does not seem to support this interpretation. Recent survey evidence shows that, among the native-born, issues of greater sexual equality are expressed almost as strongly, although in less ideological phrases, by working class women as by the middle class. One reason is that they are even more likely to be faced with the danger of doing two jobs unassisted, housekeeping and half the bread-winning. Working class children are even more likely to break from the guidance of the older generation if only because they do not need assistance through such a long period of education. We have no survey evidence from the late nineteenth century, but the literary sources and the fact of the close timing of fertility transition by social class suggests that the situation was not dissimilar. One reason that the working class was affected almost as early by the increasing burden of child dependency was the fact that the universal period of compulsory schooling (eight years) made up a greater fraction of the period between birth and financial independence among the working class than among the middle class. Furthermore, school teachers frequently took education to mean the inculcation of middle class ways and demand standards of clothing from their pupils that were not completely graded by their parents' ability to meet them. While the suffragette movement may have had a greater impact on relationships within the middle class than within the working class family, the reverse was probably true of the impact of the two World Wars. In any case the descriptive evidence, not only of the Depression of the 1930s but also that of the 1980s, is of working class economic distress marked by an inability to meet aspirations for children, and also of distress being caused if wives had to work. Again the language of the anguish tends to vary by social class, but the existence of different age and sex roles and the rate at which they disappeared, thus making high fertility ever more disadvantageous, seems to have been strikingly similar. Children certainly cost the poor less in absolute terms but not relative ones. Government child endowment and maternity schemes were only of significant help during the first two decades after the Second World War, and may have done something to sustain the baby boom. At other times such assistance, even for the working class families, was of much smaller impact than were the demands that the state made for greater dependency of children upon their parents.

Competing Theories

Most of the theories put forward to explain the fertility decline, its duration and its future, are not so much wrong about what they choose to explain, but are staggeringly insufficient in that they choose to explain so little. The one exception is Notestein who rightly sees it as a whole and as a movement toward individualism but who does not spell out the steps in a way that can be used for historical analysis or for prediction (except in his tenet that societies aim at sufficiently high fertility to compensate for mortality so that replacement fertility will probably eventually be achieved).

Easterlin is probably right about the post-World War II generation. They had been raised frugally and they were not particularly consumption-oriented. He completely misses the point about them wanting to build their own nests, and as early as possible. More seriously, it is not a theory but a description of an era. It probably has no predictive value. The children of the late 1970s are not being brought up with the enforced austerity of the 1930s (in spite of economic difficulties they are probably being materially more pampered than the children of the 1950s and 1960s). Only in two ways may the contemporary young be said to be more disadvantaged than those of the 1950s and 1960s, so laying the ground for an explanation based on alternating generations. First, more of their mothers go to work, but this hardly makes a parallel with the 1930s or any previous generation. Second (and Easterlin now places the stress here), they have less chance of getting a job, or at least the job they want. However, there are a whole series of difficulties here in distinguishing real alternations. Unemployment is a fraction of what it was in the 1930s, and is in fact no higher than it was in the supposedly prosperous times of the mid-1920s (and unemployment assistance is much greater). It appears to have arisen less from the capacity of the job market to expand as the cohort expands than from the employment of many more women and from attempts to employ fiscal measures to contain inflation. There is no survey information at all to show that the young now regard their situation and their consumption pattern to be so humble that they will forego consumption for reproduction; all the evidence appears to point in the opposite direction.

The Chicago Household Economists (Gary Becker, Theodore and Paul Schultz, and others) have theorized about the price of children, and whether the rich aim at more expensive children than the poor can afford. They have also described the decisions which have had to be made by the housewife and mother of the last two decades: will she follow her neighbour into the workforce or will she rear more children, or possibly read more books? They have not shown that these latter options rise in proportion to education (and, in Australia, they do not appear to do so). The theory has little application earlier than the 1960s, when the great majority of housewives felt that they should stay home. It has some predictive value, although the prediction seems to be for ever lower fertility. It fails completely to explain the similarity of fertility levels between different members of the primary low-fertility bloc, and the tendency of these levels to move together, unless the value of time is a completely relative concept. The work on the price of children seems to be less than helpful in explaining why the great fertility turning points operate right across societies and right across the bloc countries.

Judith Blake has emphasized the motivational factor in fertility decline in contrast to that of contraceptive technology which she ascribed to Norman Ryder and Charles Westoff (Blake and Das Gupta, 1975). Everything said here is, of course, on the side of the primacy of motivation, but it is argued, first, that one must be able to identify the precise target of the motivation and why it has arisen at that particular time and, second, that the motivation may take into account the problems of using contraception or of the effects of using contraception both in terms of relations with one's spouse and one's parents. My interpretation of the Ryder-Westoff position (Westoff, 1973) is that they would accept much of that proposition.

Geoffrey Hawthorn has begun to formulate a theory of social converg-ence amongst the young of the bloc "in aspirations for time and money, more generally, for a form of life which was previously unavailable to all but an extremely small proportion of privileged people at this point in the life cycle", resulting in options other than being parents (or parents of a large brood) and hence in declining fertility (Hawthorn, in press). It is doubtful whether convergence is the underlying mechanism, even for the 1970s. In Australia it is clear that one clue to the nature of the demographic transition—one that suggests succession—is the fact that the poorer of one generation did not behave like the rich of the previous generation. The gap in fertility behaviour was only a few years when fertility began declining a century ago (Ruzicka and Caldwell, 1977, pp. 171–176) and has been a shorter period still in every subsequent movement (Caldwell and Ware, 1973). The theory has its attractions for explaining the 1970s, once the young had reached the stage where this option was open to them, but it is of little value for explaining the behavioural change of the previous one hundred years.

The Possibility of a General Theory

This paper has attempted to move towards a general theory of fertility which can be employed not only to explain the onset of fertility decline but its subsequent extent and timing. To what degree can this be said to have been successful?

The theory in its most generalized form, namely that an economy based very largely on family production will be characterized by high fertility and that eventually a society based on the labour market—whether advanced capitalism or socialism—will be characterized by low fertility, is probably unassailable. One could go further and state that in each case the fertility decision-makers had correctly discerned the kind of fertility that would serve their personal interests, even their economic interests, best. However, such a theory is of limited use for short range prediction and for explaining the timing of fertility decline.

The theory also states that the returns to the decision-makers, particularly the patriarch, are ensured in familial production by the specific relations of production, characterized by marked inequality by age and sex. Such inequality at the family level is not needed to ensure the success of labour market production or to create a chain of command—in fact the system works better if both employment and consumption goods can be offered to all on a competitive basis. When a substantial measure of equality is achieved within the family and society, large families will inevitably be an economic burden. With the rise of labour market production, fertility did not immediately decline, partly because adults, and especially male adults, had much still to gain by retaining most of the inegalitarian age and sex structure, and partly because wives and children still produced household goods and services in the traditional way.

Given the production system of the primary low-fertility bloc countries in the late nineteenth century any crisis that produced a major movement towards greater equality by age and sex in consumption patterns (and, by sex, in reproductive decision-making patterns) probably would have begun fertility decline. If the suffragette movement had accompanied its demand for votes with a stronger demand for decision-making equality especially in the reproductive field, for more equal consumption and for more sharing of bread-winning, fertility may have declined slowly from this cause alone. This did not happen, largely because the industrial system was not yet in a position to offer sufficient employment or to replace household services. Thus, the first great crisis occurred in terms of age equality and was brought to a head by the movement to universal schooling, which the industrial system could afford. One could attempt a specific postulate: it is unlikely that constant high fertility will be maintained for longer than a few years in any society where most adult males work for wages once universal schooling for a minimum of 6–8 years is enforced and this is accompanied (as was the case in the primary low-fertility bloc, and is usually the case elsewhere) by other legislation implying child dependency. The latter proviso, for instance, did not hold in Prussia of the early nineteenth century, while many Third World countries do not make compulsory education laws effective when they exist. The paradoxical situation emerged where greater child dependency also meant greater consumption equality. In this sense, the onset of fertility decline can probably be predicted, but the question remains as to whether the speed of the decline can be forecast.

Mass wars, with their necessary appeal for social mobilization, clearly reduce age inequalities (and some aspects of sex segregation while strengthening others). Until the First World War most primary low-fertility bloc countries had either never experienced such a war or had not done so for a long period. The exceptions are France during the Napoleonic Wars and the United States during the Civil War, both countries where there appears to have been some subsequent continuing fertility decline. The wars could not have been timed (although the form they took depended on the ability of the industrial system to sustain them), but, had the First World War occurred a generation earlier, fertility probably would have declined faster. Research in Korea during the 1960s revealed a widespread belief that the military convulsions of the 1950s had changed family and social relations in a way that was fundamentally responsible for allowing the fertility decline of the following decade (Caldwell and Caldwell, unpublished research notes).

It would be satisfying if one could postulate a necessary order between age and sex crises, but much of the ordering seems to have a fortuitous element. Nevertheless, the post-World War Two demand by young females for an equal but different role and the post-Vietnam War demand for an equal and similar role were accelerated by the fact of those conflicts.

The crises, then, have accelerated fertility decline, but they themselves were not the product of demographic change. One should not go further and claim that acceleration could have been ever greater with ever more crises. That would obscure the stage element in fertility decline. Children partly demanded more equality only when fertility decline had produced families with so few of them that they enjoyed a scarcity value. The suburbs became lonely and forced young women into the labour market only when these small families grew up. The acceptance of the contraceptive and sexual revolutions were interrelated and took time, partly because they often involved changes over more than one generation with older parents accepting without fierce struggle behavioural changes amongst their children just reaching adulthood.

In these circumstances the changes of the last hundred years have hardly been surprisingly slow. It is improbable that any set of circumstances would, for instance, have fitted them into a single generation. Fast changes of that kind are more likely among successor societies borrowing experience and social patterns from the primary low-fertility bloc.

The Future

In the long social and demographic transition every generation has felt that a lengthy period of transition has been completed, that social change could go no further, and usually, that fertility could not fall much further. Classical demographic transition theory assumed that replacement level was the end product of the transition, and that is assumed by the members of Z.P.G., by United Nations (1974a) analyses of the size of global population when the stationary state is achieved, and, in Australia, by the Report of the National Population Inquiry.[9]

Yet there is nothing in the analysis above to suggest any reason why there should be such a floor to fertility decline. Even contemporary demographic statistics seem to argue otherwise, Ruzicka showed that after 10 years of marriage the 1955-7 and 1962-3 marriage cohorts recorded 6% of wives with no births and 15% with one (Caldwell et al., 1976, p. 22); A. H. Pollard employed 1973 parity progression ratios to argue that contemporary fertility behaviour implied that the proportion of females remaining childless or eventually bearing one child would be 22% and 6% respectively (Pollard, 1974).[10] If the remainder were to converge on a parity of two, there would be

[9] Volume 1, especially Chapter 7, "Projections for Australia", pp. 255-314, fertility assumptions II, III, and IV.

[10] The use of cross-sectional data at a time of rapid change may overstate the childless, but Ruzicka has shown that by 1978, only 50% of couples who had been married for three years had any children at all (Ruzicka and Caldwell, in press).

continuing fertility decline. The argument of a replacement balance implies that the remainder will average above two, that it is society as a whole that, in some mystic way, seeks a balance.

The other argument that can be posed for a replacement floor is that of historical experience: fertility rose in the 1930s after net reproduction rates fell just below unity, and the present fertility decline seems to be bottoming out. The impression provided by the Depression years is false: the net production rate in Australia fell not only to unity but even to 0·939, but this is the appearance given by cross-sectional data, for no cohort averaged completed family size below 2·4 and no cohort of married women below 2·7. The present appearance of having reached a floor—one below long-term replacement level it might be noted—is a reflection of the fact that the decline in numbers of births appears to be ceasing, a temporary effect deriving from adult female age structure. There is certainly a slowing in the decline in fertility rates, but that decline has not ceased. More importantly, in a situation where the major force depressing fertility is the conflict between female work aspirations and childbearing, such a slow-down might be anticipated in economic circumstances where the unemployment rate for females under 25 years is 15%.

However, the thesis argued here is that the driving force in social and demographic change is still the reduction in age and sex difference demanded by the egalitarian ethic. Furthermore, in the decades immediately ahead the sex battle is likely to be fought mostly in the work place, partly because the cultural contrast between bread-winners and others was never erased and partly because the mainstream of the Women's Movement has reasserted it at almost nineteenth century strength. The age battle is likely to take ever more the form of resistance to what remains of older generation disapproval of *de facto* marriage, casual sexual relations, homosexuality and lesbianism, divorce, young mothers working through their children's infancy, and the lack of grandchildren. Youth victory on every one of these fronts is likely to depress fertility. Nor is there any evidence that the suburban home is likely to become less lonely for the young wife caring for children there.

There are possible pronatalist forces, although, at this time, they look likely to be weaker during the rest of this century.

The first is a governmental reaction to potential fertility decline. So far it has been at a surprisingly low level in the primary low-fertility bloc countries, largely because of a feeling of inconsistency over expressing concern over population explosion abroad and population implosion at home at the same time. But there are already signs of coming governmental reactions, possibly arguing the need for fertility convergence between industrialized and non-industrialized countries. Certainly, in terms of constructing the necessary ideologies, there are already family sociologists waiting to be the heroes of the hour. Western governments will inevitably become more interested in recent experiences in Eastern Europe where government intervention in Czechoslovakia apparently has raised fertility above replacement level,[11] but whether the same measures will work in the primary low-fertility bloc, or continue to work in Eastern Europe, is open to a good deal of doubt. Certainly the history outlined in this paper owed very little to the action of governments (except that democratic electorates often discouraged governments from making the sale of contraceptives illegal and ultimately encouraged them to liberalize abortion rules).

There are other possibilities, of which the most likely is a more sustained revolt against the work ethic and bourgeois lifetime goals, being in essence an age revolt, and being brought into existence by another major crisis, a decades-long malfunctioning of the world economy. (We will omit the discussion of the potential impact of World War III). In these circumstances there could be more emphasis on reproducing one's own social unit.

However, my best guess, based on the above analysis, is for declining population in all bloc countries by the early twenty-first century (except for those with net immigration, which will perhaps become a common feature) and in the world as a whole—a much more industrialized world—by the end of that century.

---

[11] See Frejka (1980). Increases in fertility have also occurred recently in the German Democratic Republic, Hungary, Poland and Romania. See United Nations (1976), Table 22 and (1979).

E

Specific Difficulties

9

The failure of theories of social and economic change to explain demographic change: puzzles of modernization or Westernization

Perhaps the most extraordinary aspect of demography is its intellectual isolation. This arises not only from the defensive stance that most social sciences adopt on their borders or from demographers' lack of expertise in contiguous disciplines, but the fact that these other disciplines concerned with social change often appear to have little to offer. Demographers look at works on social and economic change expecting to find explanations for the onset of fertility transition or of such steepness in mortality decline that cannot be explained by technological or environmental innovation, only to discover that these issues are all but ignored.

One reaction—and one which has come close to dominating modern demography—is to decide that the great demographic changes were phenomena that occurred largely within a demographic context and can be explained by indices that demographers are most competent to measure. This solution is a peculiarly satisfactory one from the viewpoint of the profession, maximizing the use of existing skills. It has permitted the World Fertility Survey to develop a Core Questionnaire (1975)[1] which seeks masses of demographic data and little other information so that inevitably demographic phenomena will be largely explained in terms of other demographic change (and probably correctly, within the limited range allowed for the explanation). It has encouraged demographers to seek explanations of fertility change in terms of shifting attitudes—of ideal family size, reproductive norms, and so on—even when there was little satisfactory

[1] The only socioeconomic questions are on education, literacy, residence at 12 years of age (countryside, town, city) and work histories of respondent and husband. The exception to the generalization is the fairly detailed work history for the two spouses.

evidence that movement in ideals and norms preceded behavioural changes, let alone that the origins of such change lay in them.

An alternative reaction, probably the dominant view in the other social sciences, is that demography has little that needs explanation; indeed that there is really no such discipline but merely an area of behaviour where the measurement of change should be encouraged by persons with adequate statistical techniques. Mortality decline was always desired and occurred when the means were available, while replacement and survival, rather than high fertility, had always been the reproductive aim. I believe that the mortality transition can be shown to have had social as well as technological roots (Caldwell, 1979), but will concentrate here on the issue that is potentially much more challenging to the adequacy of socioeconomic change theory, that of the onset of fertility transition.

It can be argued that nothing much happened, that the death rate fell and so did the birth rate, leaving the surviving family at much the same size (Lewis, 1955, p. 311).[2] The truth is probably rather that something very significant happened when sustained fertility decline occured, perhaps the most fundamental social change in history, and that the instinct of most demographers is right in feeling that they are the custodians of a great truth and that explanations of social change which cannot account for fertility decline are inadequate.

Certainly, any comparison of the experience of the post-fertility-decline population with that during the decades or generations immediately preceding the transiton, demonstrates a marked contrast. Australian women who married a generation before the beginning of fertility decline averaged seven births, reared six children, brought five to adulthood, and were accompanied into old age by four or five.[3] The American experience was undoubtedly similar. In England of the late eighteenth century, a hundred years before the transition, women who married bore on average six children, raised four to five through childhood, and brought four to adulthood and three to their old age. This concentration on the erosion of the family helps to give a less than whole picture of the change. One reason is that reproduction was not merely for support in old age; even in economic terms young children provided help. Another reason is that socially it is far off the mark. The pre-transitional family was dominated by reproduction as contemporary descriptions and novels well attest. Even a woman who would enter old age with only three or four surviving children, would have experienced around seven pregnancies and births, and would have at least

[2] See also Davis (1977), p. 172, where it is argued that movements of this type mean that it would be "better to compute a child rate than a birth rate, because people do not desire births but children".

[3] Sources and estimates are from: Ruzicka and Caldwell (1977); Caldwell and Ruzicka (1977); Keyfitz and Flieger (1968); Coale and Demeny (1966).

begun rearing six or seven children with their infancies and childhoods, and possibly deaths, overlapping through twenty to twenty-five years or probably the great majority of the married life that she and her husband would spend together. Nor was this a temporary phenomenon. In European settlement areas overseas birth rates remained far above death rates for centuries; this is the experience from which Malthus drew his lesson, and he drew it at the close of the eighteenth rather than the nineteenth century. There was, until the late nineteenth century, no move to change this position even in those societies which were sufficiently removed from their more traditional roots to have been described as "born modern".[4] In Australia the daughters of those who married in the 1870s bearing seven children and rearing five or six to adulthood, bore five around the turn of the century and reared four to adulthood, while the granddaughters in the 1930s bore three and usually reared three.

The nature of the family and the household had changed dramatically. In the most traditional parts of the contemporary world—in, for instance, the rural areas of Sahelian Africa where the annual rate of natural increase may still be only 1% in spite of early marriage and virtually unrestricted fertility—the family is characterized more than in any other way by children, by their births, their growing-up and their deaths. This is not so in post-transitional societies. Something epoch-making happened for good and sufficient reasons, and any explanation of change which ignores or fails to explain the fertility transition is almost certainly wrong.

This paper has two interrelated aims. The first is to evaluate the most influential contemporary theories of change by the criterion just proffered and to search for an explanation and solution. The second is to ascertain whether they are broad enough to explain the diffusion of demographic change as part of a more general process of social diffusion. It will be maintained that the formation of a global society is at least as much a reality as the formation of a global economy and that this is far from being a simple process of the latter dictating the former; indeed it will be argued that a global demography is being established.

The more detailed attention will be paid to those who have put forward in recent times comprehensive theories of change which appear to have had a substantial impact on the contemporary global change is interpreted. On the social, psychological and attitudinal side, this includes Daniel Lerner (1964), Alex Inkeles in Smith and Inkeles (1966); Inkeles (1969); Inkeles and Miller (1974); Inkeles and Smith (1974); and Everett Hagen (1962). From the more economic viewpoint it includes Arthur Lewis (1955), Walt Rostow (1956, 1960 and 1964) and Gunnar Myrdal (1968), and Theodore Schultz (1973) representing the Chicago household economists. In addition

---

[4] A description used by Shorter (1976), p. 14.

some attention will be paid to a score of others, some profound but without equal public or cross-disciplinary impact.[5]

This is not an exercise of marginal significance to demographic theory. On the contrary, the enquiry should be central. There cannot be two adequate and different explanations of the broad sweep of social change. If the major theories of social and economic change do not easily explain both the fact and timing of fertility decline, then the theories themselves are probably not merely deficient but wrong. Similarly, little trust can be put in a narrow explanation of demographic change that cannot be expanded to explain the other major social transformations that occurred around the same time.

There is a real need to concentrate on several of the main change theorists. Collectively, their way of looking at the problem has had a major impact on demographers trained in either sociology or economics. Without this backing, there probably would have been a much greater reluctance to accept the concept of changing ideal family size as of fundamental importance, indeed as being anything but a symptom.

One of the basic weaknesses of contemporary social science is its desire to seek only positive results, and its feeling that it is time-wasting to point to the significance of what is absent rather than what is present. The following analysis will, on the contrary, devote much of its attention to the absence of adequate explanations of fertility decline, on the grounds that this omission is not merely fortuitous but is evidence of fundamental error in the explanation of social and economic change as well and to the need for recognizing that a separate theory of demographic change is a meaningless and dangerous concept.

The Explanations Offered for Fertility Decline

Lerner, in spite of all his emphasis on "psychic mobility", not only offers no explanation for fertility decline, but fails to mention its occurrence. Nowhere in "The Passing of Traditional Society" is high fertility referred to as a characteristic of traditional society. One explanation is, of course, that he was analysing the Middle East during the 1950s, at a time when moderate family size was a characteristic of only elite groups probably confined largely to urban areas of Lebanon and Western Turkey.[6] Nevertheless, the failure

[5] These include Bellah (1969); Bendix (1964 and 1967); Black (1966); Black *et al.* (1975); Clark (1967); Crook (1978); Davis (1962); Deutsch (1961); Eisenstadt (1966); Feldman and Hurn (1966); Foster (1973); Kahl (1968); Kellert *et al.* (1967); Levy (1966); McClelland (1963 and 1966); Mannheim (1940); Moore and Feldman (1960); Moore (1961); Portes (1973); Schnaiberg (1970); Weiner (1966).

[6] "The passing of the Traditional Society" was first published in 1958. The first Middle Eastern study to identify groups with lower fertility was Yaukey (1961). Lerner's questionnaire seeks information at the end under the heading of "Respondent's Personal Characteristics", on the number of children, and ages of eldest and youngest child, but the material is not employed in the analysis.

to discuss the possibility of declining fertility, and the circumstances that might give rise to it, is surprising in view of the discussion by demographers during the 1950s of hypothesized relationships between fertility and development. (Hatt, 1952; Milbank Memorial Fund, 1954.)

Hagen, in his 1962 book *On the Theory of Social Change: How Economic Growth Begins*, ignored fertility altogether both in traditional society, which he otherwise treats in detail, and in the society that follows.

Inkeles, in a series of publications spanning over a decade from 1966 and written either on his own or together with Smith or Miller, nowhere really discusses why modernization might penalize the highly fertile in a way that traditional society would not. The closest Inkeles and Smith came to it was in a single passage published in 1966:

> "we assumed that modernity would emerge as a complex but coherent set of psychic dispositions manifested in *general* qualities such as a sense of efficacy, readiness for new experience, and interest in planning, linked, in turn, to certain dispositions to act in *institutional relations* (their italics)—as in being an active citizen, valuing science, maintaining one's autonomy in kinship matters, and *accepting birth control* (my italics) . . . we assumed these personal qualities would be the end product of certainly early and late socialization experiences such as education, urban experience, and work in modern organizations such as the factory" p. 355.

On reporting on the completed research project in six developing countries, i.e. Argentina, Chile, East Pakistan (Bangladesh), India, Israel and Nigeria, in *"Becoming Modern"* the only references in the index to fertility decline were under the heading "Birth control, attitudes toward". There were 12 references of this kind but most were still in the form of planning hypotheses or justifications for questions asked or scales employed. The most specific was: "Although birth control depends in great measure on scientific technology and on particular practices guided by that technology, even the most spectacular advances in science, such as new contraceptive pills, cannot have the desired effect except as they may be supported by the motive to use them and by patterns of interpersonal relations that make that motivation effective. To assess attitudes in this area, therefore, we inquired into our respondents' ideas of the ideal number of children and into their readiness to limit that number under various conditions" (Inkeles and Smith, 1974, p. 27). The only argument that was not attitudinal was the intriguing reference to "patterns of interpersonal relations", but what was meant is apparently fully covered a few pages later in the statement, "Men more independent of the extended family might well also be more interested in practicing birth control" (ibid., p. 32). The findings appear briefly in several references to "modern characteristics, such as favouring birth control" (ibid., p. 84), and a longer statement about the educated: "They valued science more, accepted change more rapidly, and were more prepared to limit the number of children they would have. In short, by virtue of having had more formal schooling, their personal character was decidedly more modern" (ibid., p. 143). It is a case of viewpoint (even toward family size) rather than behaviour, and of opinions rather than of material circumstances.

The economists do not lean much further towards economic determinism. Lewis, in his 1955 study, "The Theory of Economic Growth", backed three different possibilities without appearing to regard them as in any way alternatives, but rather being additive in nature. The first was admittedly economic but of unknown nature: "We do not know what caused this decline [in fertility]. We assume, and argue, that it followed inevitably from the process of economic growth, and that it will therefore be repeated in all countries as they undergo the same processes, but we have no certainty that things will turn out this way" (p. 311). The second was demographic determinism in the form of mortality decline: "It is pretty safe to assume that the fall in the birth rate is due to a change of attitude towards childbearing and not merely to new techniques of birth control. What brought this change of attitude? Probably the most important reason is simply the fall in the death rate" (ibid.). The third was the removal of the Notesteinian props when this became prudent: "Sooner or later the disadvantages of a rapidly growing population become obvious to the leaders of the community, and the religious precepts urging maximum childbearing are dropped" (ibid., p. 312). The implied argument seems to be that high fertility was never economically advantageous for those individuals or societies accidentally achieving fertility beyond that needed for survival, but that high fertility had to be encouraged to ensure that all societies and nearly all families physically survived. Because fertility beyond replacement (or perhaps even fertility at or below this level) was not economically advantageous to the family (and was probably disadvantageous) religious exhortation was needed to prevent fertility control being practiced. When mortality declined, and the danger of not surviving (at least at the societal level) had passed, priority could be given to the economic disadvantages of high fertility, which had been there all along and had plagued those sections of the community with below average child mortality, and the religious sanctions on fertility control were relaxed with the result that fertility control was practiced and the birth rate declined.

Rostow published a paper on "The Take-off into Self-Sustained Growth" in 1956 which was expanded into "The Stages of Economic Growth" in 1960. There was only one reference to the cause of the fertility decline: "The view towards the having of children—initially the residual blessing and affirmation of immortality in a hard life of relatively fixed horizons—must change in ways which ultimately yield a decline in the birth-rate, as the possibility of progress and the decline in the need for unskilled farm labour create a new calculus" (1960, p. 19). The argument is that large numbers of children (or at least large numbers of children with no skills or little education) are a disadvantage to the family once the economy attains sustained economic growth. Presumably they are earlier less of a disadvantage, although the possibility that they might have been no economic disadvantage (or even a positive advantage) seems to be nullified by referring exclusively to the problems of survival and company in traditional society. He makes no attempt to explain the curious fact that Britain, the United States and Germany experienced take-offs considerably before the onset of fertility decline, Britain a quarter of a century earlier.

Myrdal, in 1957 in his "Economic Theory and Under-Developed Regions" made repeated references to fertility decline and birth control, but always as something that had happened, and hence had economic and social consequences, in the West, and was needed elsewhere. However, in the three-volume "Asian Drama: An Inquiry into the Poverty of Nations", published in 1968, there are four references to fertility decline giving a hint of an explanation for its occurrence.

"The prospects for a spontaneous spread of contraceptive practices [in South Asia] cannot be discussed by analogy to Western experience. The progressive reduction of fertility in the West, particularly since the last quarter of the nineteenth century, was indeed the consequence of widespread spontaneous adoption of birth control practices. But it occurred in an economic, social and cultural context so different from South Asia's that any comparison is pointless. Even without considering birth control as a simple function of levels of income and living, it must be recalled that its spread on a significant scale in the West began only when those levels were much higher than they can be expected to be in the near future in South Asian countries, under even the most optimistic assumptions. As for industrialization and urbanization, literacy, education level, and a rationalist culture in general, the differences are equally great" (p. 1443). "It is more relevant to study such fertility differentials as may exist within individual South Asian countries, between groups differing in, say, income and education . . . as to the possibilities for a spontaneous spread of birth control through a rise in income, education, and the like for the masses of the people" (p. 1445). Next, we are told of the possible consequences "if fertility tended to decline in response to economic growth . . ." (p. 1447). Finally, the conclusion is drawn that, "as yet only a very few people in South Asia are awake to the advantage of birth control for the individual family" (p. 1447).

The references to "a rationalist culture" and "being awake to the advantages of birth control" certainly imply that high fertility, or at least an above average number of surviving children, is economically disadvantageous even in traditional, subsistence, agrarian societies. The engine for change is economic growth and it works through education, literacy and urbanization, which produce enlightened or rational people capable of calculating where their future advantage lies.

In the introduction to a volume devoted to the new household economists, Theodore Schultz explained that "in thinking about the economics of fertility, social cost and benefits aside, the analytical key in determining the value of children to their parents is in the interactions between the supply and demand factors that influence these family decisions" (Schultz, 1973, p. S3). "A very young child is highly labour-intensive in terms of cost, and the rewards are wholly psychic in terms of utility. As a child becomes a teenager, the additional cost borne by the parents involves less labour intensiveness and the rewards, especially in poor countries, consist in increasing part of useful work that the teenager performs . . . in reality each consumer service has two prices attached to it: (1) a money price, as in traditional theory of consumer choice, and (2) a time cost of acquiring the consumer goods and processing them in the household; and the time cost that is involved in consuming the services obtained from this household activity. It is obvious that bearing a child and caring for the infant child are normally highly labour-intensive activities on the part of the mother. What has not been clear is the difference in the value of time of mothers in bearing and rearing children associated with the difference in the human capital of mothers. The studies (that follow) contribute substantially in clarifying this relationship" (pp. S5–S6). However, most do not contribute to understanding either the economics of pretransitional societies or the changes leading to the onset of fertility decline because the emphasis is on the contemporary United States. There is certainly the implication here that there are societies where high fertility could be economically rewarding, although the following statement casts some doubt on whether Schultz himself would agree: "the decline in child mortality underway in most poor countries is in all probability an important variable to which parents are responding with lags as they become informed and are prepared to act, given the state of information that is relevant to their fertility decisions" (pp. S9–S10). There is certainly a tool here for constructing and testing a theory of the destabilization of the stable high fertility situation, given that the problems of dealing with parental time consumption in work and child-care situations very different from the United States could be overcome. So far this has not been done, and members of the group have been largely content to work on aggregate economic and social indices which establish that massive—and, presumably, eventually decisive—change is occurring, (T. P. Schultz, 1973) or on theoretical constructs for such analysis (De Tray, 1973) without demonstrating the sequence of household changes that leads to high fertility becoming economically disadvantageous or that determines the timing of that event, two essential requirements for a satisfactory theory of the initiation of fertility transition.[7]

Elsewhere[8] there is practically nothing in the way of explanation. In the work within the *Social mobilization* tradition, extending from Karl Mannheim (1940) through Karl Deutsch (1961), there appears to be only a solitary comment from C. E. Black: "In the advanced countries, as a result both of external pressures and of changes in family practices, the birth rate has been significantly reduced" (1966, p. 23). The emphasis, as in the whole tradition, is on migration weakening kinship bonds, without much explanation of the mechanics, except distance, and none referring to fertility change. Wilbert Moore had put this into words in 1961: "Although the links between economic development and smaller families are not fully established, it appears clear that they center in part on the institutionalization of mobility, in part an emphasis on familial (as distinct from extended kinship) values themselves" (p. 77). None of the work of Reinhard Bendix (1964 and 1967) attempts to explain fertility decline, nor do the 25 scholars assembled by Myron Weiner in "Modernization: The Dynamics of Growth" (1966). Marion Levy, in his double volume on "Modernization and the Structure of Society", says only: "Even if we found a way to control the birth rate tomorrow by methods inoffensive to the people concerned, those methods would not preserve the general structures of relatively nonmodernized societies in their previous forms" (1966, p. 127). Colin Clark, in 1967 in Population Growth and Land Use, said much on the impact of demographic change, but explained the fertility component of that change only in the following way: "In the 'nuclear' family the upbringing of an additional child is felt as a much greater burden than in the 'extended' family, even though, objectively, the nuclear family's economic resources may be much higher than the other's" (p. 187). It is more a question of where the burden lies than of the nature of the existence of the burden. Subsequently, in the modernizing society with nuclear families those desiring upward mobility feel, in accordance with Arsene Dumont's theory of capillarity, a very real burden (Clark, 1967, pp. 186–187)—but this explains the process of fertility decline, not its origin.

There is little point in carrying this essentially negative analysis any further. The central point is that there is no detailed theory attempting to explain the beginning of fertility transition in either social change or economic change theory. There are assertions that fertility control would economically be a good thing for the wider community that go back to Malthus' race between population and food, but no explanation of the

---

[7] An attempt at a theoretical approach to these problems is Ben-Porath (1979).
[8] Including the works cited in Footnote 5, p. 272.

changes that lead individuals to restrict fertility. Nor is there any satisfactory analysis of the economics of societies with stable high fertility—the way nearly the whole human race has lived until the last hundred years. The important point is that fertility decline is all but ignored. If this is because it is unimportant or mechanically inevitable, then the field of demography is hardly worth sustaining. If it is because it cannot be easily explained, then the theories of change are inadequate not merely for the purposes of the demographer but in themselves.

The passing references—a few paragraphs in thousands of pages—to the origins of the fertility decline attribute it to mortality decline (without discussing whether high fertility was ever advantageous in itself), growing rationalism, the nuclearization of the family (usually in terms of shedding the shared load, and almost never in terms of changed power structures and decision-making mechanisms), changing attitudes to family size related to all the foregoing reasons, a new awareness or availability of contraception, and, amongst the household economists only, a changing economic calculus. Except for the last, these are mostly just intellectual crumbs from the demographers' table, picked up undigested in passing—Frank Notestein (1945 and 1953) on religious and social supports for high fertility, Kingsley Davis (1955) on the traditional family, the KAP surveys on ideal family size and knowledge of contraception, and so on.

There has been, then, no theory of fertility decline outside the field of demography, and demographers are ill-equipped to be given sole responsibility for erecting such theory for two reasons. The first is that the existence of the discipline encourages them to seek demographic reasons—or, at least, reasons that demographers can measure with their usual tools—for demographic phenomena. The second, and most important, is that the existence of the discipline encourages them to explain only demographic change. No theory of change is adequate that does not simultaneously explain the whole range of social, economic and demographic change (or at least provide a framework for so doing).

For the demographer, a central question is the reason for the failure of contemporary change theory.

Toward an Explanation for the Failure of Contemporary Change Theory

The failure of change theories largely arises from the period in which they were evolved and the virtues of those who created them. Their publication (or, in the case of Inkeles and Smith, the underlying research) was in the late 1950s and 1960s, the great era of international tension and of technical aid.

They are obsessed not only with change, but with the virtues of change, not only with the advantages of being "modern" but with the characteristics (almost the "virtues") of *modern man*.

This led to the error that vitiated them, and that defied all the rules of scientific method and what should be social scientific method. So keen were they to examine where social change was leading that they took practically no interest in what was changing and where rapid change had begun.[9] They took only passing, and usually pejorative interest, in traditional society, and hence cut themselves off from any chance of observing the onset of change or explaining it. Often the traditional society, far from attracting research interest, seemed almost repellent (the following references all coming from a single paragraph by Inkeles and Smith):

> "Men and women tied by the binding obligations of powerful extended kinship systems . . . Some have tried to win more freedom . . . They have sought to replace a closed world, in which their lives tread the narrowest circles . . . From a desperate clinging to fixed ways of doing things . . . fear of strangers and hostility to those very different from themselves . . . rigidity and closed-mindedness . . . passivity, fatalism, and the subordination of self to an immutable and inscrutable higher order" (pp. 4–5).

George Foster wrote, "Throughout history people in traditional societies have accepted these conditions because they knew nothing else" (1973, p. 2). Some of this reaction was the result of sociologists accustomed to industrialized countries suddenly working, often briefly, in one, or a whole range, of Third World countries (anthropological literature has few parallels with the above). Some lay deep in Europe's own change from familial production—the basic theme of Marx and Durkheim—and in the circumstances of North America's settlement by migrants and often by Protestants.

A central aspect of the inadequate treatment given to the traditional society was a failure to discuss adequately its economic base, and hence to its modes of production and other circumstances which determine whether reproduction is economically advantageous or not. Foster outlined the nature of traditional society with no reference to familial production (p. 1). Hagen, with a far deeper knowledge of traditional society than most change theorists, nevertheless, sought the mainsprings of behaviour elsewhere: "To the peasant, life is a mystery in a profound sense in which it is not a mystery to modern man . . . The major aspects of his personality, and the relationships within his community, I hypothesize, are closely related to this

---

[9] There has been protest at studying "modernization" without an adequate study of society at the beginning of the specified period and from a "neo-evolutionist" point of view. Cf. Bendix (1967), Smith (1973) and Feldman and Hurn (1966). However, the writers do not mention demographic change.

sense of impotence" (1962, p. 65).

There is, in fact, a concentration on personality change, which often seems to go as far as implying that individuals could always have lived different ways of life merely by opting to so do, whether or not the needed economic and social institutions for the new way of life had yet come into existence. Hagen wrote that, "Traditionalism . . . is a state [of mind] that may characterize any society" (p. 58). This view has clearly been an influence on the demographers' penchant for measuring ideal family size as a primary determinant of behavioural change. A central issue with regard to this paper, although its discussion will be left until near the end, is whether the behaviour measured by "change" researchers of this type is really an index of personality at all.

Lerner identified "mobile man" who could "identify with new aspects of environment" because of "empathy" or "the capacity to see oneself in the other fellow's situation" (1964, pp. 49–50).[10] Geographical mobility was at first the necessary catalyst but this was increasingly displaced by "psychic mobility" as "radio, film and television climax the evolution set in motion by Gutenberg" (p. 53). In the field the differences between traditional, transitional and modern man could be measured by the construction of scales compounded from responses to questionnaires, although (and the reason will be suggested later) the key opinion, potency and happiness scales failed to display differences of the magnitude apparently anticipated (pp. 99–102). Significantly Lerner also gave strong support to two methods of analysing change which may ultimately be proved to generate an illusory picture of what causes what, cross-cultural comparisons and the search for variables which move together to a statistically significant extent: "Our analysis of statistical data on 73 countries around the world confirmed this view of modernization as a 'systemic' process. The demographic, economic, political, communication and cultural 'sectors' of a modernizing society grow together and this joint growth occurs in regular phases" (p. 401).

Inkeles (and Smith, and Miller) also adopted "the sociopsychological approach to modernization which treats it mainly as a process of change in ways of perceiving, expressing and valuing. The modern is defined as a mode of individual functioning, a set of dispositions to act in certain ways" (Inkeles and Smith, 1974 p. 16). A modern man is "an informed participant citizen", with a "marked sense of personal efficacy", "highly independent and autonomous in his relations to traditional sources of influence especially when making basic decisions about the conduct of personal affairs", "ready for new experiences and ideas" and "relatively

---

[10] The concept of empathy is taken from the fields of psychology and history (cf. Collingwood, 1946), where it referred to projection and understanding but not to behavioural change.

open-minded and cognitively flexible" (p. 290). With regard to measuring the degree of change, the "solution to the problem was to derive a list of modern *personal* qualities from the presumed requirements of daily living in a modern and complex *society*, and, in particular, from the demands made on a worker or staff member in a modern industrial establishment" (p. 18). They also "started . . . with the conviction that men are not born modern, but are made so by their life experience" (p. 5), and subsequently claimed to have shown that men may become modern in adulthood (p. 303), in fact that late socialization explains as much as early socialization (Inkeles, 1969, pp. 216–217).

This approach was not marginal, but tended to represent the mainstream (and has strongly influenced demographers). As early as 1935 Mannheim had been arguing that "a transformation of society is inconceivable without the transformation of the human personality" (1940, p. 15). In the early 1960s David McClelland (1963 and 1966) was measuring the "impulse to economic growth" by the index nAch or the "need for achievement", calculated from literature from the time of archaic Greece and from children's readers in the contemporary developed and Third World. Hagen (1962, p. 97) was searching for the innovational and authoritarian personalities that determine the likelihood of the succeeding generation having a need for achievement. Kellert, Williams, Whyte and Alberti were in Peru, defining modernization as the "conflict between people who want to do things in the old ways and those who want to do things in the new ways", and accordingly trying to distinguish a "group with old customs" from "a group with modern ideas" (1967, pp. 407–408). Black was also arguing the partial replacement among modernizing influences of physical migration by "the people's heightened awareness, through vastly expanded means of communication" (1966, p. 24). Joseph Kahl argued that the fundamental motive force was the "modernization of values" (1968, pp. 6–8), and when he found a difference between reported ideal family size in Mexico and Brazil during the 1960s, he wrote: "I suspect that these differences are related to some old traditions within the Portuguese and Spanish cultures that were transferred to the New World, and possibly to some differences between the Negro contribution in Brazil and that of the Indian in Mexico" (p. 79). Amongst the economists, Rostow argued not the changing economy but the necessary new ideas of national dignity, private property, the general welfare and a better life for children (1960, p. 6). "New types of enterprising men come forward—in the private economy, in government, or both—willing to mobilize savings and to take risks in pursuit of profit or modernization (pp. 6–7). This happens most often now because of "external intrusions": these invasions—literal or figurative—shocked the traditional society and began or hastened its undoing; but they also set in mind ideas and sentiments which initiated the process by which a modern alternative to the traditional society was constructed out of the old culture" (p. 6).

Fundamental Problems in Change Theory

Change theory of this type raises difficulties for understanding general social and economic change and hence its demographic component. Five problems will be examined here. Much of the discussion cannot be focused on demographic change because change theory so rarely mentions fertility transition. But an anlysis of its problems does throw light on why this omission occurs.

(1) *The neglect of fundamental institutional change*

For most of human history the family, in its wider or narrower sense, has been the subsistence producing and consuming unit. Individuals with other ideas about how and where they wanted to live, far from creating modern society, would usually have faced disaster. Familial production of this kind, like the succeeding capitalist production, was governed by a set of rules in conformity with the power structure. Although these were usually obeyed, always supported by adage and custom, and often incorporated into religion, scepticism or hostility with regard to them usually did not create alternative employment—when migration to seek non-familial employment became possible on a considerable scale the world was already changing. The family power structure, and the respect it demanded, was maintained by access to land (or areas in which to hunt and forage). For reasons discussed in Chapters 4, 5 and 7 fertility is likely to remain high in societies of this kind. Such societies could be stable without central governments; indeed the demands of governments posed some threat to the familial morality that justified the family power structure (see Chapter 10). Where such government existed, its power structure tended to be modelled on the family, and governing elites were small (partly because the surplus of production over subsistence needs was small). Where capitalist production emerges, only a government can enforce law and morality to allow it to operate.

The emphasis on personality, attitudes and behaviour misleads us about the fundamental changes, even though it might tell us something about a transient persistence in the rules or superstructure (but see below) which explained a relatively short persistence in some behavioural patterns such as unrestricted fertility.[11]

[11] Cf. generally Portes (1973), especially p. 33; and, on the persistence of high fertility, Chapter 5 and Caldwell (1977a).

First, it misconstrues the basic nature of a society based on familial production, especially the fundamental importance of land and the lack of other employment or access to food and other requisites. Thus Hagen reported with seeming surprise, "the ownership, or if this is not possible, the proprietorship, of land is more vital to the peasant than perhaps any other aspect of his material life" (1962, p. 63). "Such a thing as an *individual* business venture is virtually unknown. Every economic act is taken in the name of the family and the associates in economic activity are members of the family" (p. 65). Foster reported that, "The demands of urbanization, industrialization, and a monetary economy usually are *uncongenial* to the extended family groupings of subsistence peoples" (1973, p. 59), and that "the factors that determine these motivations are cultural, social and psychological" (p. 5).

Often it is the power structure or relations of production that are seen almost as optional choices. Hagen (1962) wrote: "The (Burmese) family is a unit created to serve the needs of the father" (p. 161). "As the child grows, if he is a boy he becomes more of a rival to his father. Hence the father finds that the time has come for training, and he consistently quiets, subdues, and represses the child" (p. 145). (This) "also is in accord with the need dominance of parents. Their world image and their need dominance interact, each reinforcing the other" (p. 146). One must conclude that the hierarchical structure of authority and power in traditional societies has been so stable because the simple folk as well as the elite accepted it. The simple folk must feel satisfaction in depending for decisions and direction on individuals above them" (pp. 71–72). "If a hierarchical authoritarian social structure persists for centuries (as it has in traditional societies), it must be concluded that the members of the society found it satisfactory, and did so because in childhood they found such a structure of relationships the best solution to the problems they faced" (p. 6).

Even the emergence of the State is often seen almost as a choice. "A modern *nation* needs participating citizens, men and women who take an active interest in public affairs and who exercise their rights and perform their duties as members of a community larger than that of the kinship network and immediate geographic locality" (Inkeles and Smith, 1974, p. 4). "Where traditionalism is present . . . behaviour is governed by custom, not law" (Hagen, 1962, pp. 55–62). The sequence is wrong. It sounds as if an interest within the traditional family in national and international affairs produces a new economy and new state apparatus (indeed this is the only interpretation possible of the stress that both Lerner and Inkeles place on the significance of opinions on these matters), rather than a non-familial economy bringing employees out into a world where these matters are now important to them. It is, indeed, curious what interest has been aroused by Lerner's Turkish peasant who declared, "My God! How can you ask such a thing? How can I . . . I cannot . . . president of Turkey . . . master of the whole world?" (1964, p. 3), and by Inkeles' Pakistani farmer who punctuated the interview by declaring, "I am but a foolish man; what can I say?" (Inkeles and Smith, 1974, p. 78).

Unwilling to give priority to changes in the modes of production, attitudinal and behavioural change theorists are almost forced to explain change in terms of social deviance, often ignoring the range of deviance and of specialized roles and occupations existing over eons in stable traditional societies. Hagen decided that the basic cause of change "is the perception on the part of the members of some social group that their purposes and values in life are not respected by groups in the society whom they respect and whose esteem they value (1962, p. 185). Nigel Crook (1978) showed that such an approach could be used to provide a theoretical framework for a micro-study investigating fertility decline in a single Indian village, only provided firstly that one assumed economic change that affected the cost of children, and hence secondly relinquished any claim to be investigating the origin of economic change and the total succession of events precipitating fertility decline. "What is crucial then is the distribution of potential deviants in the village" (p. 206).

Often the stresses perceived in traditional society (which does indeed have stresses even if in a stable situation that has only a potential for inducing change) are largely those of transitional society where familial production and its morality have already been substantially eroded. Clearly this was the case of Lerner's traditional village before transition, Balgat, eight kilometres from Ankara, and soon to be denuded of its land by the growth of the city (1964, pp. 19–42). Indeed his dichotomies between traditional and modern are largely the contrasts between living within a system of familial production and living outside it: village versus town, land versus cash, illiteracy versus enlightenment(!), resignation versus ambition, and piety versus excitement (p. 44).

(2) An Emphasis on Simultaneous Data and a Neglect of History

Change theorists concentrate almost entirely on changing societies. Neither they nor demographers ever devote sufficient time to determining how stable traditional societies of familial production and high fertility work. Most analysis is done from cross-sectional data on the assumption of a linear continuity of attitudes and behaviour. This has been hailed as a decisive advance: "A new spirit was abroad in the 1960s which was more eclectic, less ideological, more interdisciplinary. The lead was taken by economists in the study of what they called development or growth. Relying heavily on factor analysis, they sought to identify the common socioeconomic characteristics of the 'advanced' countries and to discover the common paths, if any, that had led to economic growth" (Inkeles, 1977, p. 136). Such an approach could not of course identify paths let alone origins. However, Kahl (1968) maintained that such analysis could establish that socioeconomic status was the primary determinant of the *emergence* of modern attitudes. Allan Schnaiberg claimed, "We can certainly link modernism as a whole to the process of urbanization, the spread of education and literacy, and presumably the development of an industrial urban base" (1970, p. 419).

There has been counterattack. Bendix wrote of the "oversimplification (resulting) from heavily ideological interpretations of the contrast between tradition and modernity, and from undue generalizations of the European experience" (1967, p. 293), and argued that "studies of social change are not possible without a 'before-and-after' model of the social structure in question" (p. 317). Feldman and Hurn charged that "while most of the sociological assertions about modernization employ a rhetoric of behaviour, the data are hardly ever observations of behavioural changes" (1966, p. 379), and that "they are almost never longtitudinal data" (p. 379, fn. 5).

A telling defence is that society before change cannot be located, that there are no origins, but only mile-posts. This should not, of course, prevent real comparisons over time or more thoroughgoing investigations of the natures of societies characterized by very different levels of familial production (cross-cultural comparisons are much more dangerous because cultural phenomena really are being compared across cultures). However, such investigations really should be possible—and should be a gift to all change theory—of fertility decline. We do have origins. Almost within living memory, fertility nearly everywhere was as high as it had ever been, and this is still the case over much of the Third World. We should be able to investigate stable high fertility in its own right and not as an anomaly that has resisted change.

There is another problem in using cross-sectional data to interpret change which is serious, although neglected, and may help to explain a good deal of the misunderstanding of the mechanism of change. Most of the interpretation is based on being able to prove a statistically significant difference between the behaviour of two or more groups—or rather of two or more temporary subdivisions of the respondents divided for this purpose by a single characteristic or by a set of characteristics, taken really, one at a time. There are several drawbacks. First, the respondents may be divisible into quite different groups by each apparently significant characteristic, and the compound formed hypothetically by combining the most modernized and most traditional characteristics may not represent real groups of importance in the community. Secondly, those characteristics which yield the most significantly diverse distributions may merely be relatively superficial characteristics determined by deeper underlying characteristics. For instance, whether the respondents had arranged marriages or not (often used as an explanatory variable when examining the likelihood of using contraception) may largely reflect whether they came from a family farm or business or not and hence whether the control of the younger generation was vitally important to the parents or not. Thirdly, some characteristics are chosen for analysis (or, more often, for data collection in the first place) and others forgotten according to an underlying—and often hidden and unstated—hypothesis or according to what other researchers have collected and found significant according to their unstated hypotheses (a kind of accelerator principle operates). Fourthly, and perhaps most seriously, if the sample is large enough even small differences can be described as "highly significant" (and ironically researchers argue with funding organizations for larger samples just so small differences can be so described). Thus the importance of the duration of education is said to be proved if 70% of persons with secondary education do something compared with only 67% of persons with primary education (one needs around 3500 respondents with such schooling to show significance at the 5% level and 7000 at the 1% level).[12] The real significance is, of course, that most persons with both primary and secondary education do behave in this way, while another important point is that substantial minorities of both groups do not. If both proportions are rising with time (as they did, for instance, with contraceptive use in the West, then the real point may be that the time lag is only two years) (Caldwell and Ware, 1973, Table 8, p. 23). Fifthly, this kind of research approach apparently allows researchers from the West to transfer their expertise immediately to Third World countries, and to write subsequent reports as if the data analysis by standard methods either spoke for itself or was subject to a universal interpretation with, at the most, a few footnotes to show that historical or anthropological sources had been glanced at. All these points suggest that fundamental misunderstandings can arise about the nature of social change and its origins. That these approaches are used can be confirmed by leafing through the pages of any social science journal which gives some interest to the Third World and which has a leaning towards the analysis of large data sets rather than an historical, theoretical or anthropological approach (in the population field, the journal *Demography*, strongly influenced by those with a background in "quantitative" sociology, is an example).

(3) The Scales Employed
Even if one were not worried about the nature of change, or the concepts

[12] These are minimum sample sizes because it is assumed that all respondents belong to one or the other of the two categories and that the sizes of the two categories are similar.

used to define and measure it, one might well stop short at accepting the findings of the scales commonly employed. For instance, Stephenson reports that he accepts the Smith-Inkeles definition of modernization, but denies that their own scales have in any way measured it (1968, p. 267, fn. 15). I agree with his criticism, partly agree with his reservations about persons from one culture devising scales for another culture (p. 268), let alone a set of them, and then totally disagree with his own definition upon which his measures are based. That definition is: "Modernization is the movement of persons or groups along a cultural dimension from what is defined by the cultural norms as traditional toward what is defined by the same culture as modern. Those values defined in the local culture as traditional comprise what may be called traditionalism; those defined as modernism constitute modernism" (p. 268). Until recently, truly traditional societies had little idea what was modern, only what was either deviant or delinquent. Even now much depends on whether they take the word "modern" or its translation to be used in an approving or disapproving sense. If in the former sense (and sometimes in the latter sense) it will probably be taken to mean *Western*, or just *American*. In any case the answers will probably be as superficial—and will certainly be entirely attitudinal and behavioural, revealing nothing about the fundamental forces of change in the society—as those from an American or European respondent would be. The responses in some societies might emphasize what the powerful do, and in others what the young do, even if this has not meant in the past that the poor or the young once they have grown older subsequently act the same way. Feldman and Hurn complained, "The stage to which they belong is typically judged by their occupation" (1966, p. 381). The problem about the improved scales is that they make judgements based on a great number of measures worse than occupation. In fact occupation, or at least the setting of that occupation within a production mode, may be the only appropriate measure.

Certainly the contents of the scales are alarming to any demographer who intends to use them as an independent measure of the restriction of fertility according to placing on a traditional–modern continuum. The narrower reason is that they are not independent of fertility, and accordingly inevitably tend to move with fertility decline. Indeed, when Inkeles attempted in 1969 to set down the personality qualities which identify modern man, the first quality to be listed was "openness to new experience, both with people and with new ways of doing things such as *attempting to control births*" (p. 210). The Inkeles and Smith core attitude scale (OM–1) includes ideal family size, and attitudes to both birth control and the oral contraceptive. Indeed, the latter question incorporates the assumption that there is always a negative relationship between high fertility and economic well-being and begins by informing the respondent: "A man and his wife have several children. This is as many as they can afford. . .". Their expanded attitude scale (OM–2) includes in addition a question on the number of children you would have if you were well off (and tells the respondent that there is a relationship between economic condition and ability to educate children and implies an obligation to educate them), a question on whether one would follow the lead of a government advising the limitation of the size of the family (it is apparently modern to bow to the Government) and a question on the relative responsibility of each spouse when practicing contraception (1974, pp. 329–330). The broader reason is that this is only one set of questions among a series of sets on an interrelated complex of attitudinal and behavioural changes which often tend to move together. There are other sets of questions on matters almost inextricably related to the value of children and the likelihood that fertility control will prove advantageous: kinship obligations (two questions in the core and three more in the expanded scale); women's rights (seven in the core and three more in the expanded scale); ageing and the aged (one in the core and an extra one in the expanded scale). The other 23 sets of questions, ranging from *active public participation* to *citizenship* and from *dignity* to *time valuation*, have exactly the same drawbacks. They gauge certain changes at a certain point in time. They explain nothing about the origin of change or about the force that keeps it moving. Masses of questions do offer evidence on the change from familial production to employment on the non-familial capitalist labour market but they are never interpreted this way (all but one of the *dignity* questions are either about the patriarch's economic relations or those involving control of his wife or son or about labour control relationships in factories). There is nothing in the analysis suggesting that fundamental transformations in the economy are of importance (except for their environmental impact, such as the experience of working in a factory). The basic explanation for change is on the role of the media in providing individuals with greater data banks of information, with little concern for the fact that information that is significant in one way of life may not be in another.

The emphasis on Inkeles and Smith here does not arise from their weaknesses, but because of their influence (on demographers as well as other social scientists) and because of the details they have provided about their methodology and viewpoint. In fact most other attempts to scale social change have also concentrated on the results rather than the forces of change. An investigation of traditional behaviour amongst Chinese in Hong Kong (Dawson *et al.*, 1971) scaled and analysed attitudes to family size, parental desire for sons, chastity as a supreme virtue, gifts in social and interpersonal relations, brideprice, parental discipline, the higher status of males, polygamy, respect for the aged, husband dominance and paternal government without mentioning the functions of these institutions in traditional familial production, without indeed mentioning such activities except for questions on "farming as an honourable institution". Sometimes scaling concentrates on a single theme, said to be the basic mechanism for change, such as the investigation of the decline of cooperation and the rise of competitiveness carried out by Meeker (1970) in Liberia and by Bethlehem (1975) in Zambia.

(4) The Neglect of Cultural Diffusion: Modernization versus Westernization

Much attention is given to the formation of a global economy, and very little to the establishment of a global society. Cultural diffusion is a part of everyday experience and concern from Western Europe to remote parts of the Third World. But it is not a significant element in social change theory. This may be very misleading in terms of the anticipated rate of change and of the timing of such events as the onset of fertility decline.

Modernization is that degree of social change which inevitably accompanies economic change because the new economic order demands it—anything less would be grossly inefficient and even chaotic. The factory hand, at least during his working hours, must obey his boss and not seek guidance from his father, and he must obey the factory's or the government's rules about not stealing the equipment even if the possession of such equipment would please his father and benefit the whole family (this is an idealized model—reality will be discussed in the next section). *Westernization* is the social change over and above this which results from importing aspects of the Western way of life. There is a huge indeterminant middle ground, because Western ways of life, though imported because newspapers say they are more fashionable or missionaries more virtuous, have been more honed to an industrial way of life (or at least one centring on non-familial production) and may fit in better with the new economic system and may raise individual productivity at the same level of capital investment. In this sense the West, and especially its Anglo-Saxon part has been largely modernized (although there has also been a complex pattern of cultural diffusion), while Westernization has been an important aspect of the Third World experience. Thus behaviour patterns, which are only dictated over the long-term by economic change, may move at a faster rate relative to economic change than occurred in the West—children may become economically disadvantageous and fertility may fall at an earlier time.

The study of these different rates, and of the cultural diffusion which gives rise to them, would seem to be basic to a study of social change—particularly among those concentrating on attitudinal and concomitant behavioural change. No such emphases have appeared, for complex reasons.

Marx in his earlier writing was clearly willing to regard the superstructure as only loosely tied to the dictates of the changing modes of production (1975), but later opted for more direct economic determinism and downplayed the role of both social and economic diffusion even in Western Europe (1976, vol. 1, pp. 90–91). In fact the reasons for down-playing diffusion have often been ideological and even almost political. Lerner, who, from every description, clearly regards the cultural flow from the West as being of fundamental importance in the Middle East (for instance, "The nations of the North Atlantic area first developed the social processes . . . by which this state of mind ("modernity") came to prevail (1964, p. viii). From the West came the stimuli which undermined traditional society in the Middle East; for the reconstruction of a modern society that will operate efficiently in the world today, the West is still a useful model") (p. ix) shies away from any definition along these lines: "modernization appears as Westernization by historical coincidence . . . The Western model must . . . be freed from the constraints of ethnocentrism in order to function effectively" (pp. viii–ix). "Any label that today localizes the process is bound to be parochial. For Middle Easterners more than ever want the modern package, but reject the label 'made in U.S.A.' (or, for that matter, 'made in U.S.S.R.'). We speak, nowadays, of modernization" (p. 45). Inkeles seems to waver between considering Westernization a tactless concept and a wrong one. "Some may, therefore, insist that such individuals (ones who score high on the OM scales) have become 'Westernized', or at least more like Westerners. I prefer to think of them as having become more modern, because I personally find it more appropriate to think of the qualities which make up the modernity syndrome as not being the distinctive property of any single cultural tradition . . . I see little to be gained by spilling a great deal of ink over the issue. It seems much less important to settle the issue of whether individual modernity is Western or not than it is to decide what consequences follow from its spread" (1977, p. 145). He adds, "some sort of psychological Westernization may be a practical necessity for any country which seeks to modernize its institutions . . . Each nation and each people should be free to make the choice either to import the set of institutions which are generally considered to be modern, to live as they have always lived, to borrow some other pattern, or to invent wholly new institutional patterns of their own" (p. 146). This seems clear enough but then follows an extraordinary attestation of psychological and attitudinal autonomy: "Imperialism can export Coca-Cola, blue jeans, Hollywood movies, and capital-intensive production. But it cannot export individual modernity. Individual modernity may develop as a response to prior colonial action, but, being built into the psyches of the people, it must of necessity be a native product, home grown, no matter how foreign was the origin of the seed" (p. 146). Black, in a search for "the characteristics of modernity that may be assumed to be of universal validity" (1966, p. 4), and agreeing that cultural diffusion is important (p. 6), then defines modernization so as to lose any meaning beyond "change" and to avoid the issue of how much follows inevitably from the arrival of new economic institutions: "The advantage of a term such as 'modernization' is not only that it has a broader scope than 'Westernization', 'Europeanization', 'industrialization', or even 'progress', but also that it is less encumbered with accretions of meaning" (pp. 7–8). The fact of the matter is that the clarification of exactly what has happened and is still happening is of vital importance. In the demographic field it helps to provide an answer to the question as to whether Third World countries have to attain the levels of urbanization, non-agricultural employment and real per capita income of Britain of a century ago before they can expect fertility to decline or whether the fact that it has already declined elsewhere is of significance, either because the practice and its ethos can be imported or because some predetermining social change can be unwittingly or wittingly imported.

Not all treatments of change restrict social change to meeting the minimum needs of economic change or being dictated by economic change. Some suggest a certain primacy for social change, which implies a far greater potential significance for Westernization. Feldman and Hurn averred that, "Modernization refers to those social changes that generate institutions and organizations like those found in advanced industrial countries" (1966, p. 378), and Davis that, "economic modernization requires a large amount of individual movement in the social hierarchy" (1962, p. 67). Inkeles and Smith avoided explaining the impact of schooling in terms of an imported, and hence Westernizing, message, and the impact of factories merely in terms of a new set of rules or relationships for a new mode of production by treating both as institutions inevitably imparting implicit lessons not designed purposively. The school changed the personality by reward and punishment, exemplification, modelling and generalization (1974, pp. 139), while adults were imbued with new personal qualities from the "requirements of daily living in a modern and complex *society*, and, in particular, from the demands made on a worker or staff member in a modern industrial establishment" (p. 18).

What occurred in Europe and what is happening in the contemporary Third World is complex with everywhere differences in accent because of specific cultural contexts. Bendix (1967) has argued that the European change was far more complex, riddled with idiosyncracies derived from European history, than the historical models of it, let alone those derivations employed by change theorists. One reason for debate, even for denying Westernization when it is patently there, has been that the cultural changes are more painful and from the individual's viewpoint more basic than the economic ones; as Robert Bellah wrote, "Modernization, whatever else it involves, is always a moral and religious problem" (1969, p. 37)—one of values and meanings. Both what is exported and what is imported are far from being general products suited exactly to the economic situation: "We cannot easily separate modernity and tradition from some *specific* tradition and some *specific* modernity . . . The modern comes to the traditional society as a particular culture with its own traditions" (Gusfield, 1967, p. 361)—and that, in terms of current Westernization, includes contemporary Western traditions about intergenerational relations and about family limitation.

No real attempt can be made to explore individual examples of change, but passing reference might be made to two cases, Sri Lanka which appears to have experienced more social than economic change, and where mortality and fertility have both experienced substantial declines, and Japan, the first non-Western country to industrialize and to attain low birth rates. Much remains to be done to explain change in Sri Lanka (Ames, 1972–3; Gooneratne, 1968), but the evidence is growing, and it points to massive Westernization, such as is found in many oceanic islands (Caldwell *et al.*, 1980) and, to a somewhat lesser extent, in Kerala. Michael Ames concludes that, "Ceylon has become Westernized in institutions, values and aspirations without a corresponding degree of economic modernization" (1972–3, p. 143) in a situation where "Christianity was freely identified with the scientific civilization of the west, in fact as its wellspring" (p. 152), and where the proportion of literate males and females in 1900 was similar to the pattern in India and Pakistan in 1961, while the proportion attending school in 1930 paralleled Indonesia in 1961 (p. 168). He details how easy it is to identify a movement as largely indigenous or anti-Westernization when the impact is Westernizing by analysing the nature of the Buddhist revival from the second half of the nineteenth century: "The ways in which Buddhists responded to the threat of Westernization were obviously influenced by the very things against which they reacted . . . They copied, or reasserted, their own Buddhist counterparts of the dominant western attitudes: the belligerent puritanism, the individualism, this-worldly activism, technological rationalism, scepticism and utilitarianism of the Christians" (p. 160). Japan is of interest because the same history can be seen as one of indigenous change with little Westernization (Hagen, 1962, p. 25; Fuse, 1975, pp. 2–3; Eisenstadt, 1966, p. 78) or as one where Western influence was decisive (Hara, 1977; Jansen and Stone, 1967, p. 229; Bellah, 1969, pp. 37 and 45). Hagen goes so far as to survey the experience of Japan, India, China and Indonesia in terms of social and economic change and then to conclude, "Clearly the effects of contact with Western knowledge, disruption of traditional culture, and availability of resources either were irrelevant or were nullified by other influences" (1962, p. 25)—and this from a major change theorist.

(5) Change in Personality, Attitude, Behaviour or the Rules?

This is the fundamental question and is all but ignored. It has enormous significance for demographic behaviour and for social change theory. If much of the behaviour and attitudes measured are merely what the actors do or say in a specific economic context, then the social change scales are meaningless except as evidence of that context. The same is true for measurements of demographic behaviour. This examination begins to focus some of the worries raised in the previous sections.

Massive changes in economic relationships have occurred over much of the world. In traditional societies of the past, perhaps 90% of the population were peasants (Black, 1966, pp. 20–21), and many of the remainder were merchants or craftsmen who used their families for production in the same way as do peasants. This world has passed, and in much of the Third World two-fifths of occupations are for wages usually paid by non-relatives.[13] Familial production was governed by rules which tended to benefit the powerful—the old and the male—and these rules were embedded in morality and theology (see Chapters 5 and 7). In non-familial production, people had different relationships and espoused different moralties.

But this is a model. Bendix (1967) has warned that real Europe was never as simple as this, and neither is the contemporary Third World. Great numbers of people live not in one or other of these two systems but in both either simultaneously or in alternation. For generations the assertion, that "separation has taken place first, and perhaps most dramatically, between family and economic occupational roles" (Eisenstadt, 1966, p. 3), is not generally true. It is also not true that "the chance to get ahead by dint of effort rather than by virtue of birth stimulates people to work harder" (Davis, 1962, p. 68); they work in the different contexts within the rules and according to the pressures applied and the rewards offered. Even in a traditional society, men behaved in a different way, according to a different morality, when they were in the King's Army than when they were back with kinsfolk on the farm. There is much to the charge that in change theory, "Rural populations are perceived as stereotypically traditional, and urban populations as sterotypically modern [while] transitional populations are thought to be marginal, subject to strains, anomic, etc." (Feldman and Hurn, 1966, p. 381).

[13] Calculated from International Labour Office (1978), Table 2A, based on data for 26 countries, not including India, China or most African states.

In point of fact descriptions of the more varied real world often emphasize our societies and individuals can live in two worlds. In neither Mexico nor India is the Great Tradition a feature only of the towns and the Little Tradition of the villages: Pauline Kolenda has demonstrated very well why the version of Hinduism aimed at solving more immediate wants and fears meets most of the needs of the rural population, but how the version that surveys the eons past and ahead is known and can be adjusted to by the rural–urban migrant or the boy upwardly mobile through school (1964; cf. also Bendix, 1967, pp. 313–314). Gusfield makes the point also about India, "Almost always the Indian intellectual speaks a regional language as his mother tongue, is steeped in classic Sanskrit literature, and is deeply tied to an extended family. Parental arrangement is still the very dominant mode of marital selection, and he is often married to a highly traditional wife" (1967, p. 359). Crook's village deviants (1978) were there even in the stable village; most villagers were probably deviant in some way, and nearly all could be deviant if a different situation offered itself. Lerner's people of Balgat had not had a personality change in those four short years from 1950 to 1954 (1964, pp. 19–42) not even modern communications could do that. It was merely that a different situation had offered itself (and, if one takes that standpoint, the whole book can be read differently).

The most important different situation is a job on the open labour market in contrast to working within the family system. But the immediate contrast for the individual is usually not the one of full transition from one system to the other; that is the course of the whole society over generations. It is not the case that the lingering elements of the old way of life "constitute a serious deterrent to the introduction of new and improved production techniques, since a progressive individual's greater income may be drained away in maintaining traditional forms of hospitality and help to relatives" (Foster, 1973, p. 60). Except in conditions of very rapid economic change this is an unreal situation. The usual one in Africa and South Asia is described by Moore and Feldman, "In many cases the real problem, which has not been given adequate recognition, is that industrialization in developing areas has not given workers sufficient opportunity to make a clean break with the past. The industrial worker is unwilling to give up even the meagre economic and emotional security offered by the family, tribe, or village for low wages, inadequate housing, insecure job tenure, separation from family, poor supervision, language difficulties, racial discrimination, and lack of status and sense of belonging" (1960, pp. 300–301). Claude Meillassoux has emphasized that the wages are often low because the familial support is available (1972, p. 102). The actual position is even more complex than this. Industry would not exist in some areas but for the fact that the family system allows low wages to be paid. The fact that the workers live between two worlds—two sets of economic rules—allows them to bend both sets: they need not be quite so deferential to the patriarch and they can be somewhat casual about obeying the boss's instructions to be at work punctually every day. This quite conscious optimizing of their life style makes them more traditional on the Inkeles-Smith scale (they fail all the Time Valuation questions, as well as most of the Work Commitment, Aspirations, Efficacy and Planning ones) (1974, pp. 319–347). Often both individuals and families live in both the old and new systems getting what they can from each. There is usually not even a conflict in values; the system of values from one world is used to maximize returns from the other (Gusfield, 1967, pp. 354–355). The patriarch emphasizes the duty to the older generation and the son who has a job in town gives not only deference but a sizeable amount of his earnings. The son's job is threatened or he faces an unwanted transfer, and the patriarch talks to a neighbour so that the latter's son, who has a key post in the employing organization, takes action to remove the threat.

The essential point is that in much of our present world, where transition is still occurring from familial production to a completely non-familial system, people can, and do, live and work in both systems, with an awareness and a respect for the moral orders of each system. In the West this has been going on for centuries; the male household head goes out to work, espousing to his fellow workers a certain morality and world view appropriate to their working together in the market place, and then he returns home where his wife (and, until this century, his children) are producing domestic goods and services in a system of familial production which he encourages by a philosophy of family virtue, loyalty, and gratitude, quite different from the morality he expects to bind himself and his employer (see Chapter 5, pp. 173). This is not hypocrisy; people regard the morality as being suited to the mode of production. In the Third World, one often seems to meet a different man, a much more traditional one, if after knowing him while employed in the town, one searches him out, after his sacking, back in the village, living in the extended family compound and working beside his brothers and under his father on a subsistence farm. He will talk in a different way than he did in the town, and may even voice different views (even in private—although it should be noted that most survey interviews in the Third World are not carried out in private).

I am not arguing that a man back in the village reverts completely to his former unawareness of the outside world. In the village the people who have worked in the town are distinguishable from those who have not (Caldwell, 1969, p. 200) (although they often only parade their knowledge of the outside world to a visitor from that world). But these are almost parlour tricks. The important point is that they have not forgotten the lifestyle and the priorities of the village. They can fit back into it again without clumsiness and usually without resentment. They know the advantages of the town job, but they usually will not begin even to weaken the links with the family unless they are completely convinced that a town job is assured for a lifetime and that the extended family can no longer help or hinder.

In the town a man sees and hears things not heard in the village. He has to answer more quickly and often make decisions at his job especially if it is an unsupervised one; at home in the village such quickness and the taking on of such responsibility would justifiably make his brothers and father suspicious. In the town he must put on a show of working hard; in the village he must put on a show of deferring to age and experience. In the town he must sound as if community or national interests come first, and in the village as if family ones do. In the town he must talk to strangers; politics is one possibility, partly because it is a common experience, and partly because government does have a greater bearing on the lives of townsmen. But, and this is the crucial point, is it not these discussions or the fact that he knows the President's name that propelled him towards acquiring his town job; he knows these things because they are relevant once he has a town job. Nor will this knowledge make him overthrow the familial morality of the village if he has to work there.

How are these transition circumstances seen by the change theorists? Inkeles and Smith "proposed, then, to classify as modern those personal qualities which are likely to be inculcated by participation in large-scale modern productive enterprises such as the factory, and, perhaps more critical, which may be required of the workers and the staff if the factory is to operate efficiently and effectively" (1974, p. 19). They noted that, "In actual fact, the personal qualities *defined as modern* in many different researches show a remarkable degree of overlap. Variants on the themes of fatalism, empathy, efficacy, innovativeness, flexibility, achievement, orientation, information, and active citizenship abound. Almost as frequently . . . stress, alienation and anomie" (Inkeles, 1977, p. 144). In other words, people in town jobs behave the way they are expected to do, and, if they are rural–urban migrants, show the strains exhibited by most displaced persons. These characteristics were measured by batteries of questions which did little more than confirm the two different ways. Sometimes they showed an appaling inability to empathise with traditional familial production and its morality, such as the preliminary sentence in an Inkeles and Smith question on Kinship Obligations: "Some people say that a boy should be taught to give preference to a friend or relative, even when others have *a more rightful claim*" (Inkeles and Smith, 1974, p. 333).

What did they find? Inkeles and Smith found that, "A good deal was foreshadowed by whether a man was born in the countryside or in the city" (p. 282), and that "the UNIs (those in urban non-industrial employment) consistently outperformed (i.e. gave fewer "traditional" responses) the cultivators, who provided our baseline of *disadvantage*" (p. 214). One might conclude that this shows that those born in the countryside are more likely still to have links with familial agriculture and to express views showing those links. But the conclusions drawn were that, "To some extent, the rural setting from the start, inculcates traditional attitudes" (p. 282), that farming gives a man "little opportunity to develop his modernity" (p. 283), and that "few things in the nature of their work stimulated them to new ways of looking at things, to a heightened sense of personal efficacy, or to any of the other changes which would have made them more modern" (p. 285). These conclusions were drawn in spite of the discovery that the type of home and school background was not very important (p. 236ff.), and the "important surprise . . . that the men in certain non-industrial occupations, such as cabdrivers, newspaper vendors, barbers, and street hawkers, showed rather more modernity than we had assumed" (p. 304)—i.e. the uneducated in non-familial employment. They were drawn also in spite of the finding that people could become "modern in adult life by accepting a factory job" (p. 303). Some of the findings on information, taken by the researchers to be significant, showed how little "information" means except in its job and lifestyle context: workers in fairly large, and often unionized, factories were shown to be more likely to have heard of Moscow than were village farmers (p. 214). Even Lerner's happiness index (1964, pp. 398–399), which he used to establish that the traditional man was less happy, is at one with fatalism scales; there are good reasons in the traditional family why individuals should not announce their success too jubilantly or create too much fuss about disasters, even the death of children.

The important point is that questions of this kind measure the occupational transition by measuring many things that move at the same time. They do not predict the future. They do not explain the changes except that they appear to be associated with movement from traditional familial farming. They do not explain why such movement is occurring, and they certainly do not add to our knowledge that fertility decline is likely to start at some time in that process, let alone what determines the timing.

The Mutual Contributions and Potential Contributions of Social and Economic Change Theories and Demographic Change Theories

Any hope that demographers might have that they could understand more about the onset of fertility decline if they delved deeper into the explanations offered by social and economic change theory for the onset of change is likely to be dashed. Such theory has very little to say about fertility decline, not because it is not thought to be important, but because the theory does not begin to have the apparatus for dealing with the problem—or, indeed, for other problems of social and economic change. The theorists' approach is wrong in the failure both to research pre-existing society and in the emphasis on attitudes and deviance. Among the social change theorists this is probably explained by a desire to use only the tools of their own disciplines (sociology and social psychology) and by a social engineer's excitement in producing modern man—people like us. A similar excitement seems to have motivated the economic change theorists.

There is unlikely to be much understanding of the onset of change until we know a great deal more about the traditional family and about familial production, mostly in peasant farming but also in traditional artisan and commercial groups. Economic anthropologists have done something on exchange relationships but much less on relative labour inputs and consumption patterns within the family that is the essence of this mode of production. Other anthropologists have devoted a great deal of attention to kinship relations, but very little to the internal power structure within the family and the decision-making apparatus which determines individuals' "standards of living". The field of peasant studies has devoted more attention to political movements than to the nature of the peasant economy. Work is not only needed on the age-old peasant family economy, but on families with members working partly outside them, or working wholly outside them for some periods only. Work is needed on the Western family, especially in the nineteenth century, and perhaps on the Middle Eastern urban family today, to discover the economic and demographic implications of marked divisions of labour by sex and generation with the females, and perhaps the young males, providing labour for the household as a subsistence production unit.

This is the route the demographer must also follow. It is pointless to go along with the social change theorists in emphasizing the measurement of changing ideal family size and attitudes to contraception. Even the measurement of fertility and contraception change is merely confirmation that something more fundamental in the society is also changing.

There is almost certainly only one way forward, and that is to assume (and attempt to prove) that the economic advantages of high fertility have declined. We need to note such findings as those of Saad Gadalla (1978, pp. 194–219) in rural Egypt that economic reasons dominate both high fertility motives and low fertility ones and that a shift toward desiring low fertility has been occasioned by an almost silent but complex economic change:

"The villagers are aware of the increased costs of food, clothing, medical care, and education which they are providing their children. They even frequently compare how little it used to cost their own parents to feed and clothe them with what it costs today. They also compare how limited and simple their needs were and how diverse and complicated their children's needs are now. They realize that everyday general expenses are much higher year after year. In short, they are sensitive to the economic costs of rearing children, aware that a large family costs more to support and maintain than a small one, and encountering much more economic difficulty in raising their families than did their parents and grandparents" (p. 117).

We need to investigate that increasing difficulty very carefully for some of the changes are subtle. I have used the term "net wealth flows" in Chapter 4, to try to define the net difficulty—the losses minus the gains from children—and have attempted to show just how complex the impact of the education factor is (Caldwell, 1979).

I believe that we will be able to show that the fertility decline occurred because children changed from being on the whole an economic advantage to an economic disadvantage. I do not think that anyone has been able to show that peasant families, practicing subsistence agriculture, are relatively disadvantaged by large families, at least from the vantage point of the patriarch, or other decision-maker, and when the balance sheet is worked out over a lifetime—our evidence seems to point in the opposite direction. But adequate research on this point is not the end of the road. We must examine the economics of the transitional family—of the returns to the patriarch and to the son who works in the town, of their continued economic relationship, and of what it economically implies for the fertility of both father and son. Under what conditions will the son, or the grandson, restrict his fertility? In extended families how are fertility decisions made, for clearly it is the economic context of the fertility decision-maker we must keep in mind? I believe that we will ultimately show that the driving force of change in the worthwhileness of high fertility is the change from one mode of production to another—from familial to capitalist production—but that the point at which high fertility (or all fertility) becomes uneconomic can vary by decades, and perhaps in parts of the historic West, by generations, according to such social factors as whether children are taught to work hard and live austerely or not and according to whether mass education upsets the ability to maintain their hard working and relatively austere consumption situation. It is because of slippage of this order that the differentiation between minimum home-grown change and Westernization becomes important.

If demographers can tease out something close to the full pattern, they can teach change theorists a great deal more than the value of the scraps of theory and conventional belief that they have already presented. Ironically, they might also move economic change theorists more toward economic analysis, and might convince them that one of the great changes in human relations occurred in the transition from familial to non-familial production, a change suitably attested by the one significant transition in family size.

The point here is not that some demographers have not been working along the right lines, but that their canvases have not been large enough. Freedman in the early 1960s concluded that the explanation of fertility decline lay in the fact that "industrial urbanization was associated with a much more complex division of labour" (1961–62, p. 56). Lorimer, in 1965, had attempted to demonstrate how transition from agrarian to industrial production changed the balance of production over consumption through the life cycle in such a way as to make children a greater economic burden (1967, pp. 92–95) but he failed to grapple with the problem of how internal family relationships might yield very different consumption patterns (taking consumption in its broadest sense) by age and sex in different societies. Others have noted the relationship between economic change—or rising income—and fertility decline, sometimes cautiously postulating the major impact to come through such secondary factors as rising education and declining mortality (Simon, 1974).

Nevetheless, a full satisfactory theory of demographic transition is unlikely to be distinguishable from a fully satisfactory theory of social and economic change from a system of familial productive to one of non familial production. In neither case will the theory be adequate unless it can explain not merely the fact of fertility decline but the timing of its onset. Nor will it be satisfactory if it appears to deal with autonomous economies or societies, and fails to explain the role of exportable change. Demographers and others would almost certainly find it of great value to concentrate more on the intrafamilial social and economic relationships associated with different modes of production and to examine the effect on the value of children of changes in these relationships.

10

Mass education as a determinant of the timing of fertility decline

This article proposes mechanisms through which mass education produces declines in fertility and reviews the evidence, both in the nineteenth century demographic transition in the West and in contemporary developing countries, for such a relationship. It is argued that the primary determinant of the timing of the onset of the fertility transition is the effect of mass education on the family economy. The direction of the wealth flow between generations is changed with the introduction of mass education, at least partly because the relationships between members of the family are transformed as the morality governing those relationships changes.

The attainment of low fertility and the ability to erect and sustain massive educational systems are ultimately dependent on major economic changes; but the timing of such economic change is not necessarily closely related to the timing of alterations in the social structure that are sufficient to initiate new patterns of fertility behaviour.

Traditional family-based production is inevitably characterized by high fertility; and a fully developed system of capitalist production, with most production arising from wage labour offered to individuals within the family by outsiders, is ultimately just as inevitably characterized by low fertility (see Chapter 7). However, the timing of the transition between a condition in which high fertility is not an economic burden for economic and reproductive decision makers to one in which it clearly is a burden is not merely dependent on the rate of economic or occupational change, but on the nature of the cultural superstructure and the family economics that superstructure helps to determine (see Chapters 4 and 5).

Family production works within a framework of family morality, which enjoins children to work hard, demand little, and respect the authority of the old. Under this system, the patriarch, as head of the family, exercises authority. Children are employed from an early age and are valued as an addition to the work force. The flow of wealth is upward from children to parents and even grandparents, and high fertility is profitable, at least in the long run, to the parents. In that the social structure supports economic realities, the achievement by parents of large families is additionally rewarded by being regarded as honourable and a fulfillment of parents' duty to their elders. This morality (and the concomitant high fertility) can long survive the growth of a substantial capitalist labour market, partly because it is supported by public religion and private adage, and partly because the parental generation continues to benefit from it, especially when most domestic production of goods and services is subsistence production by wives and children. What the family morality cannot survive and is ultimately supplanted by is a new, community morality that is eventually necessary for fully developed non-family production (whether described as capitalist or socialist), and that is taught, explicitly and implicitly, by national education systems.

Like the timing of fertility decline, the timing of mass schooling is not completely economically determined. Britain could have supported a large educational system, had it been so inclined, in the first quarter of the nineteenth century instead of the last. In the great educational debate about the need for universal schooling in the West in the nineteenth century, not even employers claimed that the demand for educated labour exceeded the supply. The battle for universal schooling was won on three issues, in the following order of importance: first, the case for greater social justice and for a ladder for gifted individuals from poverty to middle-class comfort; second, the argument that the necessary underpinning for democracy was a fully educated electorate; and third, the need for national power and progress sustained by an educational system that would not waste hidden talents (Tyack, 1976, p. 356; Lawson and Silver, 1973, pp. 267–363; Leybourne and White, 1940, pp. 17–28). Most British politicians correctly assumed that universal schooling would inevitably closely follow the enfranchisement in 1867 of the urban working class. Attitudes toward the contemporary developing world have not been very different—humanity and justice demand schooling for all. As early as 1951, UNESCO proclaimed "the general principle of the necessity of instituting systems of compulsory, free, and universal education in all countries, whether self-governing or not" (UNITED Nations, 1951).

Most developing countries display strong associations between the fact of education and the level of education achieved, on the one hand, and a range of demographic behaviour, on the other. In Ghana, propensity for rural–urban migration is largely determined by the duration of education; in Nigeria, the single most important determinant of a child's chance of survival is its mother's level of education (Caldwell, 1968b and 1979). In countries in the early stages of fertility transition or apparently nearing fertility decline, the most marked fertility differentials appear to be educational ones.[1] In developing countries or states that have achieved universal education ahead of the level of economic development that usually accompanies it—Sri Lanka, Kerala, and a range of insular micro-states—fertility transition has been dramatic. These findings were once frequently taken as being largely reflections of such other socio-economic conditions as household income, but there now appears to be increasing recognition of the possibility that education itself may be of fundamental significance.

The Argument

The greatest impact of education is not direct but through the restructuring of family relationships and, hence, family economies and the direction of the net wealth flow. It is postulated here that education has its impact on fertility through at least five mechanisms:

First, it reduces the child's potential for work inside and outside the home. This occurs not merely because certain hours are subtracted from the day by school attendance and homework, but, perhaps more importantly, for two other reasons. The child is frequently alienated from those traditional chores that he feels to be at odds with his new learning and status. Parents, other adults, and even siblings may share some of these feelings and either fail to enforce traditional work or positively discourage it. Parents may feel that the child should retain all its energies for succeeding at school; they may feel that traditional familial work does not befit a person who is headed for nontraditional employment and status; they may be apprehensive of alienating the affection of a child who is so demonstrably going to be successful in the new, outside world.

---

[1] Fertility differentials by education can be found in some pretransition or early transition societies, but, in keeping with the argument in this paper, they are slight. On India, see Driver (1963), Table 88, p. 99; Dandekar and Dandekar (1953), pp. 65–66; United Nations (1961), pp. 121–123. On Ghana, see Gaisie (1975), pp. 343–344. On Nigeria, see Sembajwe (1981); Dow and Benjamin (1975), pp. 434–435; Dankoussou et al. (1975), p. 689; Courel and Pool (1975) pp. 741–743. Even desired family-size differentials tend to be small. On India, see United Nations (1961). In societies undergoing rapid fertility transition, differentials in fertility can be quite large, even if the time lag is not very great. On Taiwan, see Freedman et al. (1972 and 1976); Freedman and Takeshita (1969), p. 99. On Chile, see Tabah and Samuel (1962), p. 280. On Lebanon, see Chamie (1977), p. 379. In late-transition or post-transitional societies the differentials in fertility or desired family size can range from nonexistent to quite marked. On the United States, see Rindfuss (1975), pp. 24 and 27. On Eastern Europe, see Frenkel (1976). These data support the hypothesis that the onset of fertility transition is a movement that affects the whole society at much the same time, although exhibiting leading and lagging social elements during the period of change.

Second, education increases the cost of children far beyond the fees, uniforms, and stationery demanded by the school. Schools place indirect demands on families to provide children with better clothing, better appearance (even extending to feeding), and extras that will enable the child to participate equally with other school children. But costs go beyond this. School children demand more of their parents than do their illiterate siblings fully enmeshed in the traditional family system and morality. They ask for food and other things in the house in a way that is unprecedented, and they ask for expenditures outside. Their authority is the new authority of the school, and their guides are the nontraditional ways of life that have been revealed. Parents regard the school child as a new and different type of child with greater needs, and fear alienating him. Parents are aware that such alienation has been made likelier because the educated child is less likely to need familial employment, and the new morality from the school (and from the outside world to which the school has provided an introduction and a feeling of membership) makes it less likely that he will as completely heed the teachings of family morality.

Third, schooling creates dependency, both within the family and within the society. In the absence of schooling, all members of the family are clearly producers—battlers in the family's struggle for survival. Children may get a disproportionately small share of the returns, but that is because they must have patience and wait, and they owe something for parental guidance and even for the gift of life. With schooling, it becomes clear that the society regards the child as a future rather than a present producer, and that it expects the family to protect the society's investment in the child for that future. Family relationships tend to adjust to this expectation. Reinforcing changes occur in the wider society: legislation to protect children typically accelerates in the first years of universal schooling. All these changes make children less productive and more costly both to the family and to the society. These changes also mean that children no longer really share responsibility for the family's survival in the present.

Fourth, schooling speeds up cultural change and creates new cultures. In the West, values of the school were clearly middle-class values, and the schools imposed as many of these on the working class as they could. However, schools induced changes in all classes, partly because, by their nature and their very existence, their agenda was so obviously that of the broad society and its economy—its capitalist economy—and not that of family production and the morality that sustained that production.

Fifth, in the contemporary developing world, the school serves as a major instrument—probably the major instrument—for propagating the values, not of the local middle class, but of the Western middle class. Little is taught or implied that is at odds with Western middle-class values, while traditional family morality is disdained or regarded as irrelevant and as part of that other nonschool, preschool—even antischool—world.

The first two postulates are widely accepted, partly because they can be seen to operate even without the recognition of a major restructuring of family morality. But it is probably the last three that have the most impact in changing family economies from a situation in which high fertility is worthwhile to one in which it is disastrous. Indeed, the significance of the changes in terms of altering the impact of fertility on parental prerogative may well be in ascending order as listed.

Several points about the nature of education should be made. The important engine of demographic change seems to be formal schooling rather than the widespread attainment of literacy without mass schooling, as occurred in the West prior to the mid-nineteenth century. Furthermore, demographic change is unlikely if the movement toward mass schooling is confined largely to males, as has been the case in parts of the Middle East. The impact of education in the West was not identical with its impact in the contemporary developing world; in the former, the importation of a different culture was a far less important aspect (and so education may have taken longer to reverse the wealth flow and required greater economic change to do so). Finally, the first generation of mass schooling usually appears to be enough to initiate fertility decline. If it does not, the second generation should prove conclusive. Educated parents tend to concede that the demands of educated children are fundamentally right, even if irritating and impoverishing. Educated mothers usually see to it that their children obtain a larger share of the family pie, and justify this to their husbands or the older generation. It seems improbable—and has yet to be demonstrated—that any society can sustain stable high fertility beyond two generations of mass schooling.

Before considering historical and contemporary evidence for education's role in initiating fertility decline, let us review the arguments of the recent literature.

Although there is a vast literature on the relationship between education and fertility, very little is strictly relevant to the argument advanced here, for three main reasons. First, most of the literature fails to concentrate on the onset of fertility transition, but confuses this issue with fertility differentials at other times, usually well on in the course of fertility decline. The examination of post-transitional fertility differentials may be of importance for predicting population growth, or even for demonstrating the different economic–demographic calculuses employed in the various social classes, but is of little value in analysing the nature of a change that has already affected all social classes. Second, the literature fails to concentrate on the onset of universal education, but usually employs indices of the proportion of educated or literate persons across a wide age range (or even includes measures of the duration of education). Third, the literature tends to concentrate far more in terms of data, and almost wholly in terms of theory, on the impact of education on the parental generation rather than on their children. It is possible to justify the standard approach by arguing that the parents, during the early period of compulsory education, can control not only their own fertility but also the regularity with which their children attend school. Such an argument ignores the impact that compulsory schooling regardless of level of daily attendance has on creating dependency and on changing social and economic relationships within the family.

Two 1979 reviews of the literature on the relation between education and fertility, by Harvey Graff and Susan Cochrane, largely fail all three tests (partly, of course, because it is not their explicit or sole aim to concentrate on the onset of fertility transition).[2] Graff's work is largely an attack on his predecessors, although he does briefly make three points of his own: the evidence for a negative relationship between the education of individuals and their fertility is not nearly as general or as strong as has often been stated; the impact of education is often specific to the society to which it is applied; education usually does not cause demographic change directly but mediates the change caused by more basic forces, apparently largely economic ones. The first argument finds support from the Australian evidence: once the Australian fertility transition was under way, the lag by level of education in reducing family size appears to have been only a year or two at most (Ruzicka and Caldwell, 1977, pp. 171–174).[3] Indeed, the fertility change appears to affect the whole society as a result of an educational transformation among all the children of the society. Graff's second argument probably does not hold good if it can be taken so far as to imply that a society can withstand the fertility transition. The historical evidence so far is all to the contrary. His third argument is not as restrictive as it first appears, and could be taken to support fully the thesis that, while the ability to erect a system of universal education and the fact of a major change in the relations of production are both products of fundamental economic change, the timing of the *onset* of fertility decline (in terms of decades, and perhaps, sometimes, generations) is more determined by the timing of the establishment of universal education—indeed education plays a mediating role.

Historians of demographic change have shown greater interest in pinpointing the beginnings of educational and demographic movements. Coale observed, "Every nation in the world today in which no more than 45% of the

---

[2] Hawthorn (1970), in a more general treatment of fertility decline, also fails these three tests.

[3] The occupational evidence for urban areas suggests that the educated led the least educated or uneducated by about three years early in the transition but that this gap subsequently widened to as much as seven years, later narrowing.

labour force is engaged in extractive industry, in which at least 90% of the children of primary school age attend school, and which is at least 50% urban has experienced a major decline in fertility. But France reduced its fertility before attaining any of these characteristics, and England had most of them before its marital fertility fell at all." (Coale, 1969, p. 18.) The measure of education is one with which this discussion sympathizes—it is certainly superior to most of the aggregate measures of education. However, it is argued below (with evidence from the studies of Coale's Princeton group) that the timing of France's fertility transition is not necessarily at odds with its achievement of universal schooling, and that the timing of the English transition is not at odds at all if we concentrate on the educational measure. Tilly, while arguing that the relationship between education and fertility decline is not necessarily as close as this paper posits, nevertheless includes a quotation from Thabault (1945) about the history of his own French village, which is very much in the spirit of wealth flows analysis: "The respect for knowledge . . . was not strong enough around 1850 (30 years before compulsory education) to push the peasants to shake off their old habits, to give up the labour of their children, or to impose on them the necessary discipline, at the cost of paying constant attention to their performance." A contemporary observer of the early Australian fertility decline recorded the views of women of reproductive age and reported that these early innovators took for granted that it was the move to universal schooling that changed the economic situation of the family and the position of children in it (Ackerman, 1913, pp. 91–93). There has also been a series of studies of relative educational and fertility differences within a single country.[4] Their evidence—usually inconclusive—is not very relevant to the argument here, partly because most use aggregate educational or literacy data across many age groups, and partly the argument here is that the attainment of universal schooling across a single nation or culture group is the force that changes intergenerational attitudes and hence economic relationships.

One study, published 40 years ago, did attempt to link the cost of education to the declining birth rate in England, but focused attention on direct costs rather than on the much more massive rises in children's costs occasioned by the transformation of economic relations within the family that accompanies mass education (Leybourne and White, 1940).

Two points are of basic importance when distinguishing between the case put here and those found in the literature. First, the new sets of family relationships and obligations, created by the fact and ethos of universal education, owe much, at least in the timing of the change, to the advent of

[4] On the United States, see Easterlin (1976); Leet (1976); Vinovskis (1976). This problem is also encountered in all studies of Princeton University's Office of Population Research project on the historical decline of European fertility, because concentration on differences between the districts of individual countries is the basic methodological approach.

education. However, this does not mean that the new familial culture, in which the wealth flows are downward, is adopted in each successive generation in proportion to the educational level attained. Once the change has taken place, it tends to become universal, and educational differentials are of little importance (and where they show up as modest fertility differentials, they may rather reflect an educational differential in the innovational adoption of new and more efficient methods of birth control). Second, from a historical point of view (and in terms of whether global fertility decline ultimately takes place or not) the pauses and apparent slight reversals in the path of fertility decline are not very important. Too many of the widely quoted economic–demographic analyses are derived from the experience of the United States during the last half-century. This was a period three-quarters of a century after nearly universal schooling had been achieved and during which the birth rate never exceeded 25 per thousand. Furthermore, a central feature of the period (and an even more central feature of the economic–demographic analyses) was the so-called baby boom, a misleading label that conveys messages that in fact are probably not real at all. The problem is that the baby boom rise in fertility was largely a compound of earlier and more nearly universal marriages in a period of imperfect contraception, of overlapping cohort reproduction with each birth cohort marrying earlier, of the fertility of some Depression and wartime marriages being delayed until after the war, and of the apparent beginning of the boom being silhouetted against the preceding lower-than-trend fertility arising from the family crises of the Depression of the 1930s (Caldwell and Ruzicka, 1977). It was not a good period from which to derive general historical lessons, and in retrospect it was only a bump in the long US, and Western, fertility decline.

The West in Retrospect

Two major points must be established—the dating of fertility decline and of the achievement of mass schooling in the West—after which the question of their possible interaction is explored.

The dating of the fertility decline has depended on our possession of better indices for measuring trends in marital fertility. Indexes of total fertility are unsuitable because they incorporate trends in the proportions married, which may vary for reasons having no relation to the pressure exerted by family size on the family economy; thus US and Australian total fertility fell through much of the nineteenth century prior to the decline in marital fertility as frontier conditions passed and as greater difficulty was encountered in the initial establishment of a household.[5] Completed marital

[5] The I_g in Australia did not begin to fall until after 1881 (hitherto it was slowly rising), but I_f fell in Victoria (where we have a complete series) by 29% in the previous two decades because I_m fell by 34% (see Caldwell and Ruzicka, 1977, Appendix A).

fertility is also not very satisfactory because the important movements in marital fertility predate the women involved reaching menopause and thus qualifying for inclusion in statistics of completed fertility. The Princeton index of marital fertility, I_g, overcomes these two difficulties (in that it restricts itself to marital fertility and provides an index of the current situation across age groups) and is now available for a growing number of countries. It has the drawback of being dependent on censuses and hence being unable to pin-point change within an intercensal period.

The evidence shows that marital fertility began to fall in England and Wales between 1871 and 1881, in the Netherlands during the same period, in Belgium between 1865 and 1880, in Germany between 1875 and 1880, in Australia between 1881 and 1891, in Italy and Spain before the end of the century, and in Portugal before the end of the World War I.[6] France appears to have experienced a long, slow decline in the I_g index, which was already as low as 0·537 in 1831 (or 80% of the level found in England and Wales in 1871) and which fell by another 8% in the next 40 years.[7] Between 1871 and 1900 it fell by another 22%, or much the same as in other parts of northern Europe and English-speaking countries of overseas European settlement. It has been suggested elsewhere that the earlier French decline in marital fertility was a different phenomenon, very possibly connected with the changing position of French wives; See Chapter 7. It is suggested here that marital fertility declined for the same reasons as in other Western countries, but did so after 1870, and hence that decline is submerged in the greater fertility declines of the late nineteenth and twentieth centuries. In spite of the frequent references to major declines in Irish fertility after the famine of the 1840s (Carr-Saunders, 1936, p. 90) the I_g index of Ireland in 1881 was similar to that found in England and Wales at that date, while its I_m index was no lower than that of Scandinavian countries (Coale, 1967, p. 209). There is no evidence of prior declines in marital fertility (I_g). In the next 30 years overall fertility (I_f) declined by 21%, but, unlike the decline in the rest of northern Europe, this was achieved wholly by a delay in marriage and a reduction in the proportions marrying. Ireland, with the Catholic Church holding strong views on the interference with fertility within marriage, was becoming northern Europe's demographic anomaly. Nevertheless, France and Ireland join the other countries of northern Europe and of English-speaking overseas European settlement (the United States, Australia, New Zealand, English-speaking Canada, and white, English-speaking South Africa) in demonstrating that some new and massive force was operating on fertility in the last third of the nineteenth century.

[6] Personal communication from William Brass, based on a chapter in press; Lesthaeghe (1977, p. 103; Knodel (1974), p. 39; Caldwell and Ruzicka (1977), Appendix B; Livi-Bacci (1971), p. 60; van de Walle (1974); Coale (1967).
[7] All data from van de Walle (1974), p. 127.

The establishment of dates for the onset of mass schooling is even more difficult. One reason is that universal education legislation in many countries was the end point of a movement over several decades to bring all children into schools, with the lagging groups being the poor, especially in rural areas. Just how many achieved some schooling and for how long is a subject of vigorous dispute, even in England where the nineteenth-century statistics are better than in most countries (West, 1965 and 1975; Lawson and Silver, 1973). During the period, most Western countries passed successive legislation making it compulsory for local government authorities to provide schools, train teachers, give financial assistance to denominational schools, and, finally, compel children (usually from age 6 or 7 to around 12) to attend school. In the earlier part of the period it was relatively easy to avoid schooling in most areas, and difficult or impossible to gain access to it in others. In another sense, too, schooling arrived slowly, for parents were not accustomed to being forced to send children to school if they needed them for work. Thus among children enrolled in school, the proportion attending daily was only 35% in the United States in 1870, rising to 41% in 1890, 53% in 1910, 68% in 1930, and 74% in 1950. The situation in Britain and Australia was very similar.[8]

In nearly all northern European countries, the United States, Australia, Canada, and New Zealand, effective compulsory schooling (in the sense that nearly all children attended school at least irregularly) for children of primary school age (6–12 years) was achieved in the period 1870–90. The exceptions are important. In Prussia, Frederick the Great instituted compulsory schooling in 1763 (and Frederick William I in areas where schools existed in 1717). While the schooling was not good—it was mostly imparted by retired military officers—it had sufficient impact to stir the rest of Europe, especially after the Franco-Prussian War of 1870, and was a much-quoted precedent in the struggle elsewhere for universal schooling. Denmark enacted compulsory education in 1739, but it was apparently not successfully enforced until the second half of the nineteenth century. Sweden apparently succeeded in introducing compulsory schooling in 1852, and this may help to explain the earlier decline in Swedish marital fertility.

In southern Europe, Italy passed compulsory schooling legislation in 1859 and Portugal a series of legislative acts beginning in 1881. Nevertheless, only Italy had most children in school in the last quarter of the century; neither Spain nor Portugal appears to have had much more than half of all children in school in the first decade of the next century. Here again the timing of the educational revolution seems to coincide with that of the fertility transition.[9]

[8] On the United States, see Tyack (1976), pp. 360–362. On Britain and Australia, see Ruzicka and Caldwell (1977), p. 22; Lawson and Silver (1973), pp 276–280; Rankin (1939), pp. 123 and 129.

[9] There is some difficulty with Spain if Livi-Bacci is correct in saying that the timing of its marital fertility transition was closer to that of Italy than that of Portugal. See Livi-Bacci (1971), p. 60

In Eastern Europe both phenomena would have to wait until after World War I. Not until then did either Russia or Poland succeed in getting more than half their children into schools (Encyclopaedia Britannica, 1953).

These changes in schooling were not the only public acts that altered the position of children, although the other legislation seems to have originated in the struggle for, and achievement of, compulsory education. In the United States, "Laws compelling school attendance were only part of an elaborate and massive transformation in the legal and social rules governing children. Children and youth came to be seen as individuals with categorical needs" (Tyack, 1976, p. 363). In Britain the Poor Law Amendment Act of 1868 made it an offence for parents to neglect to supply such "necessaries" as food, lodging, clothing, and medical aid for their children, and this was followed, at the instigation of the National Society for the Prevention of Cruelty to Children, by a spate of specific legislation beginning in 1889. In Britain such legislation had been preceded by the Factory Acts of 1833, 1844, and 1847, which limited children's working hours. That these laws did not induce fertility decline is perhaps evidence that the vital change involved the whole balance of parent–child costs and productivity, and not merely a change that affected only the first of the five postulates stated above.

A key issue is whether, in the West immediately prior to the late nineteenth century, there was in fact a family morality of the type found in traditional cultures. We have reported that Australia had a family morality, backed by the religion and outlook of the day, that enshrined the value of children living austerely and of children (and wives) working hard and being helpful without making undue complaints or demands (Ruzicka and Caldwell, 1977, Chapter 1). In a society whose standard of household comforts depended very much on labour inputs, higher fertility was not disadvantageous as long as the cost of children, relative to that of adults, did not rise, and as long as their usefulness did not decline. From nineteenth-century Russia come descriptions of traditional family morality that explicitly make the point (in other words) that adherence to these behavioural patterns would keep the wealth flow directed from children to parents; Dunn (1976) reports advice on patriarchs keeping an emotional distance from their children (as in much of the contemporary developing world) so as to ensure that the direction of the flow would not reverse. Further west, the direction of that flow was no longer so firmly fixed that the implementation of mass education could not change it. The West's egalitarian tradition and the gentleness arising out of growing affluence saw to that; there is evidence from the United States, even from the eighteenth century, that softer treatment of children was on the way (Walzer, 1976).

Family morality was not identical in every society or segment of society and was not equally affected by every type of schooling. It may not be solely the Catholic Church's stand on contraception (only markedly different from that of the Protestant churches by the 1930s) that explains the fact that the Catholic/non-Catholic fertility differential has been Australia's widest since the 1890s. In Australia the Irish Catholic population had its own denominational schools, which almost certainly taught and implied the need for more traditional (and more authoritarian) family relationships than did the state educational system. This difference in types of schooling may provide part of the explanation for the failure of universal Prussian education to reduce marital fertility. The Prussian system was a simple one, taught by men traditional and authoritarian in outlook. The children were removed from work, but schooling implied to neither children nor parents that their relative positions were changing.

What was there in Western education that could induce change? There was certainly no decision that the working class should be given middle-class expectations; there was in fact considerable discussion in the 1860s in Australia and Britain of schools suited to working-class children that would not strain the social fabric.[10] But things did not work out that way, for, as the children of the School of Barbiana demonstrated, no trained teacher or institutionalized school can have the outlook or the standards of the poor (The School of Barbiana, 1970). Indeed, schools may regard traditional working-class behaviour as the thing to be eliminated, almost as the *raison d'être* for education. Jackson and Marsden have shown that in Britain both headmasters and teachers in grammar schools try to cut their working-class children off from their own communities (1966, pp. 126–127).[11] The reading material available was from books written by the middle class about the middle class, and was saturated with wider-economy ethics about effort in the great outside world—about doing things for the good of the country rather than for the good of one's father or parents (Leeson, 1977; Darton, 1958).

What education did was partly the result of these implicit and explicit aims. It ultimately abolished the mob, the brutish poor, those vast illiterate masses that exist in the fog off centre stage in Dickens's novels, as the background in Hardy's novels, and in the fears of the well-off townsmen as described by every historian from Suetonius to Macaulay. Without question the schools took this to be a central task. They made citizens of those whose horizons had been largely confined to the family, and taught the immorality of putting family interests first. They provided a new authority and lessened the hold of the patriarch. They destroyed a family system of morality that had made high fertility no disadvantage. In a sense education demanded dependency because that made education itself more efficient.

[10] Pat Caldwell, file on the *Australasian* newspaper, Melbourne, 1865–1900.

[11] The authors "recorded a lot of evidence about the school's insensitivity and the child's hypersensitivity; the school's determination to hand on the grammar school modes, to spread its standards as the best and the only standards; and the child's awkward, clumsy and stubborn desire to preserve other ways to remain 'natural' " (p. 128).

This concept of the conflict between a wider community morality and a morality that places family interests always first is important. Absolute family priorities were always in some danger in Europe, because Christianity speaks more to the individual and less to the family than any other major religion. In the north these tendencies were strengthened by the rise of Protestantism. Family priorities have held on tenaciously in parts of the Mediterranean and in Latin America[12] indeed, this may be the major explanation of high fertility persisting longer in Latin America than the level of education might suggest.

A related problem is the persistence of high fertility in Europe, prior to the late nineteenth century, among those classes (but not every group, as the examples of the Genevese bourgeoisie and the French aristocracy show (Henry, 1965, pp. 451–452) that habitually educated their children. Ariès (1962) maintains that a concept of childhood and dependency came into existence among this group centuries ago, and that it did so precisely because of education. Nevertheless, children did not apparently become a net lifetime economic drain. It could be argued that the rich were so affluent that such losses were of no account, an argument that is blunted by the speed with which the Western rich reduced their fertility after 1870. The truth is probably that the rich of the earlier period did not suffer economically from high fertility (and did not continue to suffer for centuries without doing anything about it). The reason is probably the continuation of a strong family morality that placed family interests first. Family members helped each other, and among small, powerful elites, men needed (and gained by) trusted ambassadors; and, in a system of family morality, where could a man find trusted ambassadors except among his sons? While young, the children cost little; the austerity with which the rich often brought up their children, from the Middle Ages through the nineteenth century, was usually, by today's standards, astonishing.

The question remains as to why education did not alter the situation among the wealthy classes more rapidly. One reason is that education did not undermine patriarchal authority. Fathers, too, were educated and in exactly the same system. Educators did not bring the views and morality of another class to the pupil; indeed, the educator was most frequently a private tutor (as late as 1900, one-fifth of the students at Cambridge had previously been educated at home by private tutors (Lawson and Silver, 1973, p. 300)), usually subservient to the father and teaching his views and morality. Nor did a classical education provide much fuel for any movement to upset the family's balance of power and consumption.[13]

---

[12] On the Mediterranean, see Banfield (1958). On Latin America, compare Lomnitz (1971).

[13] Similarly, Koranic education in the contemporary world does not endanger the returns from high fertility. See P. Caldwell (1977).

The movement from a family morality to a community-wide morality was not entirely induced by the schools, although schooling immensely increased it. Subsequently, all cultural changes that made high fertility uneconomic were reinforced by a vast increase in the reading of books, newspapers, and magazines, and by the cinema, radio, and television. These media rarely gave priority to family interests. Nevertheless, most of these other influences did not compete with schooling in the nineteenth century; moreover, schooling probably exerted—as it does in the contemporary developing world—the necessary minimum change to give meaning to and create a demand for these other media.

Finally, is it possible that the real change was not the advent of mass schooling at all, but parallel and equally convulsive movements in the economy or in the reduction of mortality? There is little evidence for this in Australia: during the last 40 years of the nineteenth century the decline in mortality (including child mortality) was very moderate, as was occupational change (Ruzicka and Caldwell, 1977, p. 88). Britain by 1870 had entered the 30-year period of slow economic growth once known as "the Great Depression." Certainly, in the West, economic advance ultimately underlay the creation of mass schooling, but the advent of universal schooling determined the timing of the fertility decline. The advent of mass schooling in 15 or more countries in the late nineteenth century was close because of the transmission of the idea, while the nature of their economies and their per capita incomes varied widely. Significantly, the advent of their fertility declines was also close.

The Contemporary Developing World

Mass schooling, also as the spread of an idea, has come to much of the developing world at an earlier stage, in terms of economic structure, than it did in much of the West. It has probably much greater implications for changing family relationships and declining fertility than it had in the West. In the latter, a somewhat different culture was transmitted from one part of society to another, and ultimately certain aspects of middle-class culture were intensified and taught to the whole society. In the developing world, not only is a foreign culture being imported, but this is being done at a time when that culture has moved far toward egalitarianism within the family and toward numerous adjustments to low fertility.

The two major strains in developing-world education—the objective of instilling moral values and the importation of these values from Western culture—have their origins in the earliest colonial efforts to provide such education. In early British India, views on the role of education were often very explicit. In 1792 Charles Grant wrote that education should be used "to improve native morals" (Carnoy, 1974, p. 96). Macaulay, in his 1835 *Minute* (p. 238), asserted, "We must at present do our best to form a class who may be interpreters between us and the millions whom we govern—a class of persons Indian in blood and color, but English in tastes, in opinions, in morals and in intellect." Marx in the same year (p. 237) wrote, "England has to fulfil a double mission in India: one destructive and the other regenerating—the annihilation of old Asian society and the laying of the material foundations of Western society in Asia." (Lannoy, 1971).

In Africa there was even less doubt about promoting new moralities, for missionaries, who formed the backbone of the schooling system until the 1960s, "had come to Africa primarily to convert and civilize the heathen and to stop the slave trade" (Carnoy, 1974, p. 130). A more sympathetic observer of the missionaries comments, with regard to initiation and other *rites de passage* that were the hallmark of family morality in that they established differentiations by age and sex: "The age at which children went to school, the prevalence of mission boarding schools, and features of the initiation rites which were dangerous to health and objectionable on Christian moral grounds caused the missionaries to clash with this traditional training. The result was that it was largely abandoned by Christians." And again, more generally: "When the former training of children and young people in African societies is compared with the modern school systems now operating, certain features of the traditional patterns appear to have been abandoned, notably those which showed the close correlation between the training of personality and character and the integration and cohesion of family, clan and tribal units." (Read, 1970).[14] Sutton explained the "civilizing" role of education: "This missionary impulse made education in Western forms ancillary to religious purpose. Enough had to be taught to make Christian ideas comprehensible and to combat practices and beliefs that were regarded as barbarous or heathenish." (Sutton, 1965, p. 61). Ogunsheye, reporting somewhat ruefully on the schooling of his own people, the Yoruba of Nigeria, noted an "inevitable emphasis on English traits and individuals"; the "British put the foremost emphasis on character training" (1965, p. 130). Clearly, neither the character nor the traits were those found in traditional familial roles.

Musgrove (1952) reported of the school in which he taught in Uganda following World War II that it consciously taught European values and that it saw as part of this process the adoption of European clothing, food, and habits of punctuality. Giraure (1975) reported of the school at which he was a pupil during the 1960s in Papua New Guinea that a thoroughgoing effort was made to change his culture. He was given a new European name in the

---

[14] Quotations are from pages 275 and 274, respectively.

mission school and then required to speak only English while attending the government school. Ultimately, "we looked with horror upon the village life . . . the children returned . . . having little in common with the people among whom they were to live. The result was and still is chaos . . . juvenile delinquency . . . the breakdown of village traditions and life" (pp. 103–104). Quotations of this kind, detailing the dismantling of the pre-existing system of family relationships, would not be so telling if any participants ever told a different tale. One might anticipate the different tale with independence, but it is not so, for new nations see prosperity being built on the foundation provided by the destruction of traditional society. In modern India, where the educated are identified by "their dress, speech and manners," schooling "is now intended as a prime means of innovation, rather than as the great instrument for conservation" (Mandelbaum, 1970b).[15] In its crudest form, this goal is stated approvingly by a Westerner: "In Burma the object of education is not in doubt: Education is to serve as one of the means of social transformation from a raw material producing society where the bulk of the people had a narrow, peasant, traditional view to a diversified, somewhat industrialized society able to absorb and use the most modern of scientific knowledge: it is to build a modern nation of responsible citizens" (Nash, 1970, pp. 301–302).

There has always been some resistance or doubt. In India in the late eighteenth century, Warren Hastings and others in the East India Company banned missionary education on the grounds that it was unsettling to society. In post-World War II Uganda, schoolboys remained suspicious of European motives in providing education.[16] There is, in fact, an interesting question of why the demand for the schooling of children exists, given that it destroys a family structure of which the older generation has always approved and a family economy that brought them benefits in proportion to the number of children they had. Is education seen as a means to further social justice and mobility, the stability of the political order, and national strength, as it was in the West, or are there other attractions?

The earliest attractions toward Western education were varied. One element was virtue, because education had traditionally been a training for priestly duties. This element remains a potent force in India, where the trends toward more education and toward Sanskritization can have similar roots and appearance. Another was magical power—the ability to transcribe words into marks on paper that someone else could convert back again in another place and time. In the villages of western Uganda in the 1950s, where literacy was greatly respected, the descriptions " 'reader' and 'Christian' [were] still convertible terms."[17] In a more down-to-earth sense,

[15] Quotations are from pages 508 and 414, respectively.

[16] On India, see Carnoy (1974) p. 89. On Uganda, see Musgrove (1952), p. 248.

[17] On India, see Mandelbaum (1970b), pp. 500–520. On education as magical power, see Yates (1971), on the Congo Free State and the Belgian Congo; and Deng (1972), pp. 153–154, on the Dinka of southwestern Sudan. On Uganda, see Musgrove (1952), p. 244.

Africans wanted education in order to learn and manipulate the European secret of power (Sutton, 1965, p. 62). Jobs became increasingly important, first because they brought cash, or extra revenue, to supplement the family economy; then because individuals were deserting that economy and fending for themselves rather than for relatives; and finally because the family economy could not stand either this desertion or the competing forms of production and collapsed (Yates, 1971, pp. 161–167). Pride in children's achievements can also play a significant role (Fakhouri, 1972, p. 100), although in India a father with an unmarriable educated daughter "may be accused of sacrificing his daughter's chances in life to a mistaken whim intended to glorify his own name." (Mandelbaum, 1970a, pp. 108–109). On the other hand, in South Asia and even in Southwest Asia, there is a growing awareness that only an educated daughter can secure that desirable addition to the family—an educated son-in-law with a job in the modern sector—and that a large dowry on its own may no longer be sufficient. In South Asia even a rural family often feels the need for one educated son simply to cope with the bureaucrats (ibid., pp. 109 and 247).

The present position of education is complex and uncertain. While traditional family morality persists and the wealth flow is from the younger to the older generation, and while the educated are paid far more or have far greater access to power than the uneducated, the temptation for parents to educate their children and so obtain access to the wealth of the economy's modern sector can be immense. Yet the same education may clearly destroy the moral system that alone can guarantee the older generation large and continuing returns. It does not necessarily do so in one generation in the absence of universal education. The traditional morality can show surprising resilience, as among the Yoruba (Chapter 4, pp. 144–145; Chapter 2, p. 76; Chapter 3, p. 110) and the education of children can bring parents high rewards and can buttress high fertility.

How education can endanger the traditional system is clear enough even from the syllabuses and textbooks, and has been shown vividly by a study of infant and primary school textbooks in Ghana, Nigeria, and Kenya.[18] These books are important because they are used in schools attended by a much larger proportion of the community than are secondary schools. They are important also because they are first read when the children are young and impressionable, and when they most uncritically accept the teacher and school as new authority figures and often as superior ones with regard to knowledge about the modern world that many of the pupils will increasingly aspire to join. The messages are all the more potent because they are most

---

[18] John C. Caldwell and Pat Caldwell, "The partially hidden syllabus in infant and primary school textbooks in Ghana, Nigeria and Kenya: The family message" (in preparation, and being supplemented to include South Asia).

often found in reading primers, where the substance or attitudes are taken for truth, rather than in specialized books on society, which might be expected to point to some areas of controversy or doubt.

In the books that we studied, we found no support for such basic African traditional institutions as polygyny, unstable marriage, the condemnation of sterile women or women who repeatedly lose children, bewitchment, and, most importantly, the attitude that the needs of the family have priority over those of the community.

There was in Kenya alone, in a new series of tales from a traditional viewpoint,[19] some support (at least in stories of the past) for bride price, arranged marriage, initiation, and violence in tribal warfare. However, concessions are made to the traditional family authority structure and to the age-old upward direction of the wealth flow. Where arranged marriage and bride price exist, they merely confirm a love match already in existence—rather like the expression of parental approval of an engagement. And where a tribal conflict is plotted and carried out, it is the young man who does it while leaving his father in ignorance rather than disobeying him (Mbugua, 1971). Initiation is handled by laying stress almost solely on the joy of attaining manhood.

The school reading books generally assume that children are dependents; that the husband must farm (or work in an office) while his wife undertakes the domestic work and the children give first place to their schoolwork; that priority should be given to nation-building, citizenship, and honesty in the larger society; that children should do jobs at home to be "good" rather than as an enforceable duty to the family; that fathers are kindly and understanding rather than distant and awesome; and that parents are closer to children, and that husbands are usually closer to wives, than they are to other relatives. Children are portrayed at play; nuclear families are portrayed eating together. Drumming and traditional dance, if covered, are divorced from traditional religious rites. Extended family residence, when mentioned, coexists with nuclearization.[20] An East African first reader unintentionally brings out the magnitude of the changes with its portrayal of a family in a traditional setting behaving like members of the Western middle class: children with toys, father entertaining his young daughter, mother dapper in a clean dress. The chief thrust of school books in independent countries is exemplified by the introductory "Note to the Teacher" in a widely used Ghanaian series: "The chief aim in teaching citizenship education is to help young people become well-informed,

---

[19] The original impetus came from sessions for secondary school children written by Kenyan playwrights at the request of Radio Kenya. Other works of this type are published by Longman.

[20] As a Nigerian textbook about a Yoruba family puts it: "My grandparents live in the compound with us but in a separate house. Their house is where the elders in our village meet from time to time."

hard-working, selfless, honest and responsible citizens. With citizens such as these, a nation will be sufficiently equipped to achieve success and moral prosperity" (Olayomi, 1970; New Peak Reading Course, 1973, p. 64; Mensah, 1975).

These messages—often presented as African traditions—are remote from the family morality and lifestyle still practiced by the great majority of citizens. Yet the textbooks never give any indication that this is so: African names are used for persons, objects, and ceremonies; the illustrations show African huts, animals, and bush. But the message is contemporary Western and, if fully acted out, would certainly mean that high fertility would prove economically oppressive and that family size would eventually decline.[21]

It should be noted that syllabuses with Western messages were not merely imposed by colonialists. There has always been a strong local demand for colonial educational systems and for syllabuses identical with those in the metropolitan centres; it is partly a question of not accepting the second-best and partly one of students gaining unchallenged access to further education in the metropolises. Newly independent nations felt competitive pressures for closely paralleling the West in the nature and message of schools, and their efforts were strongly supported by international organizations. Carnoy claims, "In the nonindustrialized country, the school is an institution that not only keeps the individual from self-definition, but keeps the entire society from defining itself. The schools are an extension of the metropole structure" (1974, p. 72). That definition will in fact never hold, for schools are a mechanism for creating a Westernized global society. They do this largely unwittingly, for most educationalists take learning to be a virtue, and do not distinguish the various brands of virtue. In any case, really new workable institutions are extremely difficult to create. The West has an educational model that will inevitably be used, partly because it exists and is widely known; partly because it produces usable textbooks or textbook prototypes, syllabuses, teachers, and organizational models; and partly because it is associated with successful economic development.

The Impact of Schooling on the Developing-World Family System

The main message of the school is not spelled out in textbooks. It is assumed by teachers, pupils, and even parents. They all know that school attendance

---

[21] The message is the same among the Indians of rural Peru, where "the curriculum was oriented . . . to life in an urban metropolis, which had little meaning to the Indian child other than, perhaps, to alienate him from an agrarian existence . . . the impact the school has had seems to be in the direction of creating a hiatus between the values of the Indian child and his parents." (see Epstein, 1971, pp. 192–193).

means acceptance of a way of life at variance with the strictly traditional. Many school children no longer realize just how great that variance is or just what strictly traditional behaviour is.

Masemann (1974) reported that the hidden syllabus in the Ghanaian girls' school where she taught was the Western way of life, and said of the typical pupil:

> "She learns how to play marital, parental and occupational roles through experiencing many aspects of school life that are never made explicit in a formal curriculum. When the students write about the kind of life they expect to lead after marriage, they mention co-operation between husband and wife in financial matters, solidarity of the married couple in conflict with kin, shared responsibility for children. They feel . . . competent to 'live a modern life' and they have every intention of doing so."[22]

Several points should be noted. First, if they achieve the degree of solidarity and cooperation within marriage that they anticipate, and if they focus this on their children to the relative exclusion of their kin, then the upward wealth flow to their own parents will be greatly diminished, and the new flow over a lifetime almost certainly reversed. Second, although it is not discussed by Masemann, these students may already be making ever-stronger demands for financial support from their parents (and possibly other kin) over the strict minimum needed to keep them at school. Third, these changes in family emotional and economic relationships have not been economically determined; the economic effects—profound ones for the society and its fertility—have been purely the result of attitudinal changes arising from the intentional and unintentional Westernizing impact of their schooling.

Most developing-world societies are very much aware that schooling leads to profound social change. At early stages this is usually anticipated with apprehension.[23] Although tempted by the money and influence following in

[22] Masemann continued: "She is also expected to bring up her children with scheduled meal-times and bed-times, quite unlike the more relaxed demand-feeding and sleeping times of the more uneducated mothers. This attitude to schedule is part of the constellation of values attached to a modern industrial society, and students are expected to be socialized into valuing time as a commodity which can be wasted or put to good use and which can be turned into money."

[23] However, Margaret Mead presented a different picture of the situation on Manus Island half a century ago: "When people did not understand, when the old women shrieked at each other in the style of long ago, when middle-aged men beat their wives, when there was a poor attendance at church, when discussion in meetings was rambling and petty, the enthusiasts for the New Way would comfort themselves and each other, saying, 'When the schoolboys grow up it will be different. These others, they grew up in the old bad ways. It is not their fault that they fly into rages, they do not know how to speak in a meeting or how to treat their wives and children. But when the children grow up it will be different.' " (1956, pp. 421–422). The rages had, of course, been a method whereby the aged retained their ancient authority; the beatings of wives and children ensured patriarchal rights; but the family as the main organizational unit could be said to be waning when it was more important to exert influence in meetings or to attend church.

the wake of education, traditional families often remained justifiably apprehensive of schooling, especially for girls. In the Congo Free State during the late nineteenth century, "local people objected strenuously to sending children to the mission station because they 'came back changed' " (Yates, 1971, p. 170). Among the Dinka of the Sudan, over half a century later, "girls' education was especially abhorred because that implied turning them into town-women, immoral and unsuited for marriage" (1971, p. 153). The Dinka are not Muslim in religion, but their views are still echoed over much of the Islamic world and beyond it into village India.

There is widespread agreement that schooling at advanced levels is first and foremost a process of Westernization. Tilman (1967) wrote of the Malay College in Kuala Kangsar, Malaysia, that "by the time of graduation, its students had been throughly socialized into an upper-class English cultural environment," while Kirk-Greene (1965) reported much the same for the highly educated Hausa elite of northern Nigeria, and Sutton more generally for those receiving higher education in Africa (1965). However, the same process, although less extreme, occurs from the first days at school; the Wisers observed the effects of vestigial elementary schooling in a small village on India's Gangetic Plain 50 years ago: "The boys who know nothing beyond village routine are content. Those who have gone to school are restless. They have disassociated learning from the work their fathers have to offer them." They also reported a landowner chasing an Untouchable boy, obligated to do him services under the jajmani system, away from their classes, not because the boy had anything else to do at that time of night, but because the jajman was well aware of the alien influences transmitted by schooling and the likelihood that new attitudes would begin to change ancient lines of authority and obligation (1971, pp. 98 and 42). In Latin America, the Westernizing influence of schooling is likely to make Indian students adopt as models the lifestyles of the mestizos or ladinos. This was the major conclusion of Epstein's research in rural Peru (1971, pp. 193–198) and of Redfield's in rural Guatemala (1970, pp. 287–300). The latter, reviewing a long period of contact with the same village, wrote: "As I look at the school in the little village where I once was resident, it appears to me to play a greater part in changing the culture of the people than in handing it on from one generation to the next, although its influence in the direction of change is indirect" (p. 289).

In one sense, the attack on family morality begins with, or is paralleled by an attack on the theology that supports and justifies it. This is obvious and widely felt in Muslim societies. An imam in southern Thailand explained that "education made a man unreligious; literacy enables a man to disobey God. Civilization is antireligious" (Fraser, 1966, p. 84). "Civilization" in this sense is Westernization, culturally as well as theologically. This is less obvious in the case of more ancient religions, although these are more intimately connected with ancestral spirits and the morality of gerontratic control. Greenfield and Bruner found that illiterate children in West Africa, like their ancestors, explained a wider range of phenomena in "magical" terms—as being ordained by persons other than those present at the experiment. However, "the school suppresses this mode of thinking with astonishing absoluteness. There is not one instance of such reasoning among either bush or city Senegalese children who have been in school seven months or longer" (1966, p. 94).

Schools destroy the corporate identity of the family, especially for those members previously most submissive and most wholly contained by the family; children and women. In Mexico, "Going to school has in addition awakened new desires in children by removing them from the limited sphere of parental influence. They are no longer content to stay within patio walls at the beck and call of their mother; they urgently want to be with friends and to play after school. Play always has been, and still is, considered a possible source of danger and a waste of time by parents." (Lewis, 1960, p. 76). These problems are widespread in the developing world, with concern over the danger to the family system outweighing concern over the specific loss of time. Playing is but a symptom of a greater assault on the family's corporate identity. Literate culture often lays stress on behavioural patterns inimical to the family system, such as in its encouragement of differentiation and solitariness, whereas the oral tradition does not (Goody and Watt, 1963, pp. 336–337). Indeed, in West Africa the main limitation on the extension of rural housing seems to be not lack of labour or capital, but the lack of demand in nonliterate households for space peripheral to the centre of family activities. In India, too, education, especially when it is extended, can provide an "initial psychological impetus: a sense of individuality with a desire for greater independence. . . . [However,] the initiative for leaving the joint family often comes from the wife, whereas psychological conditioning sometimes prevents the husband from himself contemplating such a move" (Lannoy, 1971, p. 125). The wife (the daughter-in-law in the joint family) has, of course, much more to gain by such a move, and may attempt it less because she has acquired a feeling of individuality than because she has received from education a new cultural backing and a new cultural status that justifies her break with family tradition both in her own eyes and in those of her relatives-in-law (see Chapter 7). Education in India may place a man at a distance not only from his family but also from its alliances and the factions to which it adheres, thus eroding another of the values of high fertility (Mandelbaum, 1970a, p. 247).

Schooling means revolt against non-Western family relationships, although research has tended to concentrate much more on the erosion of agreement on the wife's role than on that of the child—perhaps partly because the latter is taken so much for granted. Omari, surveying secondary school pupils in Ghana over 20 years ago, found that 1% of girls desired a traditional marriage, while 86% "thought polygamy definitely backward" and 94% believed "love in marriage most important." Only 45% were certain that they would obey their parents' arrangements for marriage. "With increase in education the women fail to see the need for sharing a husband with another—apart from the fact that the thought runs anomalous to the Western ideas they have imbibed at school and abroad" (1960, pp. 203–205, 208). The strongest reaction against the education of girls in the Congo Free State and the Belgian Congo arose from the fear that girls who had been to school would revolt against arranged marriage and marriage to polygamists (Yates, 1971, pp. 168–169). The Christian church everywhere has battled polygyny, making it clear in Africa, when protesters pointed to the fact that the Old Testament recorded the institution without condemning it, that modern Christian morality means Western morality. In India there is the "fear that [a woman] will not make a proper, dutiful wife because of her schooling" (Mandelbaum, 1970a, p. 108). This chapter has concentrated on the direct impact of schooling on child–parent emotional and economic relationships whether or not husband–wife relationships have changed. Nevertheless, in the most traditional families the position of the wife of the younger generation (i.e., the mother of nonadult children) is not very different from that of the children; a change in her role is almost certain to effect a change in theirs (although the fact that children have been to school usually does not affect the role of an illiterate mother).

Fundamentally, the school attacks the traditional family's economic structure by weakening the authority of the old over the young (and of the male over the female). In Africa, where the mission and the school were for long almost indistinguishable, Yates said of the Congo that, "of course, missionary dominance meant a decrease of African political authority" and quoted the Prefect Apostolic as reported in 1905: "They [the Chiefs] sense as if by instinct that if we are successful it will mark the end of their despotic domination . . . they do not want us to speak of God, of Christ and especially of monogamy" (1971, p. 170).[24] Clignet argues that this was inevitable because of the extent to which, both in the West and in the developing world, schools have been expected to act in *loco parentis* (1975, p. 89). Schools attacked parental authority partly by providing new authority models from the West or from Westernized local people who seemed to epitomize the cultural patterns taught or implied. Indeed, the models, by their behaviour, provided much of the implicit teaching. In Burma, "The teacher is the repository of knowledge. . . . They would never

[24] Quoting Prefect Apostolic Leon Derikx at Gumbari, 30 July 1905, reported in "Mouvement des Missions Catholiques au Congo", March 1906, p. 83.

challenge [him]" (Nash, 1970, p. 307); in Masemann's school in Ghana, the teacher was the role model (1974, pp. 492–493); throughout Africa when schools first appeared, "the newly educated looked to Europeans . . . for advancement and for models of behaviour." (Sutton, 1965, p. 66). The real position is more complex even than this, for a major stabilizing force in traditional society has been the superior wisdom of the old, both occult and from long experience. The school provides the young with knowledge and skills that the old do not possess, while usually also attacking the value of traditional knowledge. This alone, during the attainment of mass schooling in the nineteenth-century West and the contemporary developing world, weakens family authority.

A Synthesis

In spite of much sophisticated analysis of "the global economy," we have hardly begun to discuss the parallel and related creation of a "global society." The movement toward a global economy makes the movement toward a global society inevitable, but such social movements as the spread of mass schooling can greatly accelerate economic change at every level from the family to the nation. With these changes will come demographic change.

The major change of demographic significance—and perhaps the most significant economic and social change—has been that from family production to capitalist production within a labour market external to the family. In the system of family production, high fertility was no disadvantage, whereas low fertility could be destructive. Family production was controlled by family morality, which gave power to the old and usually to the male, and which frequently sharply differentiated production and consumption roles by age and sex. Family morality formed the greater part of the culture (or superstructure) and often had strong religious underpinnings. The advantages that powerful family members obtained from high fertility did not pass quickly as capitalist production grew, partly because the age-old morality ensured them of more than an equal fraction of consumption and partly because family production of domestic goods and services by wives and children has waned slowly even in the most industrialized societies. Thus high fertility may continue in spite of a major decline in nondomestic family production, as long as family morality does not decay—in other words, as long as the wealth flow continues from the younger to the older generation. Family morality could hardly have decayed anywhere if family production had remained the dominant form of production worldwide. But once it began to lose its dominant position, as in the West, the new societal or capitalist morality could develop and could be exported. It is quite possible that such a morality can be at least partly grafted onto a society with a high level of family production and that it can be an element in a premature (by the precedents of Western history) fertility decline.

There have long been threats to family morality, quite apart from the development of capitalist production. These include any form of religion that is not family-centred (and even ancestral) and any form of law that is external to the family—anything, in fact, that belongs to the Great Tradition rather than the Little Tradition.[25] The least dangerous type of religion is one that enshrines the family as a necessary unit, such as Hinduism, and especially one that enshrines the sex and age segmentation of family production and addresses itself chiefly to the patriarch, as in Islam. But even these religions can become more interested in the individual, as did Buddhism in splintering from Hinduism. The greatest danger developed in the West: Judaism addressed itself to the individual as well as the family; Catholicism did not only that but did so from a huge extrafamilial, institutionalized base; Protestantism appealed almost solely to the individual (and could hardly have developed if there had not been sufficient capitalist production to have modified family morality). Any type of state organization and authority—certainly the raising of troops—offered potential danger to the uniqueness and unity of the family. This was particularly so with regard to the law, especially in the case of both the Roman law of the Republic and Empire and English common law.

The school has a very complex relation with these Great Traditions. It is another of the extrafamily institutions. But much of its impact on the family lies in the fact that it serves as a medium for these other institutions—for religion, state morality, state legal tradition, and national cultural and historical traditions. In most developing-world villages, the usual way that the first generation of school children explain the impact of education is that it makes them part of a much larger world—often they just say "of the world." Governments have always been in competition with the family for loyalty; governments that were unable to maintain a share of this loyalty ceased to function. This is particularly true in the developing world. The survival of governments depends on competition with families, and, as is clear from our analysis of school textbooks, governments regard schools as their chief instruments for teaching citizenship—for going over the heads of

[25] The Great Tradition is composed of the religious and cultural values found throughout the society and handed down as the common possession of the culture. The Great Tradition is known to the more educated or urbanized and is the tradition found generally in literature. The Little Tradition is confined to populations outside the central tradition—above all to villagers—is concerned with local gods and beliefs, and varies greatly from place to place. Robert Redfield and colleagues of the Chicago anthropology school originally applied the term to Latin America, but it is now widely used in the analysis of Indian society and is even more generally used as an analytical tool for all traditional societies.

the patriarchs and appealing directly to the children. In doing so, they inevitably emphasize the importance of the new generation and so strike yet another blow at family morality and family economics.

Nevertheless, family morality can prove remarkably resistant to change. The history of the West proves that: fertility did not fall in Britain until it was an advanced industrialized economy with only 17% of its population working in primary production and contributing less than 10% of gross national income and with 25% of its population living in centres with more than 100 000 inhabitants. However, that pattern is unlikely to repeat itself; the existence of the Western model and its spread—even when inadvertent—by national educational systems will see to that. The only exception may be the Muslim countries, where religion supports family role segmentation and where, in many cases, levels of female education are likely to remain low. The tropical African family system has so far also proved resilient, and wealth flows have continued upward even in the middle class because of a strong cultural emphasis on what the young owe to the old (partly perhaps because respect for ancestors is still prevalent) (see Chapters 2,3 and 4; Caldwell and Caldwell, 1978)[26]. In fact the traditional family expects to remain intact, and so eventually overreaches itself. It has always taken risks and has always attempted to maximize its income and resources. Hence, when an outside labour market develops, children are encouraged to earn income and bring it into the household. They are even sent to school to ensure that they can eventually earn higher incomes. Some traditional families have used their younger people to earn outside incomes for millennia (in the Middle East and the Mediterranean) while retaining control of them and their income and spending relatively little on them. This situation may disappear everywhere within the next half-century; if it does pass as quickly as this, mass schooling rather than mass industrialization will have been responsible.

The family system of morality and production has been little described and has begun to pass without even the circumstances of its passing being noted precisely because it was so all-embracing. It was not *a* morality; it was *the* morality, and hence commonsensical and unremarkable. When it does pass, within a generation or two the old morality is remembered with nostalgia; the respect for the old is remembered as childhood humility, not as the rigid system that it was. The first generation of school children who emerged from it were usually treated differently from the way earlier generations had been treated. Because of their schooling, many expected the kind of treatment they received without realizing this was an innovation, while their parents and grandparents moved, often awkwardly, to accept

[26] Of Yoruba women of completed fertility interviewed in Ibadan in 1973 and 1974–75, only 1·4% deliberately had "small" families of five or fewer live births.

and engineer this new status without realizing just how irrevocable the step was. To the researcher and to some of the teachers and other citizens, this transition was visible in the towns of Ghana 20 years ago, when many families were composed of a mixture of children who went to school and those, often somewhat older, who had not been and would never go (Caldwell, 1968a, pp. 197–209). Most parents treated school children quite differently from the way they treated their illiterate siblings,[27] and few of the school children seemed in any way aware of this. In later life, even as social scientists, they will probably be unable to recall the transition.

One can generalize further. Those who have participated in the affairs of state or the church have always been at least partly outside the confines of the sytem of family production, and they have had to modify its morality. This is also true of soldiers, scholars, migrants, large merchants, and anyone who employs others. Almost by definition, those who have interpreted, written, read, and challenged historical records have long been members of these numerically marginal groups. As family production and its determining morality passes, the very memories of it pass. Later generations, who live outside the system, do not regard those who were involved in family production as having been in the mainstream of history.

This brings us to an important point in the analysis of the change in relative child–adult status (and also wife–husband status) effected by education. The magnitude of the change is so great because it rests not only on what the school teaches, but also on how the educated child sees himself (especially relative to uneducated parents or siblings) and how his other relatives (especially uneducated parents or siblings) see him. These different perspectives are crucial elements in permanently changing relative intergenerational status. They are, for instance, the greatest factors in altering the relationship between an educated daughter-in-law and an uneducated mother-in-law to a point where the former can intervene individually to care for her children and to change the traditional balance of consumption and treatment within the family, with dramatic effects on child mortality (Caldwell, 1979).

There remain two problems and one essential statement.

The first problem is the distinction between the impact of education on the first generation and on subsequent generations. It has been argued here that the change resulting from education in terms of the increased cost of a child and decreased lifetime return is sufficient to cause falling fertility from the onset of mass education. This appears to have been the case in the West; within a decade of the introduction of compulsory schooling, the fertility of

[27] Of school-age children in Western Nigeria in 1973, 28% of those who did not go to school were taken to a doctor when sick, compared with 55% of school children. Changing African Family Project, Survey 2.

all occupational groups was declining (Ruzicka and Caldwell, 1977, pp. 171ff.). The pattern in the developing world may be different. In the West, a moderately high level of family morality remained so long after the development of the nonfamily labour market that a point was reached at which the chief value of children may have been their low consumption rather than their high production or return: under these conditions it may have taken very little to disturb the equilibrium. This family morality itself was, moreover, relatively weak compared with what is still found in the Middle East, Africa, or South Asia. It was already being challenged by societal morality: in spite of a proportion of parents of the generation of the 1870s and 1880s being unschooled, there was a level of literacy, numeracy, and outward-looking citizenship that affected nearly everyone. There was little equivalent in the West to the illiterate and completely traditional mothers of some of the school children in the contemporary developing world. This female illiteracy and an unquestioning, total immersion in family morality enable the patriarch to treat his wife (or wives) as one of the children and, through dominance over her, to solidify his dominance over his schooled children. A school child can falter in feeling part of a new, wider world if the father, whether educated or not, maintains his patriarchal role and the mother remains unwaveringly traditional. In this case the wealth flow may not turn downward until the second generation of mass education, when mothers as well as children are educated, and may not turn down at all if only fathers are educated and the tradition of illiterate wives persists.

A second and related problem is the distinction between education of males and females. In this regard, the key issue to explore is whether the education of the wife has a separate, interacting and compounding effect on changing family morality. Contemporaries thought such a separate effect was important in the nineteenth-century West, and it is probably important in the contemporary developing world.[28] In the traditional patriarchal family, there is undoubtedly a net wealth flow from wife to husband (and also to mother-in-law and father-in-law), which is reduced if an educated wife demands more equitable treatment or is awarded it because of the way the society views the educated. Even more important, education often leads to a strengthened bond between wife and husband, which renders the traditional family structure and its morality exceedingly difficult to maintain (see Chapters 4 and 5). Finally, educated wives, even when the child–parent wealth flow is still upward, may dislike repeated pregnancies and periods with infants and may attempt to prolong the interval between births with a consequent impact on fertility.

[28] For the nineteenth-century West, see Pat Caldwell, file on the *Australasian* newspaper, Melbourne, 1865–1900; for the contemporary developing world, see Chapter 7.

The essential statement is that the coincidental timing of the attainment of mass education and the onset of fertility decline is probably neither fortuitous nor due to a third factor dictating the exact timing of both. There are ample mechanisms to explain why mass education should have such a powerful impact on family economics. Nevertheless, the education of only half the community does not have the same effect on that half of the population, nor half the effect on the whole population. One reason is probably that, when only a fraction of the population has been to school, there remain strong forces to maintain family morality as the basic morality of the society (this may be less true in a highly stratified society). Probably a more important reason is that in such a divided society there remain very marked differentials in wages and salaries by education (especially in a highly stratified society), and an educated family can prosper. Probably these two reasons interacted in the mid-nineteenth-century West to maintain high fertility, and probably the same applies to urban Nigeria today. In Ibadan in 1973, about 40% of mothers under age 60 had been to school, while the great majority of their children—over 90% of even their dependent daughters—had attended school. Fertility was not yet falling, but this was partly explained by steep declines in the period of postnatal sexual abstinence (Caldwell and Caldwell, 1977, pp. 206–207; and 1980, Table 2). It seems highly unlikely that these daughters will be as fertile as their mothers.

There are mechanisms that can directly relate schooling to fertility decline. They are not identical in the contemporary developing world and the nineteenth-century West. The contemporary developing world has the influences experienced by the nineteenth-century West, plus the huge force of twentieth-century Westernization, especially with regard to family relationships, as taught by schools, Western example, films, newspapers, magazines, radio and television. My earlier statement of this brought protests, especially from the developed world that developing-world schools transmitted not culture but three Rs needed for economic development. That is why it has been necessary to document at some length in this paper the findings of researchers who have noted the impact of schooling. Although the evidence is scattered, the impressive point is that this long search for evidence has unearthed no findings to suggest that there was little Westernizing influence in developing-world schooling, and none to suggests that this influence was not potent in the area of family relations. Furthermore, the evidence suggests that the most potent force for change is the breadth of education (the proportion of the community receiving some schooling) rather than the depth (the average duration of schooling among those who have attended school).

This chapter was reprinted with the permission of The Population Council from John C. Caldwell, "Mass education as a determinant of the timing of fertility decline," *Population and Development Review* **6** no. 2 (June 1980): 225–255.

F

Recapitulation and Broader Implications

11

The wealth flows theory of fertility decline

The concept of "wealth flows" and the use of the concept to explain both stable high fertility and the onset of sustained fertility decline has been elaborated in earlier papers in this volume.

"Wealth flows" are defined as all the money, goods, services and guarantees that one person provides to another. The term "wealth" was used instead of "income" so as to emphasize the fact that the transactions were not all monetary; indeed at any given time they were not all material.[1] Admittedly the term is something of a misnomer in so far as "wealth" implies to an economist a stock rather than a flow.

Wealth flows analysis is fundamental to an understanding of the nature of family relationships at all times and in all places. Nevertheless, its greatest value is to be found in the analysis of the economics of familial production. Its relevance to fertility decline is found in the sense that fertility decline is the result of changes in the family's internal economic structure. Wealth flows analysis can be employed to throw light on mortality[2] and migration behaviour, and on many non-demographic phenomena.

The development of wealth flows theory lay in a nagging problem that beset two decades of field experience, both in survey results and in everyday contact. Large families did not seem to be worse off either in their contemporary condition or in their past experience of relative socioeconomic mobility.[3] Indeed, in areas where we worked, most people—and nearly everyone in rural areas—equated large families with strong, powerful and successful families. Small families, often determined by subfecundity marking a whole group of close relatives, were regarded as more likely to meet with disaster, and the local evidence appeared to confirm that this was

[1] The substitution of the term "support flows" has recently been suggested. Cf. Lesthaeghe and Wilson (1978).
[2] A partial treatment, at least in terms of changing family relations, has been undertaken in the latter part of Caldwell (1979).
[3] This was noted in data described in Caldwell (1966 and 1969).

so. Indeed there seemed to be evidence that "successful" men, the new elite, were more likely to come from families of above average size, after allowance had been made for the disproportionate numbers in the previous generation emerging from families of that size, and after standardization for socioeconomic class (Imoagene, 1976, Chapter 3).

These societies were not characterized by families of bare replacement level as a result of high fertility just compensating for high mortality. Mortality had long since fallen substantially. More significantly, even in a situation of stationary growth (such as is nearly approximated in some of the districts of Middle Africa characterized by high levels of sterility) such families have never been the rule. Very different levels of fertility and quite capricious inroads of mortality saw to it that such demographically traditional populations were characterized by both large and small surviving families. In these circumstances, the oral tradition has maintained that members of large families were fortunate because their family size ensured that they were better off. Indeed, among the Yoruba there was such identity between the terms for "large family" and "fortunate" or "well-off" family, let alone family "likely to be most prosperous" that we had difficulty in posing adequate survey questions.[4]

There is, then, a need to explain the social and economic condition of stable high fertility. Demographers have been so interested in change that they have often fallen into the trap of believing that they could explain pre-existing society in terms of the characteristics of the slowest moving segment of a society already experiencing change and could delineate the qualities of that segment by contrasting them with the qualities of the faster moving segments. In terms of social scientific method this is nonsense. We will never understand the onset of fertility decline until we understand the nature of stable high fertility societies and hence the circumstances in which destabilization can occur.

I believe that high fertility has probably been advantageous to most families over most of human history. Furthermore, the statement can be recast in terms of a tighter formulation, namely that high fertility has been economically advantageous. There are three stipulations which must be observed if the proposition is to be satisfactorily researched.

Firstly, economically advantageous means that a value can be placed upon all satisfactions—not only food but present and future safety, the pleasure of having even small things done for one, the pleasure of being able to order activity when required or desired, and so on. Secondly, the benefits and disadvantages of high fertility must be measured over the rest of a person's lifetime. Any cross-sectional measurement at a specific occasion

---

[4] i.e. in the Changing African Family Project, Nigerian Segment, Survey 2, in 1973. For a description of the project, see Okediji *et al.* (1976).

may catch the individual being investigated at a time of net disadvantage. Thirdly, this measurement in an individual's lifetime can begin and be carried forward only from the time that an individual is first in a position to make fertility decisions. Thus one cannot draw up a balance sheet from the cradle to the grave, but only from the assumption of decision-making powers to the grave. The corollary of this is that one cannot measure the returns to high fertility by adding up the condition of every member of a large family, even the children, at a given time and comparing the result with a similar calculation for a small family.

A great deal of very subtle research is required. On the first point we need to know a great deal more about the services done by members of families for each other within the family system. We also need to know the nature of risks and the value of guarantees against risk (if a reasonable premium for an insurance policy can be decided upon then this similar calculation should theoretically be possible). We also need to know how power arises from the number of people who can be influenced and what the material returns to power are.

With regard to the second stipulation we clearly need longitudinal research. We will probably have to take some risks by using as proxies retrospective information and also synthetic lifetimes made up by adding experiences of individuals of similar parity at different stages of their life cycles. Even a comparison of the history of groups of old people contrasted by parity is probably better than cross-sectional analysis of families still being formed. We attempted this approach almost twenty years ago in Ghana and came up with results close to those being argued here (Caldwell, 1966).

With regard to the third stipulation we need research that goes to the very heart of the nature of the traditional family. Who makes fertility decisions and how? What is the relation between making fertility decisions and making economic ones? The weakest aspect of the KAP surveys has been their implicit assumption that biological parents were fertility decision-makers and that the only fertility decisions were positive and initiating fertility control. I believe that it will be established that, in conditions where high fertility is either advantageous or not disadvantageous, there are powerful decision-making mechanisms operating against fertility control. It is not just meaningless tradition that there are beliefs and customs hostile to fertility control available if needed. The fact is that these controls can be operated not only by the reproductive generation but even more easily by the older generation. I am not saying that the older generation are the only fertility decision-makers and hence that the measurement of the net lifetime advantage from high fertility must be measured only from the attainment of patriarchal (or matriarchal) status. But I am saying that there is no clear-cut point where decision-making starts and where the count of the advantages and disadvantages of high fertility can begin. It is likely that the young have some influence from marriage or earlier but that this influence grows through a lifetime and hence that the count must be increasingly weighted over a lifetime. Nor is it a simple case of being able to analyse male and female lifetimes separately as if advancing age is all that matters. Clearly the balance of male and female influence in the fertility area is important and this does not remain constant over a lifetime and is also liable to change quite dramatically as the society changes.

This is a counsel of perfection but we should strive towards it in our field enquiries. In the meantime there is a good deal to be gained in terms both of extra insights and of the kind of additional analysis that can be carried out by defining stable high-fertility societies as ones where unlimited fertility is ultimately advantageous to fertility decision-makers, and societies subsequent to the onset of fertility transition as ones where this is no longer true. Indeed it would probably prove impossible to establish an adequate discipline of economic demography unless this assumption of economic rationality could be made.

When constructing a theory explaining stable high fertility and subsequent fertility decline in terms of "lifetime" net intergenerational wealth flows several more points should be emphasized.

The first is that the generations referred to in peasant societies and in labour market societies (whether capitalist or socialist) are the generations within the family. In some traditional societies the older generations may merely consist of parents and possibly grandparents, as well as parents-in-law; in others, uncles and aunts, and even great uncles or older cousins may play a role. Sometimes—and admittedly this places some strain on a strictly intergenerational approach—a rather similar role may be played by older siblings or even siblings of the opposite sex (or occasionally siblings with greater education or power in the new society). In many societies the relation of wives to their husbands is similar to that of children to fathers; this may have important demographic repercussions, for change in one set of relative positions is likely to affect the other set. In hunting and gathering societies, or in societies with some peasant production but also some continuing tribal organization, there may be a wealth flow in a small community which involves some flow from the younger generation to the older generation in general, whether relatives or not, although situations where there is not a strong orientation towards relatives are probably exceedingly rare.

The second is that the fundamental goals are social goals. There is no such thing as an economic satisfaction which is not also a social satisfaction. Economics is a way of evaluating these satisfactions and determining how they can most easily be optimized. Another grave weakness of the KAP surveys was their implicit assumption that all individuals in a family situation wanted the same thing, namely maximizing the economic condition of the nuclear family, while fearing the erosion of that family's welfare from the demands of other members of the extended family or even outsiders. There are in fact many societies in which a married man cares more about the material conditions of his parents or siblings than of his wife and children. There are societies where a man's aim is to maximize his circumstances at the expense of his wife or children. It is impossible to decide the economic rationality of fertility decisions unless one understands such social ends—for social and economic rationality are the same thing.

The third point is just how comprehensive wealth flows are. The ability of a man not to lift a finger in the house and to have his every whim satisfied immediately has been a fundamental type of wealth in most societies. So has the ability of a mother-in-law to order about her daughter-in-law even if it does not make house-keeping more efficient. There are are an indefinite range of guarantees: of help in years of scarcity or devastation, of assistance if one's neighbour raises his hand against one, of a presence that will ward off robbers (and perhaps evil spirits), of support in old age, of assistance against bureaucrats and so on. Other wealth flows are the much more obvious things of a son relieving his middle-aged father of labour (and perhaps allowing him to go more often to the coffee shop or to pontificate with his peers under the shade of a tree or on a verandah), the receipt of most of the crops harvested, and the ability to control the disposition of money earned from sales or from younger relatives working for wages.

The fourth point is that we are talking of "economic" flows—even if only the fetching of father's slippers or the guarantee of help against starvation or attack—as activities, or promised activities, or goods or money that have a material value and most of which are to some extent capable of substitution. We are not talking about *pleasure*, although the action would probably not be required and would not have a positive economic value if it did not give rise to some pleasure. The point that I am making is that I do not believe in the validity of the approach to explaining high fertility which argues that fertility will be high if the value of children, judged by *both* their economic contribution over a lifetime and the pleasure they give, is positive. I believe this to be double counting.[5] I believe that it will be shown that in societies of stable high fertility children are a lifetime net economic advantage and that pleasure in high fertility reflects this. When children are no longer an economic advantage fertility will fall, and that fall will not wait until the sum of their economic and emotional returns is negative. Once the direction of

[5] This is why I have reservations about the approach of the Value of Children Study coordinated by the East-West Population Institute, although I find their data interesting.

the wealth flow has reversed, most couples will continue to have children but they will manage to do so by receiving all the parental pleasure they desire from a smaller and more concentrated source. They will not have two or three children because this is the point where the pleasure they purchase from parenthood is equal to what that expenditure would secure in the form of substitutable pleasures. They will have that number in the full knowledge that having children is not economic, but that one's own children provide a unique form of pleasure which is not substitutable and that they can afford that expenditure for such unique pleasure. They do not have fewer because such a number would create a family which in some way would be of incomplete size and the pleasure would be somehow eroded. They do not have more because the family already has sufficient completeness and the additional expenditure would make the life of the existing family or parents markedly less satisfactory. Clearly what constitutes a complete family is a concept subject to change in social attitudes and is affected by comparison with the size of other families. It is likely to move down as children cost relatively more (as family expenditure becomes more egalitarian) and as society adjusts its views of what constitutes a complete family as a result of these pressures.

The fifth point is that there are really only two kinds of societies from a demographic viewpoint: one where unlimited fertility is an economic advantage and the other where fertility is of no economic advantage. The former is not characterized by families with an infinite number of children and the latter by families with no children for biological and psychological reasons. One society changes to the other fairly quickly and the period of transition is an unstable one. It follows that sociological analysis which attempts to establish family norms during this period of transition or economic analysis which attempts to show why a family of a certain size is a case of economic maximizing is almost certain to prove nonsensical.

The sixth point is that the reversal of the situation—the onset of fertility decline—is a reversal of the intergenerational wealth flow. This is a change of economic relationships within the family which arises from a change in the emotional balance. That is the rules about who can get what from whom (and how much) and who can tell whom to do what fundamentally alter, thus rendering high fertility (indeed any fertility) disadvantageous. Very subtle shifts in emotional relationships within the family, usually reflecting changes in society's attitudes towards male–female and parent–child relationships, can dramatically alter the direction of the wealth flow. A strengthening of spousal relationships can both weaken extended family relationships and can alter intergenerational relationships (partly because the wife's influence in parental decisions becomes more important).

A major complexity in the analysis of wealth flows in traditional society is the fact that the value of high fertility springs from two different causes with a changing balance between them over time (although this balance can suddenly revert during periods of violence). The first value of high fertility—first both in the historic sense and in the order of analysis here—is that numbers mean strength in a situation where force or factionalism is important; the second reason is that large families can yield to some of the older generation a situational advantage in terms of familial production and familial consumption. In most societies, except some tranquil legalistic industrialized societies, both values of high fertility exist side by side and even interwoven. Thus a guarantee between two persons can be a guarantee for help against either force or want. The distinction is important for the purpose of analysis but often very difficult to make.

The younger generation can provide a useful source of force both for defence against enemies and for fruitful attack upon others. In more settled conditions they can still make troublesome neighbours respectful and help to protect property from theft. A patriarch can argue his point of view with greater safety when he has a number of sons.[6] Where there is factionalism, numbers can both give the faction greater strength and purchase more influence within it. Where there are gains to be made by dominating village politics or influencing elected representatives from the area, then numbers can count. Large families are more likely to be given access to monopoly resources, or the lease of land both because they will work it more intensively and because more people will thus be beholden to the landlord, and a larger family can secure its continuity and its land and other possessions during critical periods of transition such as occur on the death of the patriarch. Large families can more readily protect their own land boundaries and trespass upon those of others, and they can also summon more witnesses and bribe more officials (or threaten them) in law suits. Inevitably, their network of alliances through marriages will be more extensive. They can more readily raise money for marriage payments, funerals, bribes, or to meet new and transient opportunities for investment. They also provide an opportunity for the division of labour not only in familial production but also in allowing the family to export one or more of its members either for more permanent employment elsewhere or to take opportunities of short-lived but worthwhile windfall gains at some distance.[7]

As peasant cultivation becomes established, gains of another type begin to become more important. These are the advantages accruing from relative positions of advantage in both family production and consumption. Familial

[6] This point is discussed in Kabwegyere and Mbula (1980).

[7] Sources here include Chapters 2, 3, 4 and 7 of this volume; the work of Mead Cain, especially Cain *et al.* (1979); the work of Barkat-E-Khuda, especially Khuda (1978); the work of A. K. M. Jalaluddin (in preparation); and Mandelbaum (1970a) and Reyna (1977).

production—usually in peasant agriculture but also among traditional merchants and artisans—is perhaps the clearest example of a pre-capitalist mode of production. Archetypically it exists when production is very largely for subsistence as has been true in most peasant societies. Unfortunately, economic anthropologists and political scientists have tended to concentrate on exchange relations beyond the family either because economic theory was more capable of coping with the phenomenon or because of a desire to analyse the political situation in terms of exploitation by outside classes. The truth probably is that even in feudal society the nature of most social relations and the prevailing morality, as well as the direction of the wealth flow and other demographic influences, is explained much more by the internal relations of the peasant families than by their social, political and economic relations to feudal proprietors. There has been a reluctance to analyse the internal relations of the family both because it is extremely difficult to do and because of the persistence of a belief about the sanctity of the family. Indeed it is in the interests of the powerful in the family to generate such a belief and commitment to family loyalty; a notion of family unity and integrity is as basic to the morality of peasant society as are similar beliefs about the nation to national states where most people work in the labour market.

But the truth of familial production is that there are major differences in power within the family and that there is exploitation involving both exploiters and exploited.[8] There is certainly potential for protest of social injustice and demand for change, but in its stable state there may be bitterness and grievance but little demand for change. One reason is that familial morality, which forms by far the greater part of articulated peasant culture, justifies the differentiations; another is that the passage of time guarantees that the exploited will become the exploiter. Most familial production is characterized by differentiation, and even segregation, by age and sex. The system is given stability by veneration for the old and greater respect for males. These positions of relative strength are institutionalized. The old derive their power from real or supposed greater experience or knowledge (even of the occult), from ownership of land and other property, from directing inheritance, from having granted life and from possessing recognized powers over behaviour and even life itself, from the control of marriage, from institutionalized weaknesses such as sibling rivalry and so on. In spite of differentials in respect to both persons and work, persons of every age and sex do have specified roles which they jealously guard and to which they force others to adhere. A man with growing sons usually does less work than he claims to do—especially if they are numerous. A woman

---

[8] See especially Chapters 5 and 7 in this volume. Attempts to measure some relevant aspects of the family are to be found in Caldwell *et al.* (1981a) and Mahmud and McIntosh (1980).

with several daughters, and above all one with daughters-in-law, will do less laborious work and instead spend her time in apparent organization. These differentials, especially by family size and by stage in family life cycle, need to be researched much more thoroughly than has yet been the case. The work is extremely difficult partly because of conventional beliefs about the superiority and inferiority of various types of work and demonstrably wrong conventional views about the energy inputs needed by various types of work. There are also conventional views about consumption deserts, often far from physiological equity, in terms of food needs (Caldwell, 1979a, and Chapter 10). Differential consumption also urgently needs adequate research.

The nature of the traditional society of familial production is of fundamental importance because it has for so long dominated much of the world's culture, and far from vestigial remnants of its morality still influence industrial society. Clearly it has critically important implications for demographic behaviour—in terms of fertility, mortality and migration. Confining our attention to fertility behaviour, high fertility is explicable much more easily in terms of economic rationality when reproductive decisions are made or influenced by those already consuming more and working less—or looking forward to soon entering this group—than would be the case in a more egalitarian family. In one sense the move towards fertility decline is explained both by a decline in the importance of familial production and a growth in internal family egalitarianism. These movements are of course related and are also related more basically (but not mechanistically tightly as will be explained below) to profound transformations in the nature of the economy.

Perhaps the main reason that the analysis of the gains from high fertility must take a life cycle approach is that fertility is essentially a form of investment for future return. Some of the return occurs surprisingly soon. Most cultures appear to have some expression like "more mouths more hands" which expresses the fact that we are dealing with a dynamic process rather than a static one. In some cultures analyses show that children do an appreciable amount of labour even from 5–9 years of age.[9] Furthermore, they do work that adults regard as demeaning and which tends to cause adults in infertile families stress if they have to do it themselves. Nevertheless, it is probably true that young children are a net drain on family resources and that, during the life cycle of the family, there come more difficult periods when small children are disproportionately represented. Where residence and labour force arrangements are of a nuclear family type this may occur early in the process of family building; in other families it may occur at a later stage when the last children have recently been born and

---

[9] I have found the work of A. O. Okore valuable. See Okore (1977 and 1978).

before all of them grow into the working age groups. At these stages per capita consumption may be relatively low. This says nothing about the value of high fertility for three reasons. The first is that the standard of living of the older decision-makers may not fall during this period. The food deficit will be entirely taken up by the children, who may, in large families, exhibit higher than average mortality but usually not so high as to completely negate the extra reproduction. The second reason is that large families often find it easier to acquire a specific possession which does not have to be multiplied on a per capita basis—a transistor radio, a concrete slab for drying cocoa, a tube well and so on. A third reason is that children are an investment in the real sense. Where there is a market for land, peasants usually have only two avenues for investment. One is land and the other is children, and the best investment is usually a mix of the two. Where land is not freehold but communally owned—or where there is an open frontier—high fertility may be the only sound investment.[10] Not only may it provide more labour, but often the fact of extra numbers is the only reason acceptable to the community for demanding family access to more land. All forms of saving for investment demand immediate deprivation for future gain. Amongst a hard-pressed agrarian population the cold-blooded failure to meet present needs in order to invest is practically impossible except in one way. That way is investing immediately in extra children whose presence cannot be gainsaid and whose feeding and other needs follow naturally as part of the family's battle through life. Indeed, in the circumstances of extended family obligations, the burden of the children in their more dependent stages might well be spread through a larger family. For this reason a biological couple might have little to gain by restricting fertility because of their being part of a larger unit often consisting at a minimum of the husband's parents and his brothers and their wives and children. But the returns during old age will not be shared as widely for, by this time, the husband's father will be dead, the economic bond between the brothers weakened, partly as a result of that death, and the original couple will now be at the apex of a new family pyramid.

The system already described can be criticized as referring only to a peasantry or to hunters and gatherers. In fact the system of family production worked very similarly amongst urban artisans and merchants who could in no way be regarded as subsistence producers. It works this way among nomads who usually have to barter or buy grains for their basic food. It even seems to have applied to richer classes whose administrative or economic activities would be better served by using members of their own family. The strength of familial morality meant that family members could

[10] In these conditions, the investment in children can be very profitable. Cf. Mendonsa (1977).

be trusted to a much greater extent than outsiders—whose chief loyalties were to their own families. In much of the contemporary world peasant proprietors who have allowed their children to go off to distant schools or urban employment feel continuing worry and uncertainty about having to employ strangers to replace family labour—there is a lack of trust, there is even danger.

This system does not collapse with the appearance of capitalism, and the labour market can be used for very long periods to supplement and even strengthen familial production. This is done by allowing, and even encouraging, younger members to earn wages. The family system continues as long as all or most of those wages are put into a common family budget largely under the control of the patriarch. The wage earner returns these wages because this is customarily expected, because he may need to fall back upon the family social security system at any time, because he has left his wife and children back on the land with his larger family, and, to some extent, because he expects his children to treat him as he has treated his family of origin. His employers support this system. Often they would not have begun production but for the fact that the family security system allows them to pay the individual worker very low wages. It is these low wages that force him to leave his wife and children with the larger family, and it is the lack of security in his employment that prevents him from breaking with his family of origin. Indeed that link gives him a certain freedom in the capitalist labour market to leave his job at will or to treat it casually. The important demographic point is that both his wife and children are largely continuing to support themselves. Even as the wage-earner becomes older and his father dies he may continue to work in the town, sending back money with specific instructions for its investment in land. Prior to this, his father may have been doing exactly the same; a recent study of a rural community in Kenya has shown that the main determinant of relative prosperity has in recent years been the ability to produce children, educate them and send them off for urban employment so that a continuous stream of money comes back for rural use (Hunt, 1979).

Ultimately the labour market (which will be treated here as capitalist production although the situation of non-familial production is not very different in socialist countries) undermines the whole system and makes high fertility—or any fertility—uneconomic. In fact the link between economic decision-making and reproductive decision-making is broken, because, even though the employer might want endless aspirants for jobs, he has not a similar control over biological parents as their own parents had. The family decision structure is shattered because support no longer depends on permission to work on the land and to receive a share of its fruits but on the individual's ability to sell his own labour power. Thus reproductive decision-making becomes identical with biological parentage even from the beginning of marriage and from the first conception. As the family tends to nucleate, emotional changes with important economic and demographic implications occur. The larger family of familial production deliberately kept weak the emotional links between spouses and even denied primacy to the emotional links between young children and their biological parents. Moralities which ensured this were necessary for the economic functioning of the larger unit, and part of that morality was the marked segmentation by sex and age. The smaller nuclear families which tended to appear as familial production declined did not have such needs and had stronger internal emotional bondings which inevitably worked towards greater egalitarianism in family consumption. Thus children (and wives) became relatively more expensive. At the same time they were likely to prove a much less rewarding investment for the future for a number of reasons. One was that parents no longer controlled the employment of adult children and hence could anticipate no certain return from them. Another was that the emotional egalitarianism within the nuclear family made it ever less likely that there would be substantial wealth flows to the older generation. Each spouse resented too much help-giving to the other spouse's parents, and each could claim that there were crying needs deserving priority not only for themselves but also for their children. Indeed, this stress on the needs of the younger generation in contrast to the very oldest generation hastened the economic egalitarianism of the young and hence made high fertility ever less rewarding.

Our lack of understanding about the persistence of high fertility in the industrialized wage-earning West of the mid-nineteenth century is based on a fundamental misunderstanding of the productive structure. The truth is that the West had become a two-tiered productive system. No longer did the family head stay at home while sending his sons off to wage employment; on the contrary he worked for wages himself. He emphasized that the labour market place was a man's world. The money coming into the household was almost entirely from his earnings and he emphasized the obligations due to this monopolistic resource as much as did the peasant patriarch emphasize his monopolistic gift of land. The system depended on a continued emphasis on segregation by sex and was clearly threatened by wives working. Much as in the pattern developed by the agrarian family once an external labour market appeared, wives sometimes worked for supplementary income as did dependent children, but their earnings largely went into a common pool mostly controlled by the patriarch (now a younger patriarch and not his ageing and often dependent father). Society and the state helped by differentiating the employment offered to women and minors and by paying them lower wages. Meanwhile the majority of the community's labour inputs (as measured by hours and physical effort) went not into the return for wages at all but into domestic production within the household carried out by wives, the children they could organize, and other unmarried female relatives. This work provided processed food, much of the clothing, a wide range of services, and the upbringing of the young. It was extremely efficient and cheap and for long the market could do little to compete. This was not merely the domestic household production of the subsistence farm—the range and quality of products had become far greater and were being produced far more cheaply than wage earners could have bought the equivalent services. The system remained stable for as long as it did because of society differentiating between "productive" work in the market place and household activities,[11] and because of a continued downgrading of the value of the latter and the actual work inputs involved. The morality (and segmentation) that supported it was obviously a variant of the original morality of total familial production.

The morality of this two-tiered system long allowed differentials in consumption which are important in explaining continued high fertility. Husbands were given better food because "they earned the wages" as well as money for outside entertainment and activities on much the same grounds; they wore better clothing because "their work demanded it". A study of nineteenth century Austrialia (see Chapter 6) has shown that children even of the middle class lived in surprising austerity; this was not taken in the conventional wisdom to be cruelty or discrimination but to be an essential part of upbringing—"not spoiling them".

The whole system was unstable for a number of reasons. One was that industry was tempted to compete in domestic production and slowly found ways of doing so, while the time would come when it would be searching for labour over and above that which could be provided by adult men—and it would offer wives higher wages while justifying the change on exactly the same grounds that home production was kept so cheap and efficient, namely that home production was an inferior kind of work. Underlying this and other changes in the internal relations of the household was the egalitarian ethic which became increasingly applied to family husband–wife and parent–child relations with the focusing of emotion within the nuclear family and with the more comfortable way of life provided by rising living standards. There was an interconnection between what wives did and what children did in domestic production—if the situation of one changed, the situation of the other was likely to be affected.

There were important alterations in these balances to which we will return, but the first massive change occurred to the position of children.

---

[11] This is still done in much labour force analysis, one justification being that the differentiation must be maintained because of the way national income is defined.

By the second half of the nineteenth century a great deal of transformation had occurred within the Western economy and to the Western family. The Australian evidence makes it very doubtful whether urban children were any longer a substantial positive economic asset, although children on farms undoubtedly were. The major factor that prevented the wealth flow from turning downward was that, prior to mass schooling, they were not much of an economic disadvantage. They were brought up frugally and were not expected to demand as much consumption as their parents, let alone their fathers. This was said to be "for their own good" and was sanctioned by religion and by a family morality which clearly still drew heavily on the morality that had been shaped in the period of familial production. It might be noted that, even in the open labour market, employers gained by having children reared in such an atmosphere—a clear case of the morality of one mode of production being employed by the next. What kept fertility high was the fact that children, in this relatively costless situation, provided a considerable input into household domestic production. In a situation where market production had barely begun to offer household services, a father with several children could find himself living in a condition of comfort, rarely lifting a hand while at home, that a childless man could not.

There seems to be some evidence contrary to this analysis. Female marriage was not early anywhere in the West; fertility had been falling in Ireland, the United States and Australia; and marital fertility was definitely declining in France. Our work leads us to believe that none of these changes will eventually be shown to have arisen from the turning of the intergenerational wealth flow downward. The Australian evidence appears to show that late female marriage was never explained until three-quarters of the way through the nineteenth century by problems of family size.[12] Rather was it what the participants continuously proclaimed, a question of the proper time to marry—that is a time when the future husband (or couple) had accumulated enough and the husband had attained a secure position so as to capitalize a small firm, namely the household of domestic production. Where female marriage was increasingly delayed—in the United States and Australia because of a retreat from frontier conditions and a relative shortage of women, and in Ireland because of specific problems in capitalizing a separate household—total fertility fell even though marital fertility did not. Indeed, the fact that high marital fertility was not an economic burden was shown by its stability in all but one country—France—until three-quarters of the way through the nineteenth century. Administrators and theorists in France, and subsequently elsewhere, believed that the French were avoiding high fertility for economic reasons. I

[12] P. Caldwell and J. C. Caldwell, "The proper time to marry in nineteenth century Australia" (project in progress).

think it highly likely that family research will eventually show that the major reason was a change in the position of the French wife. There was a move towards greater egalitarianism between the spouses and the French woman gained greater control over her own fertility, which she reduced not because of fear of the economic burden of children but because of antagonism to a great number of closely-spaced periods of pregnancy, childbirth and mothering young infants.

The high fertility situation in the West was fragile. It depended on a very considerable degree of inequality of consumption within the household at a time when adult consumption levels could be maintained by fertility reduction just as readily as by highly unequal consumption, and when, unlike the position in the peasant family, production would not suffer from such a change. There were two forces for stability which are not found in today's Third World. The first is that there were no external models of more egalitarian family consumption. The second is that the alternative method of maintaining adult consumption levels meant a resort to methods of fertility limitation which were difficult and as yet legitimized nowhere in the world. Difficult methods were of course eventually used—exemplified by the widespread employment of withdrawal, a contraceptive method unlikely to be used on any scale in any future fertility transition.

Eventually the disequilibrating mechanism arrived. It was compulsory mass schooling (see Chapter 10). In the West this probably did not reduce child productivity very much except in rural areas. However, it did a great deal to make children more costly. There were direct costs, and probably greater indirect ones, because both children and their parents saw the position of the former as having relatively changed. Children demanded more and got more. The consumption gap between the generations narrowed and high fertility became definitely disadvantageous. The battle for mass schooling created a situation where the relationship between the state and children became of great significance and education laws were only part of a mass of legislation and regulations on labour conditions and for the protection of children that created both the fact of dependency and a social atmosphere favouring it.

Once fertility began to fall it ultimately reached very low levels, in terms of historical change in a comparatively short time. The fact that the transition did not occur even more rapidly does not mean that the intergenerational wealth flow was not downward throughout the whole society. Rather should it be interpreted as a period when greater familiarization with contraception, the increasing legitimacy of its practice, and the improvement in its technology—together, ultimately with easy access to abortion and sterilization—was becoming more the pattern.[13] Over

[13] This is dealt with in Chapter 6 and in greater detail in Ruzicka and Caldwell (1977).

time the downward wealth flow probably gained ever-increasing strength and from the 1960s the position of women became an increasingly important influence.

The situation in the Third World has been different and this difference is basically explained by the movement toward a global economy and a global society. The importance of the latter has been noted much less than that of the former. Imported Western concepts of the family have come with missionaries, administrators, educational systems, and the mass media. The rights of children and of wives has been emphasized. Mass educational systems have appeared at a much earlier stage of economic development. This means that the wealth flow tended to reverse much closer to the time when familial production was breaking down. Indeed, imported concepts of the role of children may have hastened that breakdown. Furthermore, when there was some advantage in controlling fertility contraception was more easily available, often through national family planning organizations, and its use was more acceptable.

Nevertheless, even with the traditional economy beset by new external forces, the wealth flow was still remarkably resistant to reversal. One of the reasons was that the traditional family of production and consumption was able to take advantage of some of the changes. Patriarchal control often tended to remain. Younger members frequently worked for wages for at least part of the time outside the family but brought their earnings back to a common budget. Indeed the family was tempted to maximize these outside earnings by educating ever further some of its children. Often this ultimately proved to be the undoing of the system in that educated children demanded more consumption rights and once grown up might not provide the same returns to parents as children in more traditional society. While the familial morality held strong, high fertility could be rewarding over a lifetime even to urban middle class parents. In Ibadan city we found only 1% of parents deliberately restricting family size (Caldwell and Caldwell, 1978). They differed from other members of the middle class little in education or occupation. The major difference seemed to be a strengthening of the emotional nexus between the spouses, and a consequent agreement that the needs of their children came first. Their children worked less, were more likely to be taken to the doctor, and were more likely to incur a host of other expenditure. The parents realized clearly that the children were an economic loss at the time and were not likely to be an economic advantage in the future.

This brings us to a key question. When do parents know that high fertility will not be economically advantageous? Is it when the experience of a generation has already proved that the economic calculus has changed forever or is it one generation earlier? Our findings in Ibadan suggest that it may well be the latter. The first generation to expend more emotionally and materially upon their children than they demand in return realize (often almost subconsciously, without discussion, or even clearly facing the issue) that they have established precedents and attitudes within their children which will not subsequently change and hence that high fertility will not be rewarding.

The contraceptive revolution is not the same as the demographic one (see Caldwell and Caldwell, 1976). Some societies have a considerable demand for contraceptives for pre-marital or extra-marital sexual relations, or for substitution for such practices as post-natal sexual abstinence or terminal sexual abstinence (Caldwell and Caldwell, 1977; 1980). Nevertheless, familiarization with contraception means that the means are on hand immediately if fertility appears to be becoming a net lifetime burden, and even earlier if women desire to postpone the next pregnancy for reasons unconnected with ultimate family size.

We have concentrated here on the traditional patriarchal families of the agrarian Old World. In these societies the situation of children and women is often closely bound together—if one changes the other is likely to do so. However, the existing system has great stability. Such resistance to change may be found to a lesser extent in Southeast Asia where matrilocality has been common and the position of women relatively high. Children may become an economic burden at a relatively earlier stage of economic and social change.

The analysis has also concentrated on the family as a relatively autonomous institution, except to the extent that such autonomy is invaded by the demands of compulsory schooling. We may well see much greater state intervention upsetting the economic calculus by either depriving the older generation of rewards from their children or by imposing some penalty for high fertility which outweighs those rewards.

We have also ignored certain specific, but very important, models of unusual historic change. Two prime examples are Sri Lanka and Kerala where mass education came much earlier than might have been anticipated from economic indices. Both societies received social messages which otherwise would not have had the same impact; both appear to have experienced major changes in family relations; and both have experienced fertility decline earlier than macroscopic economic indices would have predicted. Almost certainly these falls were no earlier than the family economic calculus, that of net intergenerational lifetime wealth flows, would have indicated.

Wealth flows theory could be said to be economically determinist in two senses but not in a third. The first sense is that it explains fertility as declining as soon as net economic lifetime advantages from children are no longer anticipated. The second sense is that the analysis predicts that traditional familial production will always be characterized by economic advantage to high fertility and by actual high fertility except in pathological conditions or under duress from external authorities, and that non-familial production (whether capitalist or socialist) will ultimately be characterized by low fertility. The sense in which it is not as economically determinist as it might otherwise be is that it does not regard the economics of fertility as being determined at any given time directly by the means of production or the modes of production. It distinguishes two fundamental modes of production: familial and non-familial (or labour market) production. Familial production is characterized by intergenerational exploitative economic relations which favour the older generation, and by a morality that both justifies and facilitates this. Ultimately in non-familial production this morality will be replaced by another one of a more "individualistic" type. However, moralities wither only slowly, partly because some parties have economic and other interests in their retention. In the West what remained of familial morality ensured that high fertility was not economically disadvantageous long after the familial mode of production (except for household domestic production) had been massively transformed. In this sense there is an historic lag but it is not a lag in the sense that high fertility is retained once it is economically disadvantageous to the family fertility decision-makers.

Thus demographic change can be identified with fundamental social and economic change. The failure of social and economic change theory to explain the onset of fertility decline is not merely an omission but proof that those theories are insufficient to explain social and economic change (see Chapter 9).

The fundamental challenge in the demographic field is to explain the onset of fertility decline. Once such decline is established the eventual attainment of low fertility is guaranteed and analyses based on experience during that decline are of little importance and are likely to be misleading. The onset of fertility decline cannot be explained except in terms of the nature of the pre-existing stable high fertility regime and the conditions of destabilization.

These explanations will be found to be ones of fundamental economic and social change. Changes in attitudes and aspirations, in family size norms and in the acceptability of contraception will be found to be results and not causes and quite incapable of adding anything to the analysis of the onset of fertility decline.

Perhaps the most urgently needed research is that into intrafamilial economic and power relations in the traditional family characterized by familial production, and into the causes and effects of shifts within these relations. Such research has hardly begun.[14] It is of course extremely difficult, one reason being the effect on such relations of an external observer. Related to this work is the need for knowing a great deal more about the locus of economic and fertility decision-making in such families. Subsequently we also need to have such information for the successor family systems as familial production and its attendant morality was transformed with the growth of the external labour market.

[14] Some aspects of it are being attempted in the project described in Caldwell *et al.* (1981a).

12

The transition from familial to labour market production and the social implications

This Chapter examines the work patterns, family relationships and demographic behaviour found in peasant society, and then analyses the changes that occur as largely subsistence familial production gives way to market production and to employment by the labour market.

Much of the information is drawn from a study of both rural and urban families in Bangladesh (Caldwell *et al.*, 1981a), but this is supplemented with material from research in South India, the Middle East and tropical Africa. The project in Bangladesh involved recording the activities of each member of each family every day from 5 a.m. until 10 p.m. Research on work inputs carried out by recording participants' statements for short retrospective periods has become relatively common (see Chapter 2; Nag *et al.*, 1977; Changing African Family, 1974; Cain, 1977; Cain *et al.*, 1979; Boulier, 1977; Khuda, 1978). The unusual aspects of our study were that it also embraced urban populations and that it paid a great deal of attention to the initiation and supervision of work (as well as non-work activities), its location, the composition of the working group, and the ownership and disposal of the product.

The analysis assumes (and helps to substantiate) that peasant production is a distinct mode of production, the *familial mode*. It can be contrasted with the *labour market mode* of production where employment is not determined by relationship but by hire by outside individuals or institutions. This Chapter does not discuss the question as to whether there are distinct modes of production associated with shifting cultivation or hunting and gathering, where control may be exercised more by the clan or the tribal band than by relatives, and where the value of individuals may lie as much in their strength and contribution to defence as in their relative share in production and consumption. Nor does it discuss whether there are essentially different relations of production, and hence modes of production, in capitalist and socialist economies. On both points it remains agnostic and even sceptical. It does deny that there are such modes of production as the feudal mode, and regards feudal and various other economies as political and economic strategies for removing and redistributing the surplus from peasant production. The nature of that production—the way labour is organized and directed and the morality that sustains it—varies little from yeomanry to feudal employment. The latter uses the peasant family whether it regards itself as employing a single member or the whole family and production is ultimately predicated by relationships within the family and by the morality that controls those relationships.

The point being emphasized here is that there is an intricately developed mode of production, familial production, which has until recently dominated the world economy. It survives in household production in industrialized countries. The morality necessary to establish the desired relations of production has been only partly dismantled and the morality of labour market production is still only in the process of being evolved.

Familial production involves exploitation—unequal control of the product, unequal consumption, and very different degrees of power in allocating productive roles—within the family. The very examination of family exploitation is repugnant to many, largely because the morality—the cultural superstructure erected to justify the system and make it work— remains with us only partly eroded. Even Chayanov (1966a), who wrote so feelingly about the drudgery of peasant life, spoke of the family as a unit and at no stage examined differential treatment or exploitation within it. The political Left has also failed to investigate intra-familial relationships because of the political advantage in drawing attention to those who remove the peasants' surplus. Similarly, the economic anthropologists have concentrated on that surplus, in spite of the fact that it often represents only a small fraction of all production, largely because the analytical apparatus they have borrowed from the economists can cope with analysing the distribution of the surplus but is quite incapable of analysing the family's internal economic relationships.

Most of the world's culture for most of its history has been the superstructure which justifies and controls familial production. Most of peasant speech takes the form either of instructions which organize production and consumption or of conversation in terms of age and sex differences or of scandal or jokes about the partial flouting of these rules.[1] These matters are the substance of folk lore, proverb and cliche, of moral injunction and religion. This is the reason that intrafamilial exploitation is

[1] Rural conversation is being studied by J. Caldwell and P. Caldwell.

not more resented. The nature of age and sex relationships with regard to power, production and consumption is so deeply imbedded in the culture—it is in fact most of the culture—that it is taken to be either natural or divinely ordained.

Yet there is exploitation all the time. The old, and especially the male, have priority in consumption and can decide what to do. Often men do not even know how little their women have to eat because they eat first. In Bangladesh girls and young women have least access to food and other resources and, as a result, exhibit higher mortality until about thirty years of age (Ruzicka and Chowdhury, 1978, pp. 20–21).

Yet the family is rarely in a revolutionary condition and most inequalities are not resented (the situation of the daugher-in-law *vis-à-vis* the mother-in-law is an exception and frequently a cause of bitterness). One reason is the life cycle one, in that the young will soon inherit the position of the old. Another is that brothers, for instance, are usually socialized to feel more rivalry with each other than with their father—indeed even the thought of such rivalry is usually banished as unnatural or sinful. Perhaps more important is the fact that much power can be exerted by completely accepting one's specified role and by assailing those who deviate from their own roles in any way. A man who would treat his wife as more of a companion is prevented from doing so less because of his desire to exploit her to the utmost than because he would lose respect in the eyes of his peers and even of his wife (and certainly of his mother). The family system is seen at its purest in isolated rural homesteads. Life in a village adds new dimensions but usually does not weaken the system. It is true that in a village persons can seek the companionship of non-relatives but it is these companions who are usually the ones who most firmly forbid departure from established familial roles.

The family mode of production probably reached its apogee amongst peasant farmers. In such families everyone knew clearly their situational advantage and disadvantage. The power of the patriarch rested in the last analysis in his ownership or control of land, although the old have usually also made two other less convincing claims, superior knowledge and the gratitude of the young for having granted them the gift of life.

However, there have always been families without land. There have been both merchant and artisan families, found most commonly in the towns or larger villages. These have usually possessed some property necessary for their trade or craft and this served much the same role as land. They have sometimes also possessed privileged rights to undertake the work—a resource base in that a son who broke with his father could not enter the family trade. Increasingly over time there have also been landless labourers where no such lever existed, except possibly work contacts where the father's word was influential. In the whole three groups the cultural super-structure long approximated that of the peasantry, both because the latter formed the major society and because the old and the male, even if less securely based, still had situational advantages from maintaining familial morality. There were of course other groups, even fewer in number, such as rulers, aristocrats and bureaucrats who usually conformed if only for purposes of maintaining stability. There were also poorer individuals such as soldiers, but they were usually drawn from peasant families and returned to them. In more recent times life in armies has reduced familial morality to the point where soldiers may become a threat both to the peasant mode of production and also the political system controlling the labour market mode.

There are demographic implications arising from the familial mode of production. Those who gain most are at the apex of an age–sex pyramid and are in a position to benefit from high fertility and also to control reproductive behaviour. Needless to say, this control is usually by negative sanctions against birth control, normally in terms of preserving the purity of women. In fact the emphasis on the purity of women is a valuable tool for maintaining family differences. It is related also to mechanisms for keeping the emotional link between spouses weak so as to maintain the larger family unity (see Chapter 4; Gluckman, 1955) and to ensure the upward flow of wealth to the oldest generation.

Less obvious is the effect of familial production on mortality. Peasant families often exhibit high infant and child mortality. This is, of course, largely explained by their limited access to medical facilities, but it is not wholly explained this way. While it is not deliberate, it arises from the system. If children were treated as being as important as the old and were cared for so consistently, then they would less often fall sick and would less often die (Caldwell, 1979). But such a change in priorities would endanger the whole system and would be literally unthinkable. Hence, really low child mortality is usually not achieved until the familial production mode has disappeared except within the house.

The Family in Rural Bangladesh

The familial system operated in its purest form when production was almost wholly for subsistence. This is no longer true in any part of Bangladesh but all the farming families we investigated in 1978 predominantly produced food for their own consumption.

There are two other complexities about the society. First, marginal farmers and landless population now form a considerable fraction of all rural society, partly as a result of land transfer during the crises of the past decade.

Secondly, the usual segregation between the sexes is found in rather an extreme form because of the *purdah* system in this Moslem society.

The most significant finding of the research project was just how closely work inputs were related to access to resources. Adults in farming families with all but the most minimal property worked 70–80 hours a week, and this was true also of urban merchant families. In the sense that they work much shorter hours, often half to two-thirds as long, because there is no other work, both the landless rural population and the urban poor are under-employed. Where there is work on the farms, rice production takes priority, absorbing over twice as many hours of work as does housework— indeed, even women in this *purdah* society devote a minority of their working time to housework, spending more time processing the crops inside the courtyard or house or working surreptitiously in nearby fields at dusk or in the half-light of dawn.

Women work somewhat longer hours than men, partly because of the firm demands of the culture that only females should do housework and that only girls, unless there are no daughters in the family, should draw water. The situation has one rather surprising anomaly; among the richest houses males are spared some of the work because of the ability to employ labourers, while females often work uniquely long hours because houses are larger and entertaining may be greater (Khuda, 1978).

Work is segregated by sex and age to an extraordinary extent. This is sometimes obscured in survey work by using broad activity classifications. For instance, the whole family looks after cattle, but, in fact, boys watch the cows in the field, girls cut and bring home grass for them, women wash them down, and men feed them. However, if the family is small, or if there are difficulties caused by absences, sex imbalances among births, or life cycle stage, substitutions can be made. In such families in Bangladesh a boy may be seen drawing water instead of a girl, while in Africa a man may take a message instead of a boy. Such substitutions are usually felt to be very humiliating (Chapter 2) and are often avoided by adopting children or taking in suitable relatives for long periods.

Children work long hours, starting at about five years of age, reaching half of adult levels by about 10 years of age, two-thirds by 12 years and adult levels by about 14 years. Young men often work longer hours than their fathers, a fact frequently obscured by middle-aged men claiming that all their business journeys and talks are necessary—a situational advantage in the family which reaps personal advantage and which also justifies high fertility. There are two other forms of work differential. Daughters-in-law work longer hours than unmarried daughters in the same household, while unrelated live-in agricultural labourers (and servants in merchants' houses) usually work nearly all the time, often almost 100 hours per week.

It is important to note the time devoted in the peasant family to child care, because there are important demographic implications. There are two separate points. First, the time devoted mainly to child care is very small—only about 3% of all family work inputs. The reason is that there are many people around and that the child cannot do much damage to the house or to the few rather solid possessions. In any case, the hierarchy of importance within the family means that no-one thinks of devoting continuous time to a child so that every potential type of harm should be prevented from happening to him. Secondly, most child care is performed by siblings, usually by sisters, and only by brothers if there is no sister of an appropriate age.

In spite of the widespread distinction between "productive work" and housework in the analysis done by research workers[2], this distinction is largely illusory and misleading, and is usually evidence of the lingering impact of the family morality of age and sex segregation on the research worker. It is not a distinction between work that yields money and that which does not, because productive work is usually defined to include all work on crops even when most are eaten by the family. Even if it were strictly employed to separate subsistence from income-earning work, its use would still be misleading because of the extent to which various types of subsistence activity by one person can free another for income earning. In practice, the productive worker tends to be singled out as the adult male, or the person who works in the field, or the person who maintains that the product of the work is ultimately his to sell.

In the rural study we found that 8–10% of work—as measured by hours—was for money. There are complexities. The money earned by any member of the household is regarded as household money and as being under the control of the male household head. In landless families, female labourers are more likely than male labourers to be paid in kind. In any case, they may well describe their earnings as being paid to their husbands. There are many problems about who does work—he who directs it or those who work under his direction?

Beyond early childhood, males spend nearly all their working hours, and indeed most of their waking hours, outside the house. The house is not only the woman's work place—it is her place in all ways. It is a post-industrial myth that the pre-industrial family worked together. In fact, rural Bangladesh males spend most of their time outside the house with other males, usually their fathers or their sons. This has one implication of possible demographic importance: fathers, even of large families, are not affected by the presence or noise (usually, admittedly, very little) of numerous children in the house.

[2] The categorization of housework as "indirectly productive" is not much of an improvement (see Connell and Lipton, 1977, pp. 41–42).

The male working team consists most often of a man and his son, and less often of a man and more than one son. When two brothers work together they do so in the clear knowledge that one is the senior brother. However, male leisure hours are more likely to be spent with unrelated age peers. Women working in the house frequently work apart in different parts of the house but the oldest woman is almost invariably in charge.

The project investigated the initiation and direction of work. Much of this is essentially negative in that instructions are usually given only if expected work does not begin or continue. Nevertheless, a full third of all work was specifically instructed. In fact, an analysis of peasant conversation in South India showed that very little of the conversation was either general news or neutral conversation. It consisted overwhelmingly of two types: first, work instructions and nagging complaints, presumably meant to encourage the work, and, secondly, comment or scandal about those who were not doing exactly what the familial system expected (Caldwell and Caldwell, in preparation). This, then, was the spoken element of the cultural superstructure. People were asked why they did each job and again the replies were mostly of two types: first, that they would receive the family's gratitude or affection for doing the task, and, secondly, that they would be scolded or beaten if they did not do it. Clearly there is a family system.

For all work which produced a product which could be allocated for consumption, exchange or sale, the power to make such a decision and the concept of control and ownership were investigated. The power was found to lie securely in the hands of the patriarch. He regarded the product as his and saw himself as having produced it (so beware those who ask retrospective questions about production), and he saw the decisions about sale and the subsequent allocation of money as his own. Nevertheless, patriarchs also nearly all regarded such money as part of the family budget even if they allocated a disproportionate amount of it to their own needs.

The work input data was very well suited to the testing of *Chayanov's Rule* as enunciated by Marshall Sahlins (Sahlins, 1972, p. 91). It was found that, in terms of sheer numbers in the household, farming households were markedly inefficient when they had fewer than five members and average hours of work were unusually great in these circumstances. With between five and nine members, average work per head tended to decline, but beyond ten persons there was little more advantage. Most of the advantage that did accrue with numbers went to the female members of the household because of the ability of males in temporarily or permanently smaller households either to hire extra labour or to get help on a reciprocal basis (sometimes reciprocating later in the family life cycle) from relatives. Numbers had little effect on the work inputs of non-farming families.

The *Chayanov Slope* (Sahlins, 1972, pp. 108–121), measuring the balance between workers and consumers, was also examined. We actually carried out the examination in terms of the age instead of the worker–consumer balance because of our demonstration that persons of nearly every age were both workers and consumers. In farming families per capita work by age declines as the family life cycle produces a preponderance of adults. In only one other group was this phenomenon pronounced and that was amongst the modern urban elite. The reason, in the latter case, was that these families are relatively small and self-contained, obtaining little help from relatives and usually consisting of a residential nuclear family. Relatively, children help less than in other households, and therefore this group is peculiarly vulnerable to life cycle changes, so that the parents work unusually hard when the children are young but receive appreciable help from them as they grow older.

This kind of analysis helps to explain why it is in so many societies that farmers persist longest with high fertility while the modern urban elite are the first to control family size. It is not merely a matter of the latter having better education.

Living Between Modes

Much of the world's population is already caught in a transition from the familial mode to the labour market mode of production. Therefore, this transitional state is worthy of a great deal of attention although it has in fact received very little.

The earliest stage in this transition is that where the family is only indirectly employed by the market, in that they sell some of their produce. This margin of produce cannot be regarded simply as the surplus, as the money it earns is now needed for a range of conventionally indispensable expenditures. The family will tighten its belt and go hungry rather than eliminate this margin. In rural Bangladesh about 15% of the food grown was finding its way to the market. This appeared to do practically nothing to destabilize family relations and familial production. Family members did not identify this surplus as coming from any particular fraction of their individual labour. They regarded the produce that could be sold as being the fruit of the land, owned by the patriarch because he owned the land, and, to some extent, as being the result of his good direction, or of his ability to sell. The money received in return became part of the family stock, much like the food store, to be distributed by the patriarch as he saw fit. It should be added that demands for expenditure were always there and were urgent and there probably would have been a good deal of consensus about these expenditures in any case.

An apparently greater assault on the system of familial production is made when one or more members of the family work for part of their time for wages. In fact these wages, even when in cash rather than kind, do little to destabilize the situation. The earnings are regarded as family earnings under family (i.e. patriarchal) control. This is partly because family needs can be shown to be so necessitous that any failure to meet them would be regarded as an unnatural assault on the family. However, there is a more basic reason. The family farm, or even the family network of contacts, is regarded as the resource base from which the work is obtained. In rural areas, individuals are not employed as such but rather as members or representatives of families.

Seemingly the situation should change when the sons of the family migrate to the town for full-time employment. In Africa, Meillassoux (1972, p. 102) has shown that this is not so because urban employers do not have to—and do not—pay a wage that would support a family. In fact, urban employment is often capricious and not guaranteed from one time to the next. The reason that such low wages can be paid is the existence of the rural family which will take the migrant back at any time and which frequently includes his wife and children even when he is in the town. In these circumstances, the migrant can hardly break with his parents and other relatives; nor can he fail to work under his father's direction when back with the family or refuse to contribute most of his earnings to the family. The situation appears to be not dissimilar in Bangladesh and it has recently been described in very similar terms for India (Omvedt, 1980).

The position is not quite as stable amongst the landless and their smaller household numbers partly reflect the fact that adolescent or adult sons have broken with them. This is of demographic importance in that they lose control of their investment in children just as the latter have become most productive. Yet the astonishing fact is that most of the control exerted by farming families is also found amongst the landless. The reason is that even the landless family has a network of contacts for employment in rural areas and can provide a base for retreat and succour to the unsuccessful migrant in the town.

There is an important point which is almost always misunderstood, particularly by modernization theorists. There is a tendency to believe that the superstructure is an all-enveloping hypnotizing web and that everyone working in the system fully believes the entire myth. The corollary is that people pass once and for all from one mode of production to another. The truth is that many persons in the Third World work in both systems—in the town when they can secure a job and back with their family of origin when urban employment dries up. In neither situation do they appear to be like fish out of water aggressively showing their resentment. Instead, in the town they accept the employer's morality about honesty, the need for a fair day's work, and the overriding importance of the employer–employee contract; back with the family they accept the truth of all the proverbs about the need for age and sex segregation and the priority of family purposes. To a large degree they believe these different truths in their two different places without being in any way schizophrenic but regard the two different moralities—correctly—as being apposite to the two different modes of production. In fact they benefit in some ways from living in two worlds by being in a position to treat the urban employer's work times somewhat casually and also to ensure that their fathers treat them a little more carefully and with a little more respect then they would have otherwise done. The fact that African urban or mining workers could maximize their advantage in this way was often regarded by European employers as showing their incurable fecklessness and by First World sociologists as showing that they had not yet attained the psychological state of industrial man.

The Urban Situation

The parallel continuous observation of activity in Bangladesh took place in the only really large urbanized centre, the capital, Dacca. The contrasts with the rural area can be employed with care to demonstrate the differences in urban life and, especially amongst the poor, the adjustments that have to be made by rural–urban immigrant families.

Two points are of paramount importance. The first is that the urban population works on average considerably shorter hours than the rural population. The second is that just over half of all work in the city is for money—several times the fraction found in the country. Both these points require enlarging and qualifying.

The real difference in work inputs is less one of the differences between the urban and rural world views as between the resource bases. The rural landless do not work appreciably longer hours than the urban population. The merchant families of the urban traditional elite work very long hours with age and sex differentials in work strikingly similar to farming families. While urban males average only half the hours that rural males do, urban females work two-thirds the hours of their rural counterparts. The reason is that the urban house (even the poorest) is a resource base and a place where the poor can substitute labour for expenditure. In both urban and rural houses, endless housework will often take the place of quite modest alternative potential expenditure. Only a minority of work in the town is bound by an employer–employee contract, and even less by more than a casual contract. A good deal of the money earned comes from trade, some of it petty trading, or work secured on a daily or even hourly basis.

The examination of work inputs in Dacca brought out one crucially significant point. Adult males account for less than half the hours of work that yield money, and the proportion is still smaller among the rural poor who include most of the rural–urban migrants. The fraction earned by male household heads is very considerably lower than half. In these circumstances the patriarch retains (except sometimes in unemployed old age) a remarkable amount of authority, but the material basis of that authority is clearly weakened and he has to take this into account in terms of family relationships which are often less pyramidal and less dictatorial than was traditional in rural areas. Not only amongst modern elite wives, but also amongst even the wives of the urban poor, we found some money being spent by them on the grounds that it was their earnings—a phenomenon that hardly exists in rural areas. Many rural–urban migrant families are peculiarly dependent on the work of both wives and children, especially sons, when the whole family first secures an urban toehold. Because of the sanctions against females working outside the house, domestic work for others—a significant proportion of all income in Dacca—is done both by young sons, who are not constrained in this way, and by their mothers who both have the necessary skills and who are not exposed to quite such critical moral danger as unmarried adolescent girls.

Even the work in the urban informal sector is usually not part of a tightly bound system including all the family such as is found amongst farming families. Familial production certainly exists within the house, but it does not embrace the whole family, and, even amongst merchant families, younger sons are often in a position to secure full-time employment that would allow them, if they wished, to set up a separate household. Except for the very young, most of the urban population know that there is some chance that they will secure wage employment bound by the non-familial morality that such employment requires. This type of morality expressly sees itself as community and national morality, as objective and eternal, and as identifiable with the moralities taught by religion and school. It is a morality that says that priority must be given to the employer's objectives and not to the family, and it is a morality that emphasises that the agreement is with an individual and not with all members of his family. Such a situation affects an individual's behaviour and may ultimately affect his demographic performance.

Many of the measures we previously reported for rural areas are markedly different in the town. Much of the work is done on locations well away from the home and not owned by the family. Much of it is initiated by non-relatives. Little of it is done (except in the sense of bringing money home) to gain family affection, and it is spurred less by fear of physical punishment or even emotional attack than by losing employment or the possibility of greater returns in employment or promotion. Males are still found mostly outside the house during waking hours except among the modern elite. However, this exception is important, because amongst this group—those with education and working in the modern sector for wages or salaries—the male head of the household spends a considerable part of his time in the house. Inevitably, the possibility of a more companionate relationship between spouses is increased, and inevitably, too, the presence of children in the household impinges on their father.

Our observation of the use of time did reveal a major change in one type of activity between rural and urban areas, even somewhat surprisingly amongst the urban poor. The total proportion of all time spent on child care rises very greatly with the transition from rural to urban life. At the same time sibling responsibility for child care drops dramatically and mothers become overwhelmingly responsible for looking after their children. There are many reasons. If there are not greater dangers in the urban areas, there are new ones. There is a declining flow of all veneration towards the old and a greater feeling of responsibility towards children. There is another important factor which is likely, in the present debate about sex-roles, to be overlooked by social scientists from the industrialized world. Urban mothers, particularly middle class urban mothers, in the Third World are apt to regard the fact that they spend less time than others in the community on agricultural production and can instead devote more time to their children rather than delegating that task as a major social advance.[3]

There are demographic implications arising from these changes. Poor rural–urban migrants need their children to secure a purchase on town life and even to enable them to stay. The traditional elite, the merchants, organize their families much as do farmers and suffer little or not at all, from high fertility (Galal el Din, 1977). This is why simple measures of income are insufficient to determine the groups amongst whom fertility might first fall. However, the modern elite suffer from high fertility for four reasons. Their children do proportionately less work and hence are a genuine dependency burden. Second, and related to this, their small household size means that there are marked maximum and minimum periods of adult work strain during the family life cycle. Third, parents, largely mothers, undertake most of the child care. Fourth, the male household head actually spends very considerable periods within the house and is accordingly affected by the

[3] This point has been argued cogently with regard to the Sudan in a personal communication forming part of the Changing African Family correspondence by the Director of the Sudan segment, Mohamed el Awad Galal el Din (for the Changing African Family, see Okediji *et al.*, 1976)

presence of children. There can be gains too—as discussed below—from fertility, but there is every reason why fertility decline should begin amongst the modern urban elite.

Education

A complex factor related to the movement away from familial production, but by no means identical with it, is the spread of modern schooling. Our work in India has shown that schooling is least attractive to parents who have an adequate resource base for the children, largely farmers but sometimes even the traditional elite. However, the rural landless can secure very considerable advantages from the education of their children although the usual situation is that they cannot last the distance because of the immediate need for their work and because their children often have so little in the way of an educated background that they readily go to the wall in their schooling. In the towns, there is enormous pressure to keep children at school for urban earnings are usually in direct proportion to the duration of education (except amongst the merchant elite with their alternative resource base).

Education has two separate but marked effects on the transition from family to labour market production.

The first lies in the way that family economies can augment their incomes. As we have seen, family producing systems can often be supplemented by the outside earnings of junior members. There is a temptation to plan to increase those earnings by educating children. It may not even be very expensive to do this because sibling chains can be established whereby educated wage earners help their youngest siblings to stay at school.[4] The achievement of this is a tribute to the strength of familial morality. However, these kinds of families who chose to live in two worlds and to maximize their returns from two modes of production are flirting with danger because modern schooling systems almost invariably carry a Western message in favour of community morality and against familial morality (see Chapter 10). It is possible that the investment will not be adequately returned.

The second is that education is a major force in creating attitudes favouring child dependency. We divided all our Bangladesh families when choosing the original sample by their commitment to education. Those committed, especially in urban areas, regarded children's work outside schooling and homework as endangering the effort and investment already put into schooling. School children do even less work than might be anticipated by their hours spent in educational activites. In Africa it can be

[4] For Africa, see Chapter 2, p. 43.

shown that children who go to school are asked to do much less work, are treated more gently, and have more spent upon them than is the experience of their uneducated siblings (Caldwell, 1968a pp. 105–110). Schools also directly preach a message of child dependence and the fact that school children are clearly doing different things and are even dressed differently reinforces the message of dependence.

Even if schooling at first enhances the value of children, its role in making them a greater burden will inevitably become more significant as community educational levels rise, as the differential returns to education become less, and as educated children become more likely to retain a large share of their earnings. The traditional family emphasized duties to parents over those to spouses, but the message received from extended education is very different. In addition, more of the educated children are likely to survive. They are no longer treated as the least important members of the household. Research in an African city showed that children who went to school were twice as likely to be taken to medical facilities when sick as illiterate children (see Chapter 10). Moreover, this is only one measure of the extra care they receive.

A Synthesis

Although the Bangladesh peasant family is no longer a wholly subsistence producer, and although some of the children may go to school at least for a short period, the familial mode of production largely remains intact. The patriarch's sole right to control the land and his ownership of its product is undisputed. Other members of the family take it that they receive, in return for their labour, food, housing and security. If they were to demand more, the patriarch's control of resources, together with local support for his attitude, would certainly be great enough to render the challenge harmless. Even on small farms, there appears to be plenty of work to be done by intensifying labour. Work is so segregated by age and sex that very small families find their members doing work that they feel to be inappropriate and humbling. In addition, cooperation is so necessary in farming that families with fewer than five members work unusually long hours. Given that there is erosion of family numbers rising both from child mortality and from subsequent departures for marriage or work, the level of fertility needed to remain above the minimum is probably not below that which has always existed. This view is reinforced by the fact that per capita levels of work fall gently even as family size rises well above this minimum.

The key question is whether the resource base for familial production has vanished for other sections of the society. Certainly, the heads of landless families can no longer offer sufficient hours of work to keep their family members consistently employed or to provide anything above a miserable standard of living. In this case, the maintenance of the system and the unequal consumption and share of power which is its very basis depends on the refusal of farmers to provide employment to children who have broken with their families. So far, this is happening, but the system may well be challenged eventually by the growth of commercial agriculture. As these families depend for their livelihood on aggricultural labour, there are some advantages to the older generation in having a sizeable number of strong sons who not only might work longer hours but who might more easily secure employment than those whose strength has dwindled with age.

The position is more difficult still for the patriarch of a poor urban family, because, in the city, there is no real question of employers refusing jobs to unfaithful sons. However, there is still a value in family contacts for securing employment. Sons are such an important source of income that high fertility will decline only when they more consistently challenge their father's authority.

The position of the merchant elite is rather like that of the farmers except that they have a greater temptation to educate their children and so convert them into the modern elite.

Even amongst the modern elite, there are returns to high fertility as long as the familial morality holds firm. In an African city it has been shown that high fertility persists amongst most of the modern elite because they can use their position to secure high paying positions for their children and because their children still return a substantial fraction of their earnings to their parents (see Chapter 2). In other words the *wealth flow* (see Chapter 4) is still upward. Nevertheless, such family relationships are likely to be shattered earliest among the modern urban elite and it is amongst them that fertility will first decline. (There is evidence of this already, even in Dacca.)

What we have, then, is a resource base guaranteed to back up patriarchal powers and to ensure the survival of the familial mode of production only among the peasant farmers and the urban merchants. What we have elsewhere is the survival of the superstructure while the material base has changed. As long as that superstructure survives largely intact—as long as earnings are placed in a common family pool under the control of the patriarch who can decree unequal consumption—the familial system (and its high fertility) will remain intact. The superstructure still has many elements of strength—such as the control of marriage by the older generation—which we have not discussed.

Nevertheless, once the mode of production changes it is inevitable that the superstructure will eventually do so too. The capitalist employer has strong reasons for wanting to negotiate with a potential employee as an individual and not as the member of a family and to teach him while he is an employee that he is an individual. As non-familial production increases, the producers increasingly desire to expand their market by tempting individual members of the family to be consumers and not to think in family terms (Ruzicka and Caldwell, 1977; Chapter 6). For a time, of course, the patriarch can regard expenditure without his permission as immoral and purchased items as his own—thus reducing the temptation to buy—but this situation is unstable. The fact of a labour market also means the possibility of employment for family members which has not been approved by the family head and this can erode the familial system—although there remains the need for a fall-back security system. Once the resource base disappears, the spread of the educational system helps to erode the superstructure. One reason is that it fits persons for jobs of a kind that were never related to family production. However, the most important reason is that it imports many Western assumptions about family relationships that are at odds with the family system. It often implies the dependency of children. It also implies that the emotional links between spouses should be strong—stronger than their obligations to their own parents and perhaps being expressed in obligations to their children which would take priority over those to their parents. There is some evidence that middle class parents first curtail their fertility when they realize that their upbringing of their children has imparted messages which will eventually result in those children not giving economic priority to their parents (Caldwell and Caldwell, 1978, pp. 16).

The superstructure of the familial mode of production has enormous persistence. The most industrialized countries have not yet even approached the culture that will eventually be produced by the labour market mode of production. This means that it was possible to use the superstructure of the familial mode of production in an industrialized society to structure a sub-mode, a familial mode of production, within the major mode (see Chapter 5). A system developed whereby the male household head sold his labour on the outside market and so was termed the breadwinner. With some of his money he financed the subsistence household production of goods and services within his home by his wife, daughters and, to a lesser extent, his sons. Both power and consumption were shared unequally. This last form of familial production has proved unstable because the developing industrial system is inevitably tempted to offer employment to wives and to produce competing domestic goods and services for sale.

The fully developed labour market mode of production offers no rewards for high fertility or indeed for any fertility at all. When fully developed, it is doubtful whether even stationary population will be maintained. However, forms of familial production have ensured that fertility remained high in many societies long after the peasant mode of production was reduced to only a minor part of the economy. The labour market mode of production does help in the reduction of child mortality because it is not benefited by having a superstructure favouring the veneration of the old.

Finally, there is one reason for high fertility among poor populations, both rural and urban, that has not been discussed, and which can have implications for mortality as well as fertility. Children represent an investment in future labour (Caldwell, 1981). This is true not only when there are few alternative investments—the usual condition among the Third World poor—but when there are no other ways of saving. When a family is clearly in dire need, no patriarch could retain part of the income for investment rather than for meeting the current need. But, if children are already born, he can easily share the existing food among the newcomers—familial morality ensures that this can be done easily, without protest, and even without anyone analysing the situation. This will probably do something to raise mortality risks, especially among the very young who are usually at greater risk and are found well down in the priority list established by familial morality, but there will certainly be some gain in the size of the future family work force.

References

Ackermann, J. (1913). "Australia from a Woman's Point of View." Cassell, London.

Adepoju, A. (1974). *Africa* **44**, 383–396.

Alberto, J. (1976). "The Growth of the Australian Labour Force and Trends in Women's Participation." mimeo.

Ames, M. M. (1973). *Social Compass* **20**, 139–170.

Ariès, P. (1962). "Centuries of Childhood." Jonathan Cape, London.

Arnold, F. and Fawcett, J. T. (1975). "The Value of Children: A Cross-National Study, III, Hawaii." East–West Population Institute, Honolulu.

Arnold, F., Bulatao, R. A., Buripakdi, C., Chung, B. J., Fawcett, J. T., Iritani, T., Lee, S. J. and Wu, T.-S. (1975). "The Value of Children: A Cross-National Study, I, Introduction and Comparative Analysis." East-West Population Institute, Honolulu.

Arowolo, O. O. (n.d.). "Female Labour Force Participation and Fertility: The Case of Ibadan City in Nigeria." Unpublished paper.

Australia: Commonwealth Bureau of Census and Statistics (1947). "Official Year Book of the Commonwealth of Australia, No. 36, 1944–1945." Canberra.

Australia: Commonwealth Bureau of Census and Statistics (1928). "Demography Bulletin, No. 45, 1927." Canberra.

Australia: Department of Labour and National Service (1970). "Women in the Workforce, No. 9, Changing Horizons." Melbourne.

Australian Family Formation Project (1972). "Numerical and Percentage Distributions of Responses to each Question by Pre-Coded Response." Department of Demography, Australian National University, Canberra.

Banfield, E. C. (1958). "The Moral Basis of a Backward Society." The Free Press, Glencoe, UK.

Banks, J. A. (1954). "Prosperity and Parenthood: A Study of Family Planning Among the Victorian Middle Classes." Routledge and Kegan Paul, London.

Bascom, W. R. (1952). *The Journal of the Royal Anthropological Institute of Great Britain and Ireland* **82**, 63–69.

Bascom, W. R. (1969). "The Yoruba of Southwestern Nigeria." Holt, Rinehart and Winston, New York.

Baumann, H. (1928). *Africa* **1**, 289–319.

Becker, G. (1960). *In* "Demographic and Economic Change in Developed Countries" (Universities-National Bureau Committee for Economic Research), pp. 209–231. Princeton University Press, Princeton.

Bellah, R. N. (1969). *Religious Studies* **4**, 37–45.

Bendix, R. (1964). "Nation-Building and Citizenship: Studies of our Changing Social Order." Wiley, New York.

Bendix, R. (1967). *Comparative Studies in Society and History* **9**, 292–346.

Ben-Porath, Y. (1979). *In* "Economic and Demographic Change: Issues for the 1980s. Proceedings of the Conference, Helsinki 1978." Vol. 3, pp. 51–62. IUSSP, Liège.

Benston, M. (1969). *Monthly Review* **21** (4), 13–27.

Berelson, B. (1966). "Family Planning and Population Programs" (B. Berelson, ed.), pp. 655–668. University of Chicago Press, Chicago.

Béteille, A. (1974). "Six Essays in Comparative Sociology." Oxford University Press, Delhi.

Bethlehem, D. W. (1975). *International Journal of Psychology* **10**, 219–224.

Black, C. E. (1966). "The Dynamics of Modernization: A Study in Comparative History." Harper and Row, New York.

Black, C. E., Jansen, M. B., Levine, H. S. Levy, M. J. Jr., Rosovsky, H., Rozman, G., Smith, H. D. III and Starr, S. F. (1975). "Modernization of Japan and Russia: A Comparative Study." Free Press, Macmillan, New York.

Blacker, C. P. (1947). *Eugenics Review* **39**, 88–101.

Blake, J. (1968). *Population Studies* **22**, 5–25.

Blake, J. and Das Gupta, P. (1975). *Population and Development Review* **1**, 229–249.

Blumberg, R. L. and Winch, R. F. (1972). *American Journal of Sociology* **77**, 898–920.

Boserup, E. (1965). "The Conditions of Agricultural Growth: The Economics of Agrarian Change under Population Pressure." Aldine, Chicago.

Boserup, E. (1970). "Women's Role in Economic Development." Allen and Unwin, London.

Boulier, B. (1977). *Journal of Philippine Development* **4**, 195–222.

Bourgeois-Pichat, J. (1965). *In* "Population in History: Essays in Historical Demography" (D. V. Glass and D. E. C. Eversley, eds), pp. 474–506. Edward Arnold, London.

Brass, W., Coale, A. J., Demeny, P., Heisel, D. F., Lorimer, F., Romaniuk, A. and van de Walle, E. (1968). "The Demography of Tropical Africa." Princeton University Press, Princeton.

Bulatao, R. (1975). "The Value of Children: A Cross-National Study, II, Philippines." East–West Population Institute, Honolulu.

Burch, T. K. (1967). *American Sociological Review* **32**, 347–363.

Burch, T. K. (1970). *Demography* 7, 61–69.
Burch, T. K. and Gendell, M. (1971). *In* "Culture and Population: A Collection of Current Studies" (S. Polgar, ed.), pp. 87–104. Carolina Population Center, Chapel Hill.
Burridge, A. F. (1882). *Journal of the Institute of Actuaries, London* 23, 309–327.
Burridge, A. F. (1884). *Journal of the Institute of Actuaries, London* 24, 333–354.
Butlin, N. (1964). "Investment in Australian Economic Development." Cambridge University Press, Cambridge.
Butlin, N. (1970). *In* "Australian Economic Development in the Twentieth Century" (C. Forster, ed.), pp. 266–327. Allen and Unwin, Sydney.
Butz, W. P. (1972). *Rand Paper* P-4903.
Cain, M. T. (1977). *Population and Development Review* 3, 201–227.
Cain, M. T. (1978). *Population and Development Review* 4, 421–438.
Cain, M., Khanam, S. R. and Nahar, S. (1979). *Population and Development Review* 5, 405–438.
Caldwell, J. C. (1965). *Population Studies* 19, 183–199.
Caldwell, J. C. (1966). *Population Studies* 20, 5–26.
Caldwell, J. C. (1967a). *Economic Development and Cultural Change* 15, 217–238.
Caldwell, J. C. (1967b). *In* "Thailand: Social and Economic Studies in Development" (T. H. Silcock, ed.), pp. 27–64. Australian National University Press, Canberra.
Caldwell, J. C. (1968a). "Population Growth and Family Change in Africa: The New Urban Elite in Ghana." Australian National University Press, Canberra.
Caldwell, J. C. (1968b). *Population Studies* 22, 361–377.
Caldwell, J. C. (1968c). *Demography* 5, 598–619.
Caldwell, J. C. (1969). "African Rural–Urban Migration: The Movement to Ghana's Towns." Australian National University Press, Canberra, and Columbia University Press, New York.
Caldwell, J. C. (1973). *In* "Fertility and Family Formation: Australasian Bibliography and Essays" (H. Ware, ed.), pp. A3–A13. Demography Department, Australian National University, Canberra.
Caldwell, J. C. (1974). *Occasional Paper* No. 7. World Fertility Survey, Voorburg.
Caldwell, J. C. (1975a). Ed., "Population Growth and Socioeconomic Change in West Africa." Columbia University Press, New York.
Caldwell, J. C. (1975b). *In* "Population Growth and Socioeconomic Change in West Africa" (J. C. Caldwell, ed.), pp. 58–97. Columbia University Press, New York.
Caldwell, J. C. (1975c). *Studies in Family Planning* 6, 429–436.
Caldwell, J. C. (1975d). *Occasional Paper*, No. 8, Overseas Liaison Committee, Washington.
Caldwell, J. C. (1976). "The Socio-economic Explanation of High Fertility: Papers on the Yoruba Society of Nigeria." Demography Department, Australian National University, Canberra.
Caldwell, J. C. (1977a). Ed., "The Persistence of High Fertility: Population Prospects in the Third World." Demography Department, Australian National University, Canberra.
Caldwell, J. C. (1977b). *In* "The Economic and Social Supports for High Fertility" (L. T. Ruzicka, ed.), pp. 439–454. Demography Department, Australian National University, Canberra.
Caldwell, J. C. 1979. *Population Studies* 33, 395–413.

Caldwell, J. C. (1980). *In* "Living Together: Family Patterns and Lifestyles" (D. Davies, G. Caldwell, D. Boorer and M. Bennett, eds), pp. 17–25. Centre for Continuing Education, Australian National University, Canberra.

Caldwell, J. C. (1981). *Occasional Paper* No. 25, Development Studies Centre, Australian National University, Canberra.

Caldwell, J. C. forthcoming. *In* "Population of Australia" (L. G. Hopkins, ed.). United Nations Economic and Social Commission for Asia and the Pacific, Bangkok.

Caldwell, J. C. (in press). *In* "General History of Africa." (A. Boahen, ed.). UNESCO, Paris.

Caldwell, J. C. and Caldwell, P. (1976). *Journal of Biosocial Science* **8**, 347–365.

Caldwell, J. C. and Caldwell, P. (1977). *Population Studies* **31**, 193–217.

Caldwell, J. C. and Caldwell, P. (1978). *Studies in Family Planning* **9**, 2–18.

Caldwell, J. C. and Caldwell, P. (1980). *In* "Proceedings of the Conference on Population and Development in the ECWA Region, Amman, November 1978". United Nations Economic Council for West Asia, Beirut.

Caldwell, J. C. and Caldwell, P. (1981). *In* "Child-spacing in Tropical Africa: Traditions and Change" (H. J. Page and R. Lesthaeghe, eds), pp. 181–199. Academic Press, London and New York.

Caldwell, J. C. and Igun, A. (1970). *Population Studies* **24**, 21–34.

Caldwell, J. C. and Igun, A. (1972). *In* "Population Growth and Economic Development in Africa." (S. H. Ominde and C. N. Ejiogu, eds), pp. 67–76. Heinemann, London.

Caldwell, J. C. and Ruzicka, L. T. (1977). *Working Papers In Demography* **7**. Demography Department, Australian National University, Canberra.

Caldwell, J. C. and Ware, H. (1973). *Population Studies* **27**, 7–31.

Caldwell, J. C. and Ware, H. (1977). *Population Studies* **31**, 487–507.

Caldwell, J. C., Young, C., Ware, H., Lavis, D. and Davis, A.-T. (1973). *Studies in Family Planning* **4**, 49–59.

Caldwell, J. C., Campbell, D., Caldwell, P., Ruzicka, L., Cosford, W., Packer, R., Grocott, J. and Neill, M. (1976). "Towards an Understanding of Contemporary Demographic Change." Demography Department, Australian National University, Canberra.

Caldwell, J. C., Harrison, G. E. and Quiggin, P. (1980). *World Development* **8**, 953–967.

Caldwell, J. C., Jalaluddin, A. K. M., Caldwell, P. and Cosford, W. (1981a). *Working Paper* 12, Department of Demography, Australian National University, Canberra.

Caldwell, J. C., McDonald, P. F. and Ruzicka, L. T. (1981b). *In* "Nuptiality and Fertility: Proceedings of the IUSSP Seminar, Bruges, 8–11 January, 1979" (L. T. Ruzicka, ed.), pp. 211–241. Ordina Press, Liège.

Caldwell, P. (1977). *In* "The Persistence of High Fertility: Population Prospects in the Third World." (J. C. Caldwell, ed.), pp. 593–616. Demography Department, Australian National University, Canberra.

Cannon, M. (1975). "Australia in the Victorian Age." Nelson, Melbourne.

Carlsson, G. (1966). *Population Studies* **20**, 149–174.

Carnoy, M. (1974). "Education as Cultural Imperialism." Longman, New York.

Carr-Saunders, A. M. (1922). "The Population Problem: A Study in Human Evolution." Clarendon Press, Oxford.

Carr-Saunders, A. M. (1936). "World Population: Past Growth and Present Trends." Frank Cass, London.

Chamie, J. (1977). *Population Studies* **31**, 365–382.

Changing African Family (1974). "The Changing African Family, Nigerian Segment, Project 2, The Value of Children: Work Performed by Children in the Western and Lagos States of Nigeria." Demography Department, Australian National University, Canberra.

Chayanov, A. V. (1966a). In "The Theory of Peasant Economy." (D. Thorner, B. Kerblay and R. E. F. Smith, eds; A. V. Chayanov, author), pp. 1–28. American Economic Association, Richard Irwin, Homewood, Ill.

Chayanov, A. V. (1966b). In "The Theory of Peasant Economy." (D. Thorner, B. Kerblay and R. E. S. Smith, eds; A. V. Chayanov, author), pp. 29–269. American Economic Association, Richard Irwin, Homewood, Ill.

Childe, V. G. (1964). "What Happened in History." Penguin, Harmondsworth.

Chiñas, B. (1973). "The Isthmus Zapotecs: Women's Roles in Cultural Context." Holt, Rinehart and Winston, New York.

Clark, C. (1951). "The Conditions of Economic Progress." Macmillan, London.

Clark, C. (1967). "Population Growth and Land Use." Macmillan, London.

Clignet, R. (1970). "Many Wives, Many Powers: Authority and Power in Polygynous Families." Northwestern University Press, Evanston.

Clignet, R. (1975). Comparative Education Review 19, 88–104.

Coale, A. J. (1967). In "World Population Conference, 1965." Vol. 2, pp. 205–209. United Nations, New York.

Coale, A. J. (1969). In "Fertility and Family Planning: A World View." (S. J. Behrman, L. Corsa and R. Freedman, eds), pp. 3–24. University of Michigan Press, Ann Arbor.

Coale, A. J. (1973). In "International population Conference, Liège, 1973.", Vol. I, pp. 53–72. International Union for the Scientific Study of Population, Liège.

Coale, A. J. and Demeny, P. (1966). "Regional Model Life Tables and Stable Populations." Princeton University Press, Princeton.

Coale, A. J. and Hoover, E. M. (1958). "Population Growth and Economic Development in Low-income Countries: A Case Study of India's Prospects." Princeton University Press, Princeton.

Coale, A. J. and Zelnik, M. (1963). "New Estimates of Fertility and Population in the United States." Princeton University Press. Princeton.

Coale, A. J., Goldman, N. and Cho. L.-J. (1981). In "Nuptiality and Fertility: Proceedings of the IUSSP Seminar, Bruges, 8–11 January, 1979" (L. T. Ruzicka, ed.), pp. 43–60. Ordina Press, Liège.

Cochrane, S. H. (1979). "Fertility and Education: What Do We Really Know?" Johns Hopkins University Press, Baltimore.

Cohn, B. S. (1965). American Anthropologist 67, No. 5, Part 2 (Special Publication), 82–122.

Collingwood, R. G. (1946). "The Idea of History." Clarendon Press, Oxford.

Colver, A. (1963). American Sociological Review 28, 86–96.

Connell, J. and Lipton, M. (1977). "Assessing Village Labour Situations in Developing Countries." Oxford University Press, Delhi.

Coombs, L. and Fernandez, D. (1978). Demography 15, 57–73.

Cooper, N. (1969). In "It's People that Matter: Education for Social Change." (D. McLean, ed.), pp. 66–80. Angus and Robertson, Sydney.

Courel, A. and Pool, D. I. (1975). In "Population Growth and Socioeconomic Change in West Africa" (J. C. Caldwell, ed.), pp. 736–754. Columbia University Press, New York.

Crook, N. R. (1978). The Journal of Development Studies 14, 198–210.

Dalton, G. (1971) Ed., "Studies in Economic Anthropology." American Anthropological Association, Washington.

Dandekar, V. M. and Dandekar, K. (1953). "Survey of Fertility and Mortality in Poona District." Gokhale Institute of Politics and Economics, Poona.

Dankoussou, I., Diarra, S., Laya, D. and Pool, D. I. (1975). In "Population Growth and Socioeconomic Change in West Africa." (J. C. Caldwell, ed.), pp. 679–693. Columbia University Press, New York.

Darton, H. F. J. (1958). "Children's Books in England: Five Centuries of Social Life." Cambridge University Press, Cambridge.

Davis, K. (1949). "Human Society." Macmillan, New York.

Davis, K. (1955). *Eugenics Quarterly* **2**, 33–39.

Davis, K. (1962). *Population Review* **6** (2), 67–73.

Davis, K. (1977). In "Essays on Economic Development and Cultural Change" (M. Nash, ed.), pp. 159–179. University of Chicago Press, Chicago.

Davis, K. and Blake, J. (1956). *Economic Development and Cultural Change* **4**, 211–235.

Davis, N. Z. (1977). *Daedalus* **106**, 87–114.

Dawson, J. L. M., Law, H., Leung, A. and Whitney, R. E. (1971). *Journal of Cross-Cultural Psychology* **2**, 1–27.

de Beauvoir, S. (1972). "The Second Sex." Penguin, Harmondsworth.

Deng, F. M. (1972). "The Dinka of the Sudan." Holt, Rinehart and Winston, New York.

De Schlippe, P. (1956). "Shifting Cultivation in Africa: The Zande System of Agriculture." Routledge and Kegan Paul, London.

De Tray, D. N. (1973). *Journal of Political Economy* **81**, S70–S95.

Deutsch, K. W. (1961). *American Political Science Review* **55**, 493–514.

Diamond, N. (1969). "K'un Shen: A Taiwan Village." Holt, Rinehart and Winston, New York.

Douglas, A. (1978). "The Feminization of American Culture." Avon, New York.

Dow, T. E. Jr. (1967). *Demography* **4**, 780–797.

Dow, T. E., Jr. and Benjamin, E. (1975). In "Population Growth and Socioeconomic Change in West Africa" (J. C. Caldwell, ed.), pp. 427–454. Columbia University Press, New York.

Driver, E. (1963). "Differential Fertility in Central India." Princeton University Press, Princeton.

Dunn, P. (1976). In "The History of Childhood." (L. de Mause, ed.), pp. 383–405. Souvenir, London.

Easterlin, R. A. (1968). "Population, Labor Force, and Long Swings in Economic Growth: The American Experience." National Bureau of Economic Research, New York.

Easterlin, R. (1969). In "Fertility and Family Planning: A World View." (S. J. Behrman, L. Corsa and R. Freedman, eds), pp. 127–156. University of Michigan Press, Ann Arbor.

Easterlin, R. A. (1976). *Journal of American History* **63**, 600–615.

Eisenstadt, S. N. (1966). "Modernization: Protest and Change." Prentice-Hall, Englewood Cliffs.

Encyclopaedia Britannica. (1953). "Education" (Vol. 7, pp. 964–1006).

Endres, M. E. (1975). "On Defusing the Population Bomb." Halstead Press, Cambridge, Mass.

Enke, S. (1966). *Economic Journal* **76**, 44–56.

Epstein, E. H. (1971). *Comparative Education Review* 15, 188–201.

Epstein, S. (1962). "Economic Development and Social Change in South India." Manchester University Press. Manchester.

Epstein, T. S. (1967). *In* "The Craft of Social Anthropology." (A. L. Epstein, ed.), pp. 153–180. Tavistock, London.

Evans-Pritchard, E. E. (1940). "The Nuer: A Description of Livelihood and Political Institutions of a Nilotic People." Clarendon, Oxford.

Fakhouri, H. (1972). "Kafr El-Elow: An Egyptian Village in Transition." Holt, Rinehart and Winston, New York.

Fallers, L. A. and Fallers, Margaret C. (1976). *In* "Mediterranean Family Structures." (J. G. Peristiany, ed.), pp. 243–260. Cambridge University Press, Cambridge.

Fawcett, J. T. (1972). "The Satisfactions and Costs of Children: Theories, Concepts and Methods." East–West Center, Honolulu.

Fei, H.-T. (1939). "Peasant Life in China." Routledge and Kegan Paul, London.

Fei, H.-T. and Chang, C.-I. (1949). "Earthbound China: A Study of Rural Economy in Yunnan." Routledge and Kegan Paul, London.

Feldman, A. S. and Hurn, C. (1966). *Sociometry* 29, 378–395.

Fernea, E. W. (1976). "A Street in Marrakech." Anchor/Doubleday, New York.

Figes, E. (1970). "Patriarchal Attitudes." Faber and Faber, London.

Firestone, S. (1971). "The Dialectic of Sex: The Case for Feminist Revolution." Jonathan Cape, London.

Firth, R. (1967). Ed., "Themes in Economic Anthropology." Tavistock, London.

Ford, G. W. (1970). *In* "Australian Society: A Sociological Introduction." (A. F. Davies and S. Encel, eds), pp. 84–145. Cheshire, Melbourne.

Foster, G. M. (1973). "Traditional Societies and Technological Change." Harper and Row, New York.

Fraser, T. M. (1966). "Fishermen of south Thailand: The Malay Villagers." Holt, Rinehart and Winston, New York.

Freedman, D. S. (with Mueller, E.) (1974). *Occasional Paper* No. 11, World Fertility Survey, Voorburg.

Freedman, R. (1961–62). *Current Sociology* 10/11, 35–121.

Freedman, R. (1975). "The Sociology of Human Fertility: An Annotated Bibliography." The Population Council, Irvington, New York.

Freedman, R. and Coombs, L. (1974). "Cross-Cultural Comparisons: Data on Two Factors in Fertility Behavior." The Population Council, New York.

Freedman, R. and Takeshita, J. Y. (1969). "Family Planning in Taiwan: An Experiment in Social Change." Princeton University Press, Princeton.

Freedman, R., Peng, J. Y., Takeshita, Y. and Sun, T. H. (1963). *Population Studies* 16, 219–236.

Freedman, R., Coombs, L. and Chang, M.-C. (1972). *Taiwan Population Studies Working Paper* 19.

Freedman, R., Weinberger, M. B., Fan, T.-H. and Wei, S.-P. (1976). *Taiwan Population Studies Working Paper* 31.

Frejka, T. (1980). *Population and Development Review* 6, 65–93.

French, M. (1977). "The Women's Room." Sphere Books, London.

Frenkel, I. (1976). *Population Studies* 30, 35–57.

Friedan, B. (1963). "The Feminine Mystique." Victor Gollancz, London.

Fry, E. (1956). "The Condition of the Urban Wage Earning Class in Australia in the 1880s." Ph.D. thesis, Department of History, Research School of Social Sciences, Australian National University.

Fusé, T. (1975). *In* "Modernization and Stress in Japan." (T. Fusé, ed.), pp. 1–11. Brill, Leiden.

Gadalla, S. (1978). "Is There Hope? Fertility and Family Planning in a Rural Egyptian Community." American University in Cairo Press, Cairo and Carolina Population Center, University of North Carolina, Chapel Hill.

Gaisie, S. K. (1975). *In* "Population Growth and Socioeconomic Change in West Africa." (J. C. Caldwell, ed.), pp. 339–345. Columbia University Press, New York.

Galal el Din, M. el A. (1977). *In* "The Persistence of High Fertility: Population Prospects in the Third World." (J. C. Caldwell, ed.), pp. 633–658. Demography Department, Australian National University, Canberra.

Galletti, R., Baldwin, K. D. S. and Dina, I. O. (1956). "Nigerian Cocoa Farmers: An Economic Survey of Yoruba Cocoa Farming Families." Oxford University Press, Oxford.

Garlick, P. C. (1971). "African Traders and Economic Development in Ghana." Clarendon Press, Oxford.

Gille, H. and Pardoko, P. H. (1966). *In* "Family Planning and Population Programs: A Review of World Development." (B. Berelson, ed.), pp. 503–521. Chicago University Press, Chicago.

Giraure, N. (1975). *In* "Education in Melanesia." (J. Brammal and R. J. May, eds), pp. 101–104. Research School of Pacific Studies, Australian National University, Canberra and University of Papua and New Guinea, Port Moresby.

Gluckman, M. (1955). "Custom and Conflict in Africa." Basil Blackwell, Oxford.

Goode, W. (1963a). "World Revolution and Family Patterns." The Free Press, Glencoe UK.

Goode, W. J. (1963b). *In* "Industrialization and Society." (B. F. Hoselitz and W. E. Moore, eds), pp. 237–255. UNESCO, Mouton, Paris.

Goody, J. and Watt, I. (1963). *Comparative Studies in Society and History* **5**, 304–345.

Gooneratne, M. Y. (1968). *Ceylon Historical Journal* **14**.

Gore, M. S. (1968). "Urbanization and Family Change." Popular Prakashan, Bombay.

Graburn, N. H. (1971). *In* "Studies in Economic Anthropology." (G. Dalton, ed.), pp. 107–121. American Anthropological Association, Washington.

Graff, H. J. (1979). *Population and Development Review* **5**, 105–140.

Greenfield, P. M. and Bruner, J. S. (1966). *International Journal of Psychology* **1**, 89–107.

Griffiths, D. W. (1957). Ed., "Documents on the Establishment of Education in New South Wales, 1789–1880." Australian Council for Educational Research, Melbourne.

Gusfield, J. R. (1967). *American Journal of Sociology* **72**, 351–362.

Hagen, E. E. (1962). "On the Theory of Social Change: How Economic Growth Begins." Dorsey, Homewood, Ill.

Haire, N. (1943). "Sex Problems of Today." Angus and Robertson, Sydney.

Hajnal, J. (1965). *In* "Population in History: Essays in Historical Demography." (D. V. Glass and D. E. C. Eversley, eds), pp. 101–143. Arnold, London.

Hall, A. R. (1976). *Economic Record* **52**, 36–52.

Hara, Y. (1977). *The Developing Economies* **15**, 440–461.

Harrell-Bond, B. (1975). *In* "Population Growth and Socioeconomic Change in West Africa" (J. C. Caldwell, ed.), pp. 473–489. Columbia University Press, New York.

Hartmann, H. (1976). *Signs* **1**, 137–169.

Hatt, P. K. (1952). Ed., "World Population and Future Resources: Proceedings of the Second Centennial Academic Conference of Northwestern University." American Book Company, New York.

Hauser, P. M. and Duncan, O. D. (1959). *In* "The Study of Population: An Inventory and Appraisal." (P. M. Hauser and O. D. Duncan, eds), pp. 76–105. University of Chicago Press, Chicago.

Hawthorn, G. (1970). "The Sociology of Fertility." Collier-Macmillan, London.

Hawthorn, G. (1978). *Journal of Development Studies* **14**, 1–21.

Hawthorn, G. (in press). *In* "Determinants of Fertility Trends: Major Theories and New Directions for Research." (T. Mackensen and C. Höhn, eds), Ordina (for IUSSP), Liège.

Heer, D. M. and Smith, D. O. (1967). "Contributed Papers: Sydney Conference, International Union for the Scientific Study of Population, 21–25 August 1967."

Henry, L. (1956). *INED, Travaux et Documents*, Cahier No. 26. Presses Universitaires de France, Paris.

Henry, L. (1965). *In* "Population in History: Essays in Historical Demography." (D. V. Glass and D. E. C. Eversley, eds), pp. 434–456. Edward Arnold, London.

Herskovits, M. J. (1952). "Economic Anthropology: A Study in Comparative Economics." Knopf, New York.

Hicks, N. (1971). "Evidence and Opinion about the Peopling of Australia, 1890–1911." Ph.D. thesis, Demography Department, Australian National University.

Hicks, N. (1978). " 'This Sin and Scandal': Australia's Population Debate 1891–1911." Australian National University Press, Canberra.

Hill, P. (1972). "Rural Hausa: A Village and a Setting." Cambridge University Press, London.

Hill, R. (1967). *In* "Family and Fertility." (W. T. Liu, ed.), pp. 3–22. University of Notre Dame Press, Notre Dame.

Hindess, B. and Hirst, P. Q. (1975). "Pre-Capitalist Modes of Production." Routledge and Kegan Paul, London and Boston.

Hollingsworth, T. H. (1965). *In* "Population in History: Essays in Historical Demography" (D. V. Glass and D. E. C. Eversley, eds), pp. 354–378. Edward Arnold, London.

Hopen, C. E. (1958). "The Pastoral Fulbe Family in Gwandu." International African Institute, Oxford University Press, Oxford.

Hsu, F. L-K. (1943). *The American Journal of Sociology* **48**, 555–562.

Hull, T. H. and Hull, V. J. (1977). *In* "The Persistence of High Fertility: Population Prospects in the Third World." (J. C. Caldwell, ed.), pp. 827–894. Demography Department, Australian National University, Canberra.

Hunt, D. (1979). *The Journal of Peasant Studies* **6**, 247–285.

Imoagene, O. (1976). "Social Mobility in Emergent Society: A Study of the New Elite in Western Nigeria." Demography Department, Australian National University.

Inkeles, A. (1969). *American Journal of Sociology* **75**, 208–225.

Inkeles, A. (1977). *Journal of Cross-Cultural Psychology* **8**, 135–176.

Inkeles, A. and Miller, K. A. (1974). *International Journal of Sociology and the Family* **4**, 127–147.

Inkeles, A. and Smith, D. H. (1974). "Becoming Modern: Individual Change in Six Developing Countries." Heinemann, London.

International Labour Office (1978). "Yearbook of Labour Statistics 1978." Geneva.

Jackson, B. and Marsden, D. (1966). "Education and the Working Class." Penguin, Harmondsworth.

Jalaluddin, A. K. M. (in preparation). "The Value of Children in Bangladesh." Ph.D. thesis, Demography Department, Australian National University.

Jansen, M. B. and Stone, L. (1967), *Comparative Studies in Society and History* 9, 208–232.

Johnson, Allen W. (1971). *In* "Studies in Economic Anthropology" (G. Dalton, ed.), pp. 143–150. American Anthropological Association, Washington.

Jones, E. (1963). *International Social Science Journal* 15, 70–76.

Jones, E. (1971). *Population Index* 37, 301–338.

Jones, W. O. (1968). *Items*, Social Science Research Council, 22, 1–6.

Kabwegyere, T. and Mbula, J. (1980). "A Case of the Akamba of Eastern Kenya." Demography Department, Australian National University, Canberra.

Kahl, J. A. (1968). "The Measurement of Modernism: A Study of Values in Brazil and Mexico." University of Texas Press, Austin.

Kellert, S., Williams, L. K., Whyte, W. F. and Alberti, G. (1967). *Milbank Memorial Fund Quarterly* 45, 391–425.

Keyfitz, N. and Flieger, W. (1968). "World Population: An Analysis of Vital Data." University of Chicago Press, Chicago.

Khuda, B.-E-. (1978). "Labour Utilization in a Village Economy in Bangladesh." Ph.D. Thesis, Demography Department, Australian National University.

Kinch, A. (1962). *In* "Research in Family Planning." (C. V. Kiser, ed.), pp. 85–102. Princeton University Press, Princeton.

Kiray, M. (1976). *In* "Mediterranean Family Structures." (J. G. Peristiany, ed.), pp. 261–271, Cambridge University Press, Cambridge.

Kirk, D. (1966). *In* "Family Planning and Population Programs: A Review of World Developments." (B. Berelson, ed.), pp. 561–579. Chicago University Press, Chicago.

Kirk, D. (1971). *In* "Rapid Population Growth: Consequences and Policy Implications." (National Academy of Sciences), pp. 123–147. Johns Hopkins Press, Baltimore.

Kirk-Greene, A. H. M. (1965). *In* "Education and Political Development" (J. S. Coleman, ed.), pp. 372–407. Princeton University Press, Princeton.

Knodel, J. E. (1974). "The Decline of Fertility in Germany, 1871–1939." Princeton University Press, Princeton.

Kocher, J. E. (1973). "Rural Development, Income Distribution and Fertility Decline." Population Council, New York.

Kolenda, P. M. (1964). *Journal of Asian Studies* 23, 71–81.

Kubanin, M. (1931). *In* "A Systematic Sourcebook in Rural Sociology." (P. A. Sorokin, C. C. Zimmerman and C. J. Galpin, eds), Vol. 2, pp. 104–114. Russell and Russell, New York.

Kuznets, S. (1956). *Economic Development and Cultural Change* 5, 1–94.

Lang, O. (1946). "Chinese Family and Society." Yale University Press, New Haven.

Lannoy, R. (1971). "The Speaking Tree: A Study of Indian Culture and Society." Oxford University Press, London.

Laslett, P., (1972). Ed., "Household and Family in Past Time." Cambridge University Press, Cambridge.

Lawson, J. and Silver, H. (1973). "A Social History of Education in England." Methuen, London.

Leeson, R. (1977). "Children's Books and Class Society: Past and Present." Writers and Readers Publishing Co-operative, London.
Leet, D. R. (1976). *Journal of Economic History* **36**, 359–378.
Leibenstein, H. (1957). "Economic Backwardness and Economic Growth: Studies in the Theory of Economic Development." Wiley, New York.
Leibenstein, H. (1974). *Journal of Economic Literature* **12**, 457–479.
Lerner, D. (1964). "The Passing of Traditional Society: Modernizing the Middle East." The Free Press, Macmillan, New York. (First published 1958).
Lesthaeghe, R. (1977). "The Decline of Belgian Fertility, 1800–1970." Princeton University Press, Princeton.
Lesthaeghe, R. and Page, H. J. (1976). "Relating Individual Fertility to other Variables: Common Problems and Pitfalls." Paper presented to the Seminar on Marriage, Parenthood and Fertility in West Africa, Lomé, January 3–9, 1976.
Lesthaeghe, R. and Wilson, C. (1978). "Productievormen, stemgedrag en vruchtbaarheidstransitie in Westeuropeen perspectief, 1870–1930." Interuniversity Programme in Demography, Vrije Universiteit Brussel, Brussels.
Lévi-Strauss, C. (1971). *In* "Man, Culture and Society" (H. L. Shapiro, ed.), pp. 261–285. Oxford University Press, New York.
Levy, M. J. (1966). "Modernization and the Structure of Society: A Setting for International Affairs." Princeton University Press, Princeton.
Lewis, A. L. (1955). "The Theory of Economic Growth." Allen and Unwin, London.
Lewis, O. (1960). "Tepoztlán: Village in Mexico." Holt, Rinehart and Winston, New York.
Leybourne, G. C. and White, K. (1940). "Education and the Birth-Rate: A Social Dilemma." Jonathan Cape, London.
Livi-Bacci, M. (1971). "A Century of Portuguese Fertility." Princeton University Press, Princeton.
Lloyd, B. B. (1966). *In* "The New Elites of Tropical Africa." (P. C. Lloyd, ed.), pp. 163–181. International African Institute, Oxford.
Loewenthal, N. H. and David, A. S. (1972). "Social and Economic Correlates of Family Fertility: An Updated Survey of the Evidence." Center for Population Research and Services, Research Triangle Park, North Carolina.
Lomnitz, L. (1971). *In* "Studies in Economic Anthropology" (G. Dalton, ed.), pp. 93–106. American Anthropological Association, Washington.
Lorimer, F. (1954). "Culture and Human Fertility: A Study of the Relation of Cultural Conditions to Fertility in Non-industrial and Transitional Societies." UNESCO, Paris.
Lorimer, F. (1967). *In* "Proceedings of the World Population Conference, Belgrade, 30 August–10 September 1965." Vol. II, pp. 92–95. United Nations, New York.
Lucas, D. L. (1976). "The Participation of Women in the Nigerian Labour Force since the 1950's with Particular Reference to Lagos." Ph.D. thesis, University of London.
McClelland, D. C. (1963). *In* "Industrialization and Society" (B. F. Hoselitz and W. E. Moore, eds), pp. 74–96. UNESCO-Mouton, Paris.
McClelland, D. C. (1966). *In* "Modernization: The Dynamics of Growth." (M. Weiner, ed.), pp. 28–39. Basic Books, New York.
McDevitt, T. (1975). *In* "Seminar on Migration in Nigeria, Ile-Ife, May 3–5, 1975."
McDonald P. F. (1975). "Marriage in Australia: Age at Marriage and Proportions Marrying." Demography Department, Australian National University, Canberra.
McDonald, P. F. (forthcoming). *In* "Population of Australia" (L. G. Hopkins, ed.). United Nations Economic and Social Commission for Asia and the Pacific, Bangkok.

Macfarlane, A. (1978). "The Origins of English Individualism." Basil Blackwell, Oxford.

Mahmud, S. and McIntosh, J. P. (1980). *Population Studies* **34**, 500–506.

Mair, L. P. (1953). *In* "Survey of African Marriage and Family Life" (A. Phillips, ed.), pp. 1–171. Oxford University Press, London.

Mamdani, M. (1972). "The Myth of Population Control; Family, Caste and Class in an Indian Village." Monthly Review Press, New York.

Mandelbaum, D. G. (1970a). "Society in India: Continuity and Change." University of California Press, Berkeley.

Mandelbaum, D. G. (1970b). "Society in India: Change and Continuity." University of California Press, Berkeley.

Mannheim, K. (1940). "Man and Society in an Age of Reconstruction." Routledge and Kegan Paul, London. (Translated from German by Edward Shils "Mensch und Gesellschaft im Zeitalter des Umbaus", published in 1935.)

Marriott, M. (1955). Ed., "Village India: Studies in the Little Community." University of Chicago Press, Chicago.

Marshall, G. (1970). *In* "Women in the Field: Anthropological Experiences." (P. Golde, ed.), pp. 167–191. Aldine, Chicago.

Marx, K. (1975). *In* "Early Writings" (K. Marx), pp. 424–428. Penguin, Harmondsworth.

Marx, K. (1976). "Capital: A Critique of Political Economy." Penguin, Harmondsworth.

Masemann, V. (1974). *Canadian Journal of African Studies* **8**, 479–494.

Mauldin, W. P. (1965). *Studies in Family Planning* No. 7, 1–12.

Mauldin, W. P. and Berelson, B. (1977). *In* "International Population Conference Mexico, 1977", Vol. 3, pp. 163–185. International Union for the Scientific Study of Population, Liège.

Mauss, M. (1969). "The Gift: Forms and Functions of Exchange in Archaic Societies." Cohen and West, London.

Mbugua, J. N. (1971). "Mumbi's Brideprice." Longman Kenya, Nairobi.

Mead, M. (1956). "New Lives for Old: Cultural Transformation—Manus, 1928–1953." William Morrow, New York.

Meek, C. K. (1949). "Land Law and Custom in the Colonies." Oxford University Press, Oxford.

Meeker, B. F. (1970). *International Journal of Psychology* **5**, 11–19.

Meillassoux, C. (1972). *Economy and Society* **1**, 93–105.

Meillassoux, C. (1973). *The Journal of Peasant Studies* **1**, 81–90.

Mendonsa, E. (1977). *In* "The Persistence of High Fertility: Population Prospects in the Third World." (J. C. Caldwell, ed.), pp. 223–258. Demography Department, Australian National University, Canberra.

Mensah, I. D. (1975). *In* "Citizen Education for Schools" Books 1–6. Afram Publications, Accra.

Milbank Memorial Fund (1954). "The Interrelations of Demographic, Economic, and Social Problems in Selected Underdeveloped Areas." Milbank Memorial Fund, New York.

Millett, K. (1971). "Sexual Politics." Rupert Hart-Davis.

Mitchell, B. R., with Deane, P. (1962). "Abstract of British Statistics." Cambridge University Press, Cambridge.

Mitchell, J. (1971). "Woman's Estate." Penguin, Harmondsworth.

Moore, W. E. (1961). *In* "Traditions, Values and Socio-Economic Development" (R. Braibanti and J. J. Spengler, eds), pp. 57–82. Duke University Press, Durham.

Moore, W. E. and Feldman, A. S. (1961). "Labor Commitment and Social Change in Developing Areas." Social Science Research Council, New York.

Morgan, R. W. with Ohadike, P. O. (1975). *In* "Population Growth and Socioeconomic Change in West Africa." (J. C. Caldwell, ed.), pp. 187–235. Columbia University Press, New York.

Morsa, J. (1966). *In* "Family Planning and Population Programs: A Review of World Developments." (B. Berelson, ed.), pp. 581–593. Chicago University Press, Chicago.

Morton, P. (1970). *Leviathan* 2 (1), 32–37.

Mueller, E. (1972). *Population Studies* 27, 383–403.

Mueller, E. (1975). "The economic value of children in peasant agriculture." Paper presented at the Conference on Population Policy Sponsored by Resources for the Future, February 28–March 1.

Mueller, E. (1976). *In* "Population and Development: A Search for Selective Interventions." (R. Ridker, ed.), pp. 98–153.

Murdock, G. P. (1949). "Social Structure." Macmillan, New York.

Musgrove, F. (1952). *Africa* 22, 234–249.

Myrdal, G. (1957). "Economic Theory and Under-developed Regions." Duckworth, London.

Myrdal, G. (1968). "Asian Drama: An Inquiry into the Poverty of Nations." Twentieth Century Fund, Pantheon Books, Random House, New York.

Nag, M., Peet, R. C. and White, B. (1977). *In* "Proceedings of the International Population Conference: Mexico, 1977", Vol. I, pp. 123–139. International Union for the Scientific Study of Population, Liège.

Nash, M. (1970). *In* "From Child to Adult." (J. Middleton, ed.), pp. 301–313. The Natural History Press, New York.

National Population Inquiry (1975). "Population and Australia: A Demographic Analysis and Projection." Australian Government Publishing Service, Canberra.

Nelson, R. (1956). *American Economic Review* 46, 894–908. The New Peak Reading Course (1973). "New Link Reader." Oxford University Press, East African Branch, Nairobi.

Nigeria. Federal Census Office (n.d.). "Population Census, 1963: Lagos, II." Lagos.

Nigeria. Federal Census Office (n.d.). "Population Census, 1963: Western Nigeria, II." Lagos.

Nimkoff, M. F. (1965). "Comparative Family Systems." Houghton Mifflin, Boston.

Nimkoff, M. F. and Middleton, R. (1960). *The American Journal of Sociology* 66, 215–225.

Notestein, F. W. (1945). *In* "Food for the World." (T. W. Schultz, ed.), pp. 36–57. University of Chicago Press, Chicago.

Notestein, F. W. (1953). *In* "8th International Conference of Agricultural Economists, 1953." pp. 13–31. Oxford University Press, London.

Nurge, E. (1956). *The Philippines Sociological Review.*

Oeschsli, F. W. and Kirk, D. (1975). *Economic Development and Cultural Change 23*, 391–419.

Ogburn, W. F. and Nimkoff, M. F. (1955). "Technology and the Changing Family." Houghton Mifflin, Cambridge, Mass.

Ogunsheye, A. (1965). *In* "Education and Political Development" (J. S. Coleman, ed.), pp. 123–143. Princeton University Press, Princeton.

Ohlin, G. (1971). *In* "International Population Conference: London, 1969." Vol. III, pp. 1703–1728. International Union for the Scientific Study of Population, Liège.

Okediji, F. O., Caldwell, J. C., Caldwell, P. and Ware, H. (1976). *Studies in Family Planning* 7, 126–136.

Okonjo, C. (1968). *In* "The Population of Tropical Africa" (J. C. Caldwell and C. Okonjo, eds), pp. 78–96. Longman, London.

Okore, A. O. (1977). *In* "The Persistence of High Fertility: Population Prospects in the Third World." (J. C. Caldwell, ed.), pp. 313–329. Demography Department, Australian National University, Canberra.

Okore, A. O. (1978). "The Value of Children to Parents among the Ibos in Nigeria: A Case Study of Umuahia and Arochukwu in Imo State." Ph.D. thesis, Demography Department, Australian National University.

Olayomi, J. A. (1970). *In* "Civics and Social Studies for Young Nigerians." Collins, London.

Olusanya, P. O. (1969). *Studies in Family Planning* 37, 13–16.

Olusanya, P. O. (1975). *In* "Population Growth and Socioeconomic Change in West Africa" (J. C. Caldwell, ed.), pp. 254–274. Columbia University Press, New York.

Omari, T. P. (1960). *British Journal of Sociology* 11, 197–210.

Omvedt, G. (1979). *Journal of Peasant Studies* 7, 185–212.

Oppong, C. (1973). "Growing up in Dagbon." Ghana Publishing Company, Tema, Accra.

Oppong, C. (1974). *International Journal of Sociology and the Family* 4.

Oppong, C. (1975a). *Research Review*, Special Issue on Women. I.A.S., Legon.

Oppong, C. (1975b). *In* "Work in Progress Report, 2, 'Teachers' Problems'," CAFG, Legon.

Oppong, C. (1975c). "A Pilot Study of Family Systems Planning and Size in Accra: The Case of Married Nurses." Unpublished report.

Orubuloye, I. O. (1975). "Fertility and Family Limitation in Selected Rural Communities in Ekiti and Ibadan Divisions of the Western State of Nigeria, Project II: Marginals for 1,207 Yoruba Females 15–59 Years of Age." Demography Department, Australian National University, Canberra.

Orubuloye, I. O. (1981). "Abstinence as a Method of Birth Control: Fertility and Child-Spacing Practices among Rural Yoruba Women of Nigeria." Demography Department, Australian National University, Canberra.

Orubuloye, I. O. and Caldwell, J. C. (1975). *Population Studies* 29, 259–272.

Ottenberg, S. (1959). *In* "Continuity and Change in African cultures" (W. R. Bascom and M. J. Herskovits, eds), pp. 130–143. University of Chicago Press, Chicago.

Patai, R. (1971). "Society, Culture and Change in the Middle East." University of Philadelphia Press, Philadelphia.

Pell, M. B. (1867). *Transactions of the Royal Society of New South Wales for the year 1867* 1, 66–76.

Pell, M. B. (1879). *Journal of the Institute of Actuaries, London* 21, 257–282.

Peller, S. (1965). *In* "Population in History: Essays in Historical Demography." (D. V. Glass and D. E. C. Eversley, eds), pp. 87–100. Arnold, London.

Peristiany, J. G. (1976). *In* "Mediterranean Family Structures." (J. G. Peristiany, ed.), pp. 1–26. Cambridge University Press, Cambridge.

Pethe, V. P. (1964). "Demographic Profiles of an Urban Population." Popular Prakashan, Bombay.

Polanyi, K. (1968). *In* "Primitive, Archaic and Modern Economies." (G. Dalton, ed.), pp. 3–37. Doubleday, New York.

Pollard, A. H. (1974). *Institute of Actuaries of Australia and New Zealand. Transactions*, 338–373.

Portes, A. (1973). *American Journal of Sociology* **79**, 15–44.

Ranade, R. (1938). "Himself: The Autobiography of a Hindi Lady," Longmans Green, New York.

Rankin, D. H. (1939). "The History of the Development of Education in Victoria, 1836–1936: The First Centenary of Education Effort." Arrow, Melbourne.

Read, M. (1970). *In* "From Child to Adult." (J. Middleton, ed.), pp. 272–286. The Natural History Press, New York.

Redfield, R. (1930). "Tepoztlán: A Mexican Village". University of Chicago Press, Chicago.

Redfield, R. (1955). "The Little Community." Chicago University Press, Chicago.

Redfield, R. (1960). "The Little Community and Peasant Society and Culture." University of Chicago Press, Chicago.

Redfield, R. (1970). *In* "From Child to Adult." (J. Middleton, ed.), pp. 287–300. The Natural History Press, New York.

Redfield, R. and Singer, M. (1954). *Economic Development and Cultural Change* **3**, 53–73.

Reyna, S. P. (1975a). *Ethnology* **14**, 405–417.

Reyna, S. P. (1975b). *In* "Population Growth and Socioeconomic Change in West Africa." (J. C. Caldwell, ed.), pp. 582–591. Columbia University Press, New York.

Reyna, S. (1977). *In* "The Persistence of High Fertility: Population Prospects in the Third World." (J. C. Caldwell, ed.), pp. 393–425. Australian National University, Canberra.

Rich, W. (1973). "Smaller Families Through Economic Development." Overseas Development Council, Washington.

Richardson, M. (1970). "San Pedro, Colombia: Small Town in a Developing Society." Holt, Rinehart and Winston, New York.

Rindfuss, R. (1975). *Institute for Research on Poverty Discussion Papers* 263–275.

Rostow, W. W. (1956). *Economic Journal* **66**, 25–48.

Rostow, W. W. (1960). "The Stages of Economic Growth." Cambridge University Press, Cambridge.

Rostow, W. W. (1964). "The Economics of Take-Off into Sustained Growth." Macmillan, London.

Royal Commission on the Decline of the Birth Rate and on the Mortality of Infants in New South Wales (1904). "Report." New South Wales Government Printer, Sydney.

Royal Commission on Population. (1950). "Reports and Selected Papers of the Statistics Committee." H.M.S.O., London.

Russell, Josiah C. (1949). *In* "Studies in Population: Proceedings of the Annual Meeting of the Population Association of America at Princeton, New Jersey, May 1949." (G. F. Mair, ed.), pp. 103–107. Princeton University Press, Princeton.

Ruzicka, L. T. (1976). *In* "Towards an Understanding of Contemporary Demographic Change." (J. C. Caldwell, D. Campbell, P. Caldwell, L. Ruzicka, W. Cosford, R. Packer, J. Grocott and M. Neill), pp. 1–28. Demography Department, Australian National University, Canberra.

Ruzicka, L. T. (1977). Ed., "The Economic and Social Supports for High Fertility." Demography Department, Australian National University, Canberra.

Ruzicka, L. T. and Caldwell, J. C. (1977). "The End of Demographic Transition in Australia." Demography Department, Australian National University, Canberra.

Ruzicka, L. T. and Caldwell, J. C. (forthcoming). *In* "Population of Australia." (L. G. Hopkins, ed.). United Nations Economic and Social Commission for Asia and the Pacific, Bangkok.

Ruzicka, L. T. and Chowdhury, A. K. M. A. (1977–78). "Demographic Surveillance System—Matlab, Vol. 3, Vital Events and Migration." Cholera Research Laboratory, Dacca.

Ryder, N. B. (1973). *In* "Toward the End of Growth: Population in America" (C. F. Westoff, ed.), pp. 57–68. Prentice-Hall, Englewood Cliffs.

Sahlins, M. D. (1960). *In* "Essays in the Science of Culture in Honor of Leslie H. White." (G. E. Dole and R. L. Carneiro, eds) pp. 390–415. Thomas Y. Crowell, New York.

Sahlins, M. D. (1965). *In* "The Relevance of Models for Social Anthropology." (M. Banton, ed.), pp. 139–236. Tavistock, London.

Sahlins, M. (1971). *In* "Studies in Economic Anthropology." (G. Dalton, ed.), pp. 30–51. American Anthropological Association, Washington.

Sahlins, M. (1972). "Stone Age Economics." Aldine-Atherton, Chicago.

Sauvy, A. (1969). "General Theory of Population." Weidenfeld and Nicolson, London.

Schnaiberg, A. (1970). *American Journal of Sociology* **76**, 399–425.

The School of Babiana (1970). "Letter to a Teacher." Penguin, Harmondsworth.

Schultz, T. P. (1972). *In* "Economic Development and Population Growth in the Middle East." (C. A. Cooper and S. S. Alexander, eds), pp. 401–500. American Elsevier, New York.

Schultz, T. P. (1973). *Journal of Political Economy* **81**, S238–S274.

Schultz, T. W. (1973). *Journal of Political Economy* **81**, S2–S13.

Schultz, T. W. (1974). *In* "Economics of the Family: Marriage, Children, and Human Capital." (T. W. Schultz, ed.), pp. 3–22. University of Chicago Press, Chicago.

Sembajwe, I. S. L. (1981). "Fertility and Infant Mortality Amongst the Yoruba in Western Nigeria." Demography Department, Australian National University, Canberra.

Shanin, T. (1972). "The Awkward Class." Oxford University Press, Oxford.

Shorter, E. (1976). "The Making of the Modern Family." Collins, London.

Simon, J. L. (1974). "The Effects of Income on Fertility." Monograph No. 19, Carolina Population Center, Chapel Hill.

Sklar, J. (1974). *Population Studies* **28**, 231–247.

Smith, A. D. (1973). "The Concept of Social Change: A Critique of the Functionalist Theory of Social Change." Routledge and Kegan Paul, London.

Smith, D. H. and Inkeles, A. (1966). *Sociometry* **29**, 353–377.

Smith, R. T. (1968). *In* "International Encyclopaedia of the Social Sciences" (D. L. Sills, ed.), pp. 301–313. Macmillan and Free Press, New York.

Sovani, N. V. and Dandekar, K. (1955). "Fertility Survey of Nasik, Kolaba and Satara (North) Districts." Gokhale Institute of Politics and Economics, Poona.

Spencer, G. M. (1971). *Demography* **8**, 247–259.

Stephenson, J. B. (1968). *American Journal of Sociology* **74**, 265–275.

Stolnitz, G. J. (1964). *In* "Population: the Vital Revolution" (R. Freedman, ed.), pp. 30–46. Anchor Books, New York.

Stone, L. (1977). "The Family, Sex and Marriage in England, 1500–1800." Weidenfeld and Nicolson, London.

Stycos, J. M. (1964). *In* "Population: The Vital Revolution" (R. Freedman, ed.), pp. 166–177. Anchor Books, New York.

Sussman, M. B. (1953). *American Sociological Review* **18**, 22–28.

Sutton, F. X. (1965). *In* "Education and Political Development." (J. S. Coleman, ed.), pp. 51–74. Princeton University Press, Princeton.

Tabah, L. and Samuel, R. (1962). *In* "Research in Family Planning." (C. V. Kiser, ed.), pp. 263–304. Princeton University Press, Princeton.

Taueber, I. (1958). "The Population of Japan." Princeton University Press, Princeton.

Teitelbaum, M. S. (1974). *Population Studies* **28**, 329–343.

Thabault, R. (1945). Cited in C. Tilly, *History of Education Quarterly* **13**, 123.

Thadani, V. (1978). *Population and Development Review* **4**, 457–499.

Thompson, W. C. (1929). *The American Journal of Sociology* **34**, 959–975.

Thompson, W. C. (1946). "Population and Peace in the Pacific." University of Chicago Press, Chicago.

Thorner, D. (1966). *In* "The Theory of Peasant Economy." (D. Thorner, B. Kerbaly and R. E. F. Smith, eds; A. V. Chayanov, author), pp. xi–xxiii. The American Economic Association, Richard Irwin, Homewood, Ill.

Thorner, D. and Thorner, A. (1962). "Land and Labour in India." Asia Publishing House, Delhi.

Tilman, R. O. (1967). *In* "Education and Development in Southeast Asia: Symposium held in Brussels from April 19–21, 1966." (L'Institut de Sociologie), pp. 209–228. Collection du Centre D'Etude du Sud-Est Asiatique, Université Libre de Bruxelles.

Trevor, J. (1975). *In* "Population Growth and Socioeconomic Change in West Africa." (J. C. Caldwell, ed.), pp. 236–253. Columbia University Press, New York.

Trewartha, G. T. (1972). "The Less Developed Realm: A Geography of Its Population." Wiley, New York.

Trussell, J., Menken, J. and Coale, A. J. (1981) *In* "Nuptiality and Fertility: Proceedings of the IUSSP Seminar, Bruges, 8–11 January, 1979." (L. T. Ruzicka, ed.), pp. 7–27. Ordina, Liége.

Twopeny, R. E. N. (1973). "Town Life in Australia." (Facsimile edition, first published 1883). Sydney University Press, Sydney.

Tyack, D. B. (1976). *Harvard Educational Review* **46**, 355–389.

United Nations (1951). "Compulsory Education in Australia: A Study by the Australian National Co-operating Body for Education." UNESCO, Paris.

United Nations (1961). "The Mysore Population Study." ST/SOA/Ser.A/34. United Nations, New York.

United Nations (1965). "Population Bulletin of the United Nations, No. 7–1963, with Special Reference to Conditions and Trends of Fertility in the World." United Nations Department of Economic and Social Affairs, New York.

United Nations (1974a). "Concise Report on the World Population Situation in 1970–75." United Nations, New York.

United Nations (1974b). "1973 Demographic Yearbook." United Nations, New York.

United Nations (1976). "1975 Demographic Yearbook." United Nations, New York.

United Nations (1978). "Demographic Data Sheets for Countries of the Economic Commission for Western Asia, no. 2." United Nations Economic Commission for Western Asia, Beirut.

United Nations (1979). *Population and Vital Statistics Report*, Statistical Papers, Series A. Vol. 31, No. 3.

Vanden Driesen, I. H. (1971). *Africa* **41**, 42–53.

Vanden Driesen, I. H. (1972). *Africa* **42**, 44–56.

van de Walle, E. (1974). "The Female Population of France in the Nineteenth Century." Princeton University Press, Princeton.

van de Walle, E. (1975). *In* "Population Growth and Socioeconomic Change in West Africa." (J. C. Caldwell, ed.), pp. 136–152. Columbia University Press, New York.

van de Walle, E. and Knodel, J. (1967). *In* "Contributed Papers: Sydney Conference, International Union for the Scientific Study of Population, 21–25 August 1967." pp. 47–55.

Vinovskis, M. A. (1976). *Journal of Interdisciplinary History* **6**, 375–396.

Vogel, E. F. (1967). *In* "Aspects of Social Change in Modern Japan" (R. P. Dore, ed.), pp. 91–111. Princeton University Press, Princeton.

Walzer, J. F. (1976). *In* "The History of Childhood" (L. de Mause, ed.), pp. 351–382. Souvenir, London.

Ware, H. (1976). *Population Studies* **30**, 413–427.

Weber, M. (1930). "The Protestant Ethic and the Rise of Capitalism." Allen and Unwin, London.

Weiner, M. (1966). Ed., "Modernization: The Dynamics of Growth." Basic Books, New York.

West, E. G. (1965). "Education and the State: A Study in Political Economy." Institute of Economic Affairs, London.

West, E. G. (1975). "Education and the Industrial Revolution." Barnes and Noble, New York.

Westoff, C. F. (1973). "Toward the End of Growth." Prentice-Hall, Englewood Cliffs.

Wharton, C. R., Jr. (1971). *In* "Studies in Economic Anthropology." (G. Dalton, ed.), pp. 151–178. American Anthropological Association, Washington.

Wiser, W. H. and Wiser, C. V. (1971). "Behind Mud Walls, 1930–1960; with a sequel; The Village in 1970." University of California Press, Berkeley.

Wolf, E. R. (1966). "Peasants." Prentice-Hall, Englewood Cliffs.

Wolf, M. (1972). "Women and the Family in Rural Taiwan." Stanford University Press, Stanford.

World Fertility Survey (1975). "Basic Documentation, No. 1, Core Questionnaires." London.

Wray, J. D. (1971). *Reports on Population/Family Planning* **9**.

Yang, Martin (1948). "A Chinese Village: Taitou, Shantung Province." Kegan Paul, Trench and Trubner, London.

Yates B. A. (1971). *Comparative Education Review* **15**, 158–171.

Yaukey, D. (1961). "Fertility Differences in a Modernizing Country: A Survey of Lebanese Couples." Princeton University Press, Princeton.

Young, C. M. (1969). "An Analysis of the Population Growth and Mortality of Selected Birth Cohorts in Australia, with Reference to the Relationship Between Cohort and Transverse (or Calendar Year) Experience." Ph.D. thesis, Demography Department, Australian National University.

Young, C. M. (1979). *In* "Economic and Demographic Change: Issues for the 1980s. Proceedings of the Conference, Helsinki, 1978.", pp. 99–111. IUSSP, Liège.

Zaretsky, E. (1976). "Capitalism, The Family and Personal Life." Pluto, London.

Zelnik, M., Kim, Y. J. and Kantner, J. F. (1979). *Family Planning Perspectives* **11**, 177–183.